Handbook of Mood Disorders

Handbook of Mood Disorders

Edited by Leon Chapman

AMERICAN
MEDICAL PUBLISHERS
www.americanmedicalpublishers.com

American Medical Publishers,
41 Flatbush Avenue,
1st Floor, New York,
NY 11217, USA

Visit us on the World Wide Web at:
www.americanmedicalpublishers.com

ISBN: 978-1-63927-094-1

Cataloging-in-Publication Data

Handbook of mood disorders / edited by Leon Chapman.
p. cm.
Includes bibliographical references and index.
ISBN 978-1-63927-094-1
1. Affective disorders. 2. Mood (Psychology). 3. Psychology, Pathological. I. Chapman, Leon.
RC537 .H36 2022
616.852 7--dc23

Table of Contents

Preface

Every book is initially just a concept; it takes months of research and hard work to give it the final shape in which the readers receive it. In its early stages, this book also went through rigorous reviewing. The notable contributions made by experts from across the globe were first molded into patterned chapters and then arranged in a sensibly sequential manner to bring out the best results.

A mood disorder is a group of conditions which are characterized by a disturbance in the person's mood. There are two primary types of mood disorders-major depressive disorder and bipolar disorder. The major depressive disorder also known as major depression is a disorder in which a person has more than one major depressive incident. Individuals with a major depressive disorder are at increased risk for suicide. Bipolar disorder is an emotional condition that is unstable and is categorized by cycles of abnormal, persistent high and low mood. Mood disorder can be treated with the help of therapy and medications such as behavior therapy, interpersonal therapy and cognitive therapy. This book aims to shed light on some of the unexplored aspects of mood disorders and the recent researches in this field. It consists of contributions made by international experts. This book will prove to be immensely beneficial to students and researchers in this field.

It has been my immense pleasure to be a part of this project and to contribute my years of learning in such a meaningful form. I would like to take this opportunity to thank all the people who have been associated with the completion of this book at any step.

Editor

Preface

1

Psychopathological and sociodemographic features in treatment-resistant unipolar depression versus bipolar depression

Nicolas A. Nuñez[1,2], Stefano Comai[1,3], Eduard Dumitrescu[1,2], Maykel F. Ghabrash[1,2], John Tabaka[1,2], Marie Saint-Laurent[2], Stephen Vida[2], Theodore Kolivakis[2], Allan Fielding[2], Nancy Low[2], Pablo Cervantes[2], Linda Booij[1,4] and Gabriella Gobbi[1,2*]

Abstract

Background: Some authors have hypothesized that Treatment-Resistant Unipolar Depression (TRD-UP) should be considered within the bipolar spectrum disorders and that hidden bipolarity may be a risk factor for TRD-UP. However, there are neither studies comparing clinical and sociodemographic data of patients with TRD-UP versus Bipolar (BP) disorders nor are there any examining differences versus Bipolar type I (BP-I) and Bipolar type II (BP-II).

Methods: Charts analysis was conducted on 194 patients followed at the Mood Disorders Clinic of the McGill University Health Center. Sociodemographic, clinical features and depression scales were collected from patients meeting DSM-IV criteria for TRD-UP (n = 100) and BP (n = 94). Binary logistic regression analysis was conducted to examine clinical predictors independently associated with the two disorders.

Results: Compared to BP, TRD-UP patients exhibited greater severity of depression, prevalence of anxiety and panic disorders, melancholic features, Cluster-C personality disorders, later onset of depression and fewer hospitalizations. Binary logistic regression indicated that higher comorbidity with anxiety disorders, higher depression scale scores and lower global assessment of functioning (GAF) scores, and lower number of hospitalizations and psychotherapies differentiated TRD-UP from BP patients. We also found that the rate of unemployment and the number of hospitalizations for depression was higher in BP-I than in BP-II, while the rate of suicide attempts was lower in BP-I than in BP-II depressed patients.

Conclusions: These results suggest that TRD-UP constitutes a distinct psychopathological condition and not necessarily a prodromal state of BP depression.

Keywords: Treatment-resistant depression, Bipolar depression, Psychopathology, Affective disorders, Bipolar spectrum

Background

Depressive disorders are considered as one of the major worldwide public health burdens [1]. Treatment-Resistant Unipolar Depression (TRD-UP) continues to be a clinical challenge due to its heterogeneous presentation with an impact on functional impairment, declined autonomy, and poor cognitive functioning [2]. Although advances have been made to improve our psychiatric diagnostic classification systems, many intermediate phenotypes have not been accurately diagnosed and proposed predictors of treatment outcomes in depression seem controversial with remission rates remaining unchanged [3].

Over the years there has been several definitions proposed as to adequately define TRD-UP [4, 5]. TRD-UP can be defined either as the failure to respond to the first

* Correspondence: gabriella.gobbi@mcgill.ca
[1]Department of Psychiatry, Neurobiological Psychiatry Unit, McGill University Health Center (MUHC), McGill University, Room 220, 1033 Pine Avenue West,, Montreal, QC, Canada
[2]Department of Psychiatry, Mood Disorder Clinic, McGill University Health Center, McGill University, Montreal, QC, Canada

antidepressant (AD) trial [6] or two or more AD trials [7] of different classes of AD [8]. It has been described that up to 15% of patients treated for depression will fall into this category [9] and according to the Sequenced Treatment Alternatives to Relieve Depression (STAR*D) study more than 50% of depressed patients do not respond to their first AD trial [10]. However, there is currently no universal definition of TRD-UP and controversies surrounding its prevalence rates, definitions and treatment outcomes remain ambiguous [11, 12].

A number of clinical and demographic characteristics have been found to be associated with TRD-UP. These include comorbidity with anxiety panic disorder, social phobia, personality disorder, suicidal risk, melancholia, number of hospitalizations, recurrent episodes, early age of onset, total number of unresponsive treatments to antidepressants received during a lifetime [13] as well as severity of depression and having a first degree relative with an affective disorder [14].

It has been proposed that TRD-UP can be considered a "prodromal phase" of Bipolar disorder (BP) included in the bipolar spectrum disorders and a sub-threshold bipolarity or hidden bipolarity as a risk factor for TRD-UP [15]. This hypothesis has been confirmed by a recent systematic review examining possible risk factors for treatment resistance in unipolar major depression, in which, among others, the presence of a non-diagnosed bipolarity was found to be an independent risk factor for treatment resistance [16].

The diagnostic distinction between TRD-UP and BP is of paramount importance for the treatment and prognosis of depression. While TRD-UP must be treated with a combination of different classes of antidepressants (AD) or with second-generation antipsychotic (SGA) augmentation strategies [17] in BP depression, AD must be carefully used and monitored considering that they may induce a switch in mania, hypomania or symptoms such as psychomotor activation, insomnia or irritability [18, 19]. Unfortunately, it is still a challenge to accurately predict if a TRD-UP could be a masked form of BP depression.

Other studies examining the differences between UP (non-TRD) and BP depression revealed that the prevalence of characteristics such as age of onset was lower but that the total number of depressive episodes as well as the presence of a family history of depression was higher in BP than in UP depression [20–23]. Therefore, while some different characteristics between UP and BP depression have been well characterized, the different demographic, social, and clinical characteristics associated with TRD-UP versus BP depression have not yet been studied, although this early differential diagnosis is pivotal for improving diagnostic and therapeutic outcomes.

In this retrospective and observational cross-sectional chart-review study, we have examined clinical and demographic characteristics mostly associated with the diagnosis of TRD-UP or BP that have been previously described in the literature as risk factors or predictors for these disorders [14, 16, 24]. The goal was to find clinical and socio-demographical characteristics to assist clinicians to better differentiate between TRD-UP from depression as part of the bipolar spectrum disorders. As a secondary goal, given the subtypes of the bipolar spectrum, we investigated whether there were clinical and socio-demographical characteristics that differed between Bipolar Type I (BP-I) and Type II (BP-II) disorders and between them and TRD-UP.

Methods

The study was approved by the Institutional Review Board of McGill University (13–375-PSY) and was conducted in accordance with the Declaration of Helsinki and ICH Good Clinical Practice. Chart reviews were collected in the Patient Registry at the Mood Disorders Clinic (MDC) of the McGill University Health Center (MUHC). The Patient Registry at the MDC is a research database where uniform data is collected on all UP and BP disorder patients who are treated and followed at the clinic for more than 2 years (mean 7.5 years). Being a chart reviews study, the informed consent was not required.

Patients

Patients meeting the DSM-IV criteria for a major depressive episode (MDE) within a UP or BP diagnosis were included in the study [25]. The medical charts of 194 outpatients between the ages of 19–75, with a MDE and meeting DSM-IV criteria for TRD-UP (n = 100) and BP (n = 94) were reviewed. Among the BP patients, 52 were diagnosed with BP-I and 42 with BP-II. Patients with UP major depressive disorder met criteria for TRD-UP by failing at least two adequate trials with different AD in mono or combination therapy at the adequate dose and for at least three weeks [7].

The patient's diagnoses were ascertained by the Structured Clinical Interview for Diagnosis (SCID) [26] which was conducted by psychiatrists or professionals who received a training in SCID. The Maudsley Staging Method (MSM) was used to establish the severity of the TRD patients [27]. In addition, the Young Mania Rating Scale (YMRS) [28] was used to evaluate whether patients currently displayed acute hypomanic or manic symptoms and if they did not meet the criteria for a mixed episode of depression at the time of the assessment.

The inclusion criteria included patients with a diagnosis of a MDE ranging from mild to severe intensity measured by a score greater than 20 on the Montgomery–Asberg Depression Rating Scale (MADRS) and a score greater than 13 on the Hamilton-Rating Scale for Depression (HAM-D17) [29]. The duration of the current episode had to be greater than two months. Patients with a mixed episode, currently in a manic episode or with the presence of a neurological/developmental disorder and/or a mood disorder secondary to a medical condition were excluded.

Patients were selected during the phase of depression, before the administration of a stable and effective psychopharmacological treatment (treatment not changed by the psychiatrist for at least three months).

Pharmacological treatment at time of evaluation was as follows: for the TRD-UP group, 38 patients were treated with AD mono/combination therapy and 62 patients were treated with an augmentation strategy that included AD in combination with SGA (n = 49) or mood stabilizers (MS) (n = 13). In the BP group, patients were treated with MS in combination with SGA (n = 30), AD in combination with SGA and MS (n = 23), AD plus MS (n = 21), AD plus SGA (n = 10), MS monotherapy (n = 5), and SGA monotherapy (n = 5).

Clinical evaluation

A retrospective chart analysis was performed by two raters and clinical features were evaluated in the two groups. The following scales were considered for depression severity: Montgomery–Asberg Depression Rating Scale (MADRS) [30]; Clinical Global Impression-Severity of Illness (CGI-S) [31]; Quick Inventory of Depressive Symptomatology (QIDS-C16) [32] and Hamilton-Rating Scale for Depression (HAMD-17) [33].

The following patient socio-demographic information was obtained from the MDC Patient Registry: age, ethnicity, gender, marital status, employment, level of education and living arrangement as well as previous psychiatric diagnosis including Attention Deficit-Hyperactivity disorder (ADHD), alcohol or substance abuse, anxiety disorders, sleep disorders and eating disorders. Information was also collected on family history of affective disorders, age of first psychiatric consultation, age of first depressive episode and the number of depressive episodes, age of first manic episode and number of manic episodes, age of first hypomanic episode and number of hypomanic episodes. Data was also collected on the history of psychotherapy, electrical or neurological therapy, use of psychiatric services, general medical history, and number of previous suicide attempts, major depression with psychotic features, axis II, III and IV DSM-IV-TR [25] pathology, previous and current pharmacotherapy.

Patients were also assessed having depressive melancholic features and depressive atypical symptoms as defined by DSM-IV criteria [25]. Patients within the TRD-UP group had a level of resistant depression of moderate intensity according to the MSM (Mean ± SEM, 9.7 ± 0.2) and patients with BP disorders did not display current manic episodes defined by the YMRS scale (Mean ± SEM: 3.0 ± 0.7).

Reliability and inter-rater agreement for psychometric scales

A reliability analysis was performed to determine the internal consistency by means of Cronbach's alpha. Overall, we reached an acceptable reliability for all the scales (MADRS: α = 0.91; HAMD-17: α = 0.82; QIDS-C16: α = 0.77).

Inter-rater reliability was performed on a sample of 140 patients. Patients were assessed by three raters (two psychiatrists and a General Practitioner). We found moderate to good agreement (Cohen's kappa range: 0.58–0.85) [34]) (MADRS: 0.60; HAMD-17: 0.58; QIDS-C16: 0.61; CGI-S: 0.72; CGI-Global Improvement: 0.85) across all scales.

Statistical analysis

Statistical analysis was conducted using the Statistical Package for the Social Sciences (SPSS-23; SPSS Inc., Chicago, IL, USA). Data are presented as mean ± standard deviation (SD). Inter-rater reliability for individual scales was calculated using Cohen's kappa [35].

As an initial step, we considered 40 variables that were compared between TRD-UP and BP by Student's t test for continuous variables or by Pearson's chi-square (χ^2) test for categorical variables. Then, using a binary logistic regression analysis we examined which variables were specific predictors of the two affective disorders. Given the high number of variables under investigation, and to balance risk for type I and type II errors, we choose to include in the binary logistic model only those variables that in the initial step were significantly different between the two groups at an alpha level of 0.01. Moreover, we excluded from the model those variables for which few individuals ($n \leq 5$) were affected by a specific disorder in at least one of the two groups. Predictors reaching $p < 0.01$ were considered significant.

As final step, we investigated for possible differences in the clinical and demographic characteristics of TRD-UP, BP-I and BP-II patients. To examine possible differences for categorical variables, we first tested at an alpha level of 0.05 the overall 3 × 2 matrix containing all the three affective disorders. For statistically significant variables, we subsequently conducted multiple 2 × 2 cross tabulations using Pearson's chi-square (χ^2) test. For comparisons concerning continuous variables, we used the analysis of variance (ANOVA) followed by Bonferroni post-hoc test for multiple comparisons.

Results

Sociodemographic characteristics

The mean age (± SD) of the total sample was 43.6 (±14.1) years with 58.3% of the participants consisting of females ($n = 116$) and 39.2% ($n = 78$) of males. At the time of evaluation, 68.3% of the patients were unemployed ($n = 136$) and 40.1% had a single status ($n = 81$). Table 1 summarizes and compares the sociodemographic and clinical features of TRD-UP and BP patients.

Patients with TRD-UP were significantly older than BP patients (46.5 ± 13.3 vs 40.6 ± 14.3, $p = 0.003$) whereas the two groups were equally distributed in terms of gender, with a female to male ratio close to 1.5.

The prevalence of patients who were married at the time of evaluation was significantly greater in the TRD-UP group compared to the BP patients (41% vs 16%, respectively; $p < 0.001$). Similar rates of unemployment or disability were noted in the two groups (74% TRD-UP vs 66% BP, $p = 0.272$).

Clinical features and co-morbidities

BP patients had an early onset of MDE compared to TRD-UP patients (26.4 ± 9.8 vs 37.7 ± 15.3; $p < 0.001$). In line with this finding, BP patients had their first psychiatric consultation and their first psychiatric hospitalization at a younger age than TRD-UP patients ($p < 0.001$).

No differences were found between TRD-UP and BP concerning the prevalence of patients having recurrent depression (> 3 episodes) as well as the presence of comorbid substance use. However, BP patients had a higher prevalence of a history of cannabis use than TRD-UP (20% vs 6%, $p = 0.005$). The duration of the current episode of major depression was longer in BP than in TRD-UP (15.4 ± 12.1 vs 11.9 ± 11.5, $p = 0.039$).

Patients with TRD-UP showed a lower failure to different pharmacotherapies than BP patients ($p < 0.001$). Looking at the different pharmacological classes of psychotropic drugs, TRD-UP patients failed a greater number of antidepressant trials ($p = 0.009$) and a lower number of SGA ($p < 0.001$) and MS ($p < 0.001$) trials compared to BP patients.

Interestingly, the percentage of patients currently undergoing psychotherapy was significantly lower in TRD-UP than in BP patients ($p < 0.001$).

The prevalence of patients who did not have any hospitalization for depression since the first episode was greater in the TRD-UP group than in the BP group ($p < 0.001$). In contrast, BP patients showed greater prevalence of more than one hospitalization for depression since the first episode than TRD-UP ($p < 0.001$). Family history was also another characteristic that differed among the two groups. BP patients showed a higher prevalence of having at least one first-degree relative with affective disorders than TRD-UP patients ($p = 0.029$).

Of note, the prevalence of patients who had a history of suicidality was significantly higher in those affected by BP than those diagnosed with TRD-UP ($p = 0.002$). TRD-UP patients displayed higher prevalence of anxiety ($p < 0.001$) and panic ($p < 0.01$) disorders as well as depression with melancholic features ($p < 0.001$) than BP patients.

Personality disorders and medical conditions

Overall there was no difference in the prevalence of personality disorders (Axis II in DSM-IV-TR) and physical diseases (Axis III in DSM-IV-TR) between the TRD-UP and BP; however, when studying the individual clusters, TRD-UP patients had a significantly higher prevalence rate of Cluster C personality disorders (avoidant, dependent and obsessive compulsive personality) compared to BP patients ($p < 0.001$). No differences were found for Clusters A and B personality disorders.

With the exception of autoimmune diseases that were more prevalent in TRD-UP than in BP patients, there were no differences on other Axis III co-morbidities.

Depression severity and functioning

Using different psychometric scales, we examined and compared the severity of depression (MADRS, HAMD-17, QIDS-C16 and CGI-S) and the global functioning (GAF score) between TRD-UP and BP disorders. As shown in Table 2, TRD-UP patients were move severely depressed than BP patients as indicated by higher scores on MADRS, HAMD-17, QIDS-C16 and CGI-S scales ($p < 0.001$). In contrast, the global functioning of BP patients was higher than that of TRD-UP patients ($p < 0.001$).

Predicting categorical diagnosis

We used binary logistic regression to evaluate which demographic and clinical characteristics were differently associated with TRD-UP or BP (Table 3). The binary logistic regression model consisted of 11 variables involving individual characteristics (i.e., age of first depression, marital status, psychotherapy, employment status, more than one hospitalizations, first degree relatives with affective disorders), presence of comorbidities (anxiety disorders), clinical features of depressive episode (i.e., HAMD-17 score, melancholic features, number of failed pharmacotherapies) and level of overall functioning (GAF score). We excluded from the model, panic and Cluster C personality disorders since very few individuals ($n \leq 5$) were affected by these disorders in at least one of the two groups.

Our classification analysis reflected an overall goodness of fit to the data ($\chi^2 = 168.8$ $p < 0.001$ df = 11). Nagelkerke's (0.775) indicated a moderately strong relationship between predictors and variable grouping. No multicollinearity between the variables was detected (VIF range: 1.137–1.725).

Table 1 Socio-demographic and clinical characteristics of patients with TRD-UP and BP disorder ($N = 194$)

	TRD-UP ($n = 100$)	BP ($n = 94$)	Statistics
Age (Years) (Mean ± SD)	46.5 ± 13.3	40.6 ± 14.3	$t = 2.97$, $\mathbf{p = 0.003}$
Ratio of Males: Females	41:59	37:57	$\chi^2 = 0.05$, $p = 0.816$
Patients≤65 years of age	90 (90%)	91 (96%)	$\chi^2 = 3.59$, $p = 0.058$
Marital status	41 (41%)	15 (16%)	$\chi^2 = 14.79$, $\mathbf{p < 0.001}$
Unemployed/Disability sick leave	74 (74%)	62 (66%)	$\chi^2 = 1.49$, $p = 0.221$
Age of first major depressive episode (Mean ± SD)	37.7 ± 15.3	26.4 ± 9.8	$t = 6.14$, $\mathbf{p < 0.001}$
Early onset of major depressive episodes(< 25)	29 (29%)	52 (55%)	$\chi^2 = 13.80$, $\mathbf{p < 0.001}$
Age of first psychiatric consultation (Mean ± SD)	35.9 ± 15.2	24.9 ± 10.7	$t = 5.83$, $\mathbf{p < 0.001}$
Age of first psychiatric hospitalization (Mean ± SD)	40.1 ± 15.0	29.4 ± 11.7	$t = 4.15$, $\mathbf{p \leq 0.001}$
Patients with recurrent depression (> 3)	39 (39%)	47 (50%)	$\chi^2 = 2.37$, $p = 0.123$
Duration of illness-current episode (years) (Mean ± SD)	11.9 ± 11.5	15.4 ± 12.1	$t = -2.08$, $\mathbf{p = 0.039}$
Patients with comorbid substance use	27 (27%)	32 (34%)	$\chi^2 = 1.14$, $p = 0.287$
History of Alcohol use	9 (9%)	16 (17%)	$\chi^2 = 2.77$, $p = 0.096$
History of Cannabis use	6 (6%)	19 (20%)	$\chi^2 = 8.71$, $\mathbf{p = 0.003}$
History of Cocaine use	3 (3%)	3 (3%)	$\chi^2 = 0.006$, $p = 0.939$
Number of Failed pharmacotherapies (Mean ± SD)	3.6 ± 2.6	5.3 ± 2.7	$t = -4.31$, $\mathbf{p < 0.001}$
Failed antidepressant trials (Mean ± SD)	2.25 ± 1.8	1.63 ± 1.4	$t = 2.63$, $\mathbf{p = 0.009}$
Failed SGA (Mean ± SD)	0.65 ± 0.7	1.68 ± 1.2	$t = -7.17$, $\mathbf{p < 0.001}$
Failed Mood stabilizers (Mean ± SD)	0.3 ± 0.6	1.3 ± 0.9	$t = -8.55$, $\mathbf{p < 0.001}$
Patients currently having psychotherapy	41 (41%)	78 (83%)	$\chi^2 = 36.01$, $\mathbf{p < 0.001}$
Number of hospitalizations for depression since 1st episode			
None	56 (56%)	15 (16%)	$\chi^2 = 33.48$, $\mathbf{p < 0.001}$
> one	20 (20%)	60 (64%)	$\chi^2 = 38.41$, $\mathbf{p < 0.001}$
Patients with 1st degree relative with affective illness	51 (51%)	63 (67%)	$\chi^2 = 5.13$, $\mathbf{p = 0.023}$
Patients with Anxiety disorders	61 (61%)	22 (23%)	$\chi^2 = 27.97$, $\mathbf{p < 0.001}$
Patients with Panic disorders	19 (19%)	3 (3%)	$\chi^2 = 12.04$, $\mathbf{p < 0.001}$
Patients with Melancholic symptoms	74 (74%)	40 (42%)	$\chi^2 = 19.77$, $\mathbf{p < 0.001}$
Patients with Atypical symptoms	14 (14%)	25 (26%)	$\chi^2 = 4.78$, $\mathbf{p = 0.029}$
Patients with suicidal attempts	23 (23%)	42 (44%)	$\chi^2 = 10.22$, $\mathbf{p = 0.001}$
History of MDE with psychotic symptoms	27 (24%)	59 (63%)	$\chi^2 = 25.11$, $\mathbf{p < 0.001}$
Patients with Personality disorders (Axis II in DSM-IV)	44 (44%)	45 (48%)	$\chi^2 = 0.29$, $p = 0.589$
Cluster A	7 (7%)	1 (1%)	$\chi^2 = 4.31$, $\mathbf{p = 0.038}$
Cluster B	19 (19%)	16(17%)	$\chi^2 = 0.128$, $p = 0.720$
Cluster C	25 (25%)	5 (5%)	$\chi^2 = 14.36$, $\mathbf{p < 0.001}$
Patients with Medical condition potentially relevant to treatment (Axis III in DSM-IV)			
Autoimmune diseases	11 (11%)	2 (2%)	$\chi^2 = 6.101$, $\mathbf{p = 0.014}$
Cardiovascular diseases	25 (25%)	18 (19%)	$\chi^2 = 0.962$, $p = 0.327$
Chronic pain disorders	25 (25%)	15 (16%)	$\chi^2 = 2.421$, $p = 0.120$
Neurological conditions	13 (13%)	5 (5%)	$\chi^2 = 3.396$, $p = 0.065$
Metabolic disorder	10 (10%)	15 (16%)	$\chi^2 = 1.532$, $p = 0.216$

SD Standard Deviation, *TRD-UP* Treatment-Resistant Unipolar Depression, *BP* Bipolar disorder type I and type II, *MDE* Major depressive episode, *SGA* Second Generation Antipsychotics. Boldface indicates significant difference at an alpha level = 0.05

Table 2 Severity of depression and global functioning of patients with TRD-UP and BP. Data are reported as Mean ± SD

Depression severity	TRD-UP (n = 100)	BP (n = 94)	Statistics
MADRS	30.8 ± 8.95	23.2 ± 6.98	$t = 6.66$, **$p < 0.001$**
HAMD-17	23.2 ± 6.24	17.0 ± 4.61	$t = 7.92$, **$p < 0.001$**
QIDS	15.8 ± 4.26	12.7 ± 3.91	$t = 5.31$, **$p < 0.001$**
CGI-S	5.0 ± 1.21	4.3 ± 1.18	$t = 4.19$, **$p < 0.001$**
GAF	55.5 ± 10.22	60.9 ± 4.66	$t = -4.93$, **$p < 0.001$**

TRD-UP Treatment-Resistant Unipolar Depression, *BP* Bipolar disorder type I and type II, *MADRS* Montgomery–Asberg Depression Rating Scale, *CGI-S* Clinical Global Impression-Severity of Illness, *QIDS* Quick Inventory of Depressive Symptomatology, *HAM-D17* Hamilton-Rating Scale for Depression, *GAF* Global Assessment of functioning, *SD* Standard Deviation. Boldface indicates significant difference at an alpha level = 0.05

A combination of five variables (more than one hospitalization for depression, comorbidity with anxiety disorders, current psychotherapy, severity of depression (HAM-D17 score) and global functioning (GAF score) was able to significantly differentiate patients with TRD-UP from those with BP (Table 3). Of note, patients who were in psychotherapy and who had more than one hospitalization for depression had respectively 82% and 89% increased likelihood to have BP instead of TRD-UP. In contrast, the presence of a comorbidity with anxiety disorders increased by 10 times the likelihood of having a diagnosis of TRD-UP than of BP. Moreover, a lower depression severity as measured by the HAMD-17 score as well as a higher global functioning as measured by the GAF score increased the likelihood of having a diagnosis of BP instead of TRD-UP.

Sociodemographic and clinical characteristics in BP-I, BP-II and TRD-UP

As secondary aim of this study we examined the possible differences within the bipolar spectrum (BP-I vs. BP-II) and then towards TRD-UP. As reported in Table 4, we found that some sociodemographic and clinical characteristics differentiated BP-I from BP-II patients and either BP-I or BP-II from TRD-UP. BP-I but not BP-II patients were younger than TRD-UP patients ($p = 0.011$). Patients with BP-II showed a lower rate of unemployment/sick leave than TRD-UP and BP-I patients (48% vs 74% and 80%, respectively; $p < 0.001$).

The prevalence of patients who did not have any hospitalization for depression since the first episode was greater in BP-II than in BP-I ($p < 0.001$). Family history was also another characteristic that differed amongst groups. BP-II patients showed a higher prevalence of having at least one first-degree relative with affective disorders than TRD-UP patients ($p = 0.010$).

Of note, the prevalence of patients who had a history of suicidality was significantly higher in those affected by BP-II than those diagnosed with TRD-UP ($p < 0.001$) and BP-I ($p < 0.01$). We did not observed difference between BP-I and BP-II patients concerning the prevalence of comorbid substance use, of anxiety disorders, of Axis II personality disorders, and Axis III physical diseases. In addition, no difference was found between BP-I and BP-II for the levels of both depression severity and global functioning.

Table 3 Logistic regression showing odd ratios associated with TRD-UP instead of BP disorder ($N = 194$)

Variables	Coefficient B	SEM	Wald	*P* value	OR Exp(B)	OR 95% CI	
						Lower	Upper
Individual characteristics							
Age of 1st depression	−0.051	0.025	4.003	0.045	0.951	0.905	0.999
Marital status	1.583	0.701	5.108	0.024	4.872	1.234	19.235
First degree relatives with affective disorders	0.262	0.593	0.195	0.659	1.299	0.406	4.157
More than one hospitalization for depression	−2.148	0.614	12.239	**0.001**	0.177	0.035	0.389
Psychotherapy treatment	−2.232	0.699	10.190	**0.001**	0.107	0.027	0.423
History of suicide attempt	−0.135	0.625	0.047	0.829	0.874	0.257	2.974
Comorbidities							
Current anxiety disorders	2.357	0.608	15.033	**0.001**	10.560	3.208	34.763
Severity of depression							
Melancholic depressive features	0.650	0.747	0.755	0.385	1.915	0.422	8.285
Failed pharmacotherapies	0.266	0.106	6.331	0.012	1.304	1.060	1.604
HAM-D17 score	−0.193	0.067	8.208	**0.004**	0.824	0.722	0.941
Level of functioning							
Global assessment of functioning score (GAF)	0.164	0.047	11.985	**0.001**	1.178	1.074	1.293

TRD-UP Treatment-Resistant Unipolar Depression, *BP* Bipolar disorder type I and type II, *OR* Odds ratio, *CI* Confidence interval, *SEM* Standard Error of Mean. Boldface indicates significant association at an alpha level = 0.01

Table 4 Socio-demographic and clinical characteristics of patients with TRD-UP, BP-I and BP-II ($N = 194$)

	TRD-UP (n = 100)	BP-I (n = 52)	BP-II (n = 42)	Statistics
Age (Years) (Mean ± SD)	46.5 ± 13.3	$39.7 \pm 15.2^{+}$	41.7 ± 13.2	$F_{2,191} = 4.6, p = 0.011$
Ratio of Males: Females	41:59	21:31	16:26	$\chi^2 = 0.11, p = 0.949$
Patients≤65 years of age	90 (90%)	49 (94%)	42 (100%)	$\chi^2 = 4.83, p = 0.089$
Marital status	41 (41%)	8 (15%) ***	7 (17%) ***	$\chi^2 = 14.81, p = 0.001$
Unemployed/Disability sick leave	74 (74%)	42 (80%)	20 (48%)* **,###	$\chi^2 = 13.67, p = 0.001$
Age of first major depressive episode (Mean ± SD)	37.7 ± 15.3	$28.9 \pm 10.1^{+++}$	$23.2 \pm 8.6^{+++}$	$F_{2,191} = 21.0, p < 0.001$
Early onset of major depressive episodes(< 25)	29 (29%)	30 (58%) ***	22 (53%) ***	$\chi^2 = 14.07, p = 0.001$
Age of first psychiatric consultation (Mean ± SD)	35.9 ± 15.2	$24.2 \pm 10.5^{+++}$	$25.9 \pm 11.2^{+++}$	$F_{2,191} = 16.8, p < 0.001$
Age of first psychiatric hospitalization (Mean ± SD)	40.1 ± 15.0	$28.1 \pm 11.7^{+++}$	$31.3 \pm 12.6^{+}$	$F_{2,123} = 10.0, p < 0.001$
Patients with recurrent depression (> 3)	39 (39%)	27 (52%)	20 (48%)	$\chi^2 = 2.55, p = 0.279$
Duration of illness-current episode (years) (Mean ± SD)	11.2 ± 10.4	12.2 ± 11.6	16.7 ± 12.2	$F_{2,191} = 2.6, p = 0.075$
Patients with comorbid substance use	27 (27%)	20 (39%)	12 (29%)	$\chi^2 = 2.21, p = 0.331$
History of Alcohol use	9 (9%)	6 (12%)	10 (24%)	$\chi^2 = 5.89, p = 0.053$
History of Cannabis use	6 (6%)	11 (21%)	8 (19%)	$\chi^2 = 8.81, p = 0.012$
History of Cocaine use	3 (3%)	1 (2%)	2 (5%)	$\chi^2 = 0.63, p = 0.730$
Number of Failed pharmacotherapies (Mean ± SD)	3.6 ± 2.6	$5.0 \pm 2.5^{++}$	$5.6 \pm 2.8^{+++}$	$F_{2,191} = 9.9, p < 0.001$
Failed antidepressant trials (Mean ± SD)	2.5 ± 1.7	$1.35 \pm 1.4^{++}$	2.0 ± 1.4	$F_{2,191} = 5.4, p = 0.005$
Failed SGA (Mean ± SD)	0.65 ± 0.7	$1.9 \pm 1.1^{+++}$	$1.4 \pm 1.2^{+++}$	$F_{2,191} = 30.2, p < 0.001$
Failed Mood stabilizers (Mean ± SD)	0.3 ± 0.6	$1.3 \pm 0.8^{+++}$	$1.4 \pm 1.0^{+++}$	$F_{2,191} = 37.5, p < 0.001$
Patients currently having psychotherapy	41 (41%)	43 (83%) ***	35 (83%) ***	$\chi^2 = 36.01, p < 0.001$
Number of hospitalizations for depression since 1st episode				
None	56 (56%)	1 (2%) ***	14 (33%) ***, ###	$\chi^2 = 43.36, p < 0.001$
> one	20 (20%)	39 (75%) ***	21 (50%) ***	$\chi^2 = 44.41, p < 0.001$
Patients with 1st degree relative with affective illness	51 (51%)	31 (60%)	32 (76%)*	$\chi^2 = 7.76, p = 0.021$
Patients with Anxiety disorders	61 (61%)	9 (17%) ***	13 (31%) ***	$\chi^2 = 29.74, p < 0.001$
Patients with Panic disorders	19 (19%)	2 (4%) **	1 (2%) **	$\chi^2 = 12.09, p = 0.002$
Patients with Melancholic symptoms	74 (74%)	22 (42%) ***	18 (42%) ***	$\chi^2 = 19.77, p < 0.001$
Patients with Atypical symptoms	14 (14%)	11 (21%)	14 (33%)*	$\chi^2 = 6.93, p = 0.031$
Patients with suicidal attempts	23 (23%)	17 (33%)	25 (60%) ***,##	$\chi^2 = 17.73, p < 0.001$
History of MDE with psychotic symptoms	24 (24%)	16 (31%)	4 (10%)	$\chi^2 = 6.18, p = 0.045$
Patients with Personality disorders (Axis II in DSM-IV)	44 (44%)	26 (50%)	19 (45%)	$\chi^2 = 0.50, p = 0.777$
Cluster A	7 (7%)	0 (0%)	1 (2%)	$\chi^2 = 4.65, p = 0.098$
Cluster B	19 (19%)	6 (12%)	10 (24%)	$\chi^2 = 2.49, p = 0.287$
Cluster C	25 (25%)	1 (2%) ***	4 (10%) ***	$\chi^2 = 15.38, p < 0.001$
Patients with Medical condition potentially relevant to treatment (Axis III in DSM-IV)				
Autoimmune diseases	11 (11%)	2 (4%)	0 (0%)	$\chi^2 = 6.65, p = 0.036$
Cardiovascular diseases	25 (25%)	10 (20%)	8 (19%)	$\chi^2 = 0.96, p = 0.618$
Chronic pain disorders	25 (25%)	8 (15%)	7 (17%)	$\chi^2 = 2.44, p = 0.295$
Neurological conditions	13 (13%)	3 (6%)	2 (5%)	$\chi^2 = 3.42, p = 0.181$
Metabolic disorder	19 (19%)	20 (38%)*	12 (29%)	$\chi^2 = 6.83, p = 0.033$
Depression severity (Mean ± SD)				
MADRS	30.8 ± 8.9	$22.2 \pm 6.7^{+++}$	$24.3 \pm 7.2^{+++}$	$F_{2,191} = 22.7, p < 0.001$
HAMD-17	23.2 ± 6.2	$16.7 \pm 4.7^{+++}$	$17.3 \pm 4.5^{+++}$	$F_{2,191} = 30.8, p < 0.001$
QIDS	15.8 ± 4.2	$12.1 \pm 3.7^{+++}$	13.4 ± 4.0**	$F_{2,191} = 15.4, p < 0.001$

Table 4 Socio-demographic and clinical characteristics of patients with TRD-UP, BP-I and BP-II ($N = 194$) *(Continued)*

	TRD-UP (n = 100)	BP-I (n = 52)	BP-II (n = 42)	Statistics
CGI-S	5.0 ± 1.2	4.2 ± 1.3^{++}	4.3 ± 1.1^{++}	$F_{2,191} = 8.8, p < 0.001$
GAF	55.5 ± 10.2	60.9 ± 4.4^{+++}	60.3 ± 4.9^{++}	$F_{2,191} = 11.7, p < 0.001$

SD Standard Deviation, *TRD-UP* Treatment-Resistant Unipolar Depression, *BP-I* Bipolar disorder type I, *BP-II* Bipolar Disorder type II, *MDE* Major depressive episode, *SGA* Second Generation Antipsychotics
$^{*}p < 0.05$, $^{**}p < 0.01$, $^{***}p < 0.001$ versus UP-TRD; $^{\#}p < 0.05$, $^{\#\#}p < 0.01$, $^{\#\#\#}p < 0.001$ BP-I versus BP-II by Pearson's chi-square test
$^{+}p < 0.05$, $^{++}p < 0.01$, $^{+++}p < 0.001$ versus UP-TRD by One-way Anova plus Bonferroni post hoc analysis

Discussion

These results indicate that patients with TRD-UP exhibit different psychopathological features compared to depressive episodes in patients with BP, suggesting that TRD-UP is a distinct psychopathological condition and not a prodromal state of BP depression.

TRD-UP patients show higher depression severity, higher prevalence of anxiety and panic disorders and of Cluster C personality disorders, a later onset of depression and fewer hospitalizations than BP patients. Within the bipolar spectrum, BP-II patients show lower rate of unemployment and hospitalizations for depression and higher prevalence of history of suicide attempts than BP-I patients.

Using a binary logistic regression model, it was possible to distinguish TRD-UP from BP disorders. The following variables were mostly associated with TRD-UP than with BP: increased anxiety, lower score on the GAF scale, higher depression symptoms (HAMD-17 score), lower number of hospitalizations and psychotherapies.

Overall, these findings are in agreement with previous literature comparing major depressive disorder (MDD) (non-TRD) with BP [15, 36, 37]. Indeed, the higher depression severity in TRD-UP than in BP was also reported in previous studies differentiating BP from MDD (non-TRD) patients. Additionally, earlier onset of depression, a greater prevalence of family history of affective disorders and a higher rate of suicide attempts were found in BP compared with UP (non-TRD) depression [15, 36, 37].

Mitchell and Malhi [37], in an extensive review, described a higher prevalence of depressive episodes and lower functioning in BP compared with UP (non-TRD) depression. In our study, TRD-UP showed the same number of recurrent episodes but higher number of hospitalizations and a lower GAF score compared with BP, pointing out the severity of the TRD-UP condition in comparison with UP (non-TRD) and BP. The lower functioning in TRD-UP patients is in line with previous studies indicating that TRD-UP, unlike BP patients, tend to experience more unremitting depressive states and higher fluctuations with depressive symptoms despite receiving appropriate treatment [38]. Patients with BP depression showed a greater prevalence of atypical symptoms and lower prevalence of melancholic features than TRD-UP patients as previously indicated by Benazzi [39]. However, when accounting for possible confounding variables, in the binary logistic model, depression with atypical or melancholic features was not significantly associated with TRD-UP, as suggested in a previous study [40].

In TRD-UP, we found a greater prevalence of Cluster C personality disorders in keeping with Kornstein and Schneider [41] and a meta-analysis reporting that patients with affective disorders had more than 50% comorbidity with personality disorders [42].

We have shown that BP patients had a greater prevalence of metabolic disorder comorbidity compared with the TRD-UP group. These findings are in line with some studies where lifetime comorbidity in BP-I patients were reported to be between 50% up to 70% [43]. However, it cannot be ruled out that the higher rate of metabolic disease observed in BP patients was caused by the higher use of SGA in BP than in TRD-UP patients (as described in the methodology section).

Finally, patients with TRD-UP have less number of failed pharmacological trials compared to BP, especially for SGA and MS. This might be due to the polypharmacy required in BP versus TRD-UP, as previously mentioned in a youth population at risk for BP disorders [44].

Altogether, these findings suggest that TRD-UP may constitute a unique subtype of depression compared with other affective disorders, and thus depressive episodes in BP are different than those in TRD-UP. Moreover, they are in support of a bi-dimensional approach for TRD-UP and BP disorders, recognizing points of differentiation that might contribute to distinguish a diagnosis within the affective disorders. Of note, it seems that differences also exist between TRD-UP and the different sub-types of BP. Further studies with a larger sample size may allow to deeply examine the psychopathological features that may be specifically associated with either TRD-UP, BP-I or BP-II. These results could seem in apparent contrast with Angst et al. [45] arguing that a diagnostic change from depression to BP-I and BP II occurs in about 1% and 0.5% of patients per year, respectively, and supporting a spectrum theory, in which UP depression and BP depression are in a continuum spectrum [46].

In our study, we have chosen a priori patients followed in the Mood Disorders clinic for at least 2 years (mean 7.5 years), in which the possible risk of novel manic/hypomanic episode and thus consequent change in diagnosis was minimized and ruled out. This is also in agreement with a recent systematic review and meta-analysis underscoring that the rate of conversion from UP to BP disorders decreases with time reaching 0.8% in 10 years of initial diagnosis [47]. For this reason, compared to the systematic review by Bennabi et al. [16] and Dudek et al. [15], bipolarity was not a risk factor for TRD. However, in keeping with Bennabi et al. [16], comorbidity for anxiety disorders was a clear risk factors for TRD-UP.

In contrast with Cassano et al. [48] and Benazzi [23], we have not used scales such as the Structured Clinical Interview for the Mood Spectrum or the Hypomania interview guide that by characterizing threshold and subthreshold mood episodes, hypomanic or "temperamental" features related to mood dysregulation allow assessing hypomanic symptoms. This limitation has prevented us to detect if TRD-UP could also present subthreshold hypomanic symptoms. Another limitation of our study is that this is a retrospective and observational cross-sectional chart-review analysis that consequently lacks randomization and a longitudinal follow up. Prospective longitudinal studies are warranted to demonstrate that TRD will not convert in BP depression, or at least in a non-significant extent.

Despite the above-mentioned limitations, this study has several strengths: this is the first comparison study examining different clinical and sociodemographic data from an outpatient tertiary clinic for affective disorders proposing different predictors to distinguish TRD-UP from BP depression. Moreover, it adds clinical evidence towards the differentiation of TRD-UP as a unique type of depression as previously hypothesized by Fagiolini and Kupfer [49] suggesting that TRD-UP may have specific clinical characteristics, neurobiological profile, and environment in which TRD develops, requiring a combination of AD and SGA as a first-line treatment [17].

Therefore, our study supports the ancient hypothesis of K. Schneider differentiating endogenous periodic unipolar depression (a chronic condition with several episodes in lifespan, and resistant to treatment) from bipolar phasic depression (characterized by phases of mania and depression) and exogenous depression (caused by exterior factors, with less episodes during life) [50, 51].

However, to fully validate Schneider's hypothesis, these results should be replicated with larger controlled studies and include a comparison group with UP depressive patients who are not treatment resistant.

Finally, further analysis of longitudinal studies addressing neurobiological markers, clinical features between the TRD-UP and BP disorders should provide insight concerning these particular questions and evaluate the implications on pharmacological outcomes. This integrated approach will aid clinicians and researchers to disentangle initial diagnostic controversies between unipolar and bipolar spectrum improving the differential management and therapeutics of patients suffering from depression.

Conclusion

This retrospective and observational cross-sectional study shows that patients with depressive episodes in TRD-UP have a different history and distinct psychopathological features compared with BP depressive patients, thus TRD-UP constitutes a distinct psychopathological condition and not necessarily a prodromal state of BP depression. Further studies are needed to differentiate the pharmacological responses and outcomes in these distinct groups.

Abbreviations

AD: Antidepressant; ADHD: Attention Deficit-Hyperactivity disorder; ANOVA: Analysis of variance; BP: Bipolar disorder; BP-I: Bipolar Type I disorder; BP-II: Bipolar Type II disorder; CGI-S: Clinical Global Impression-Severity of Illness; DSM-IV-TR: Diagnostic and Statistical Manual of Mental Disorders, Fourth Edition. Text revision; GAF: Global assessment of functioning score; HAM-D17: Hamilton-Rating Scale for Depression; MADRS: Montgomery–Asberg Depression Rating Scale; MDC: Mood Disorders Clinic; MDD: Major depressive disorder; MDE: Major depressive episode; MS: Mood stabilizers; MSM: Maudsley Staging Method; MUHC: McGill University Health Center; QIDS-C16: Quick Inventory of Depressive Symptomatology; SCID: Structured Clinical Interview for Diagnosis; SD: Standard deviation; SEM: Standard error of the mean; SGA: Second-generation antipsychotics; STAR*D: Sequenced Treatment Alternatives to Relieve Depression; TRD-UP: Treatment-Resistant Unipolar Depression; YMRS: Young Mania Rating Scale

Acknowledgements

The authors would like to thank Rita Zakarian for proofreading the manuscript.

Funding

This research was supported by the Quebec Network on Suicide, Mood Disorders and Related Disorders, the Canadian Depression Research & Intervention Network (CDRIN), and the Graham Boeckh Foundation. Linda Booij is supported by a new investigator award from the Canadian Institutes of Health Research. Nicolas Nuñez received a fellowship from the Faculty of Medicine of McGill University. Stefano Comai is supported in part by a 2016 NARSAD Young Investigator Award from the Brain & Behavior Research Foundation.

Authors' contributions

All authors read and approved the final manuscript. NAN: collected data, created data bank, data analysis, assistance in research planning and manuscript writing; SC: data analysis, wrote the manuscript, research planning; ED: data analysis; MFG: collected data, created data bank, prepared ethical submission; JT: collected data; MSL, SV, TK, AF, NL, PC: referred patients' files; LB: data analysis; GG: wrote the manuscript, conceived the idea, research planning, supervised the team.

Consent for publication
Not applicable.

Competing interests
The authors declare that they have no competing interests.

Author details
[1]Department of Psychiatry, Neurobiological Psychiatry Unit, McGill University Health Center (MUHC), McGill University, Room 220, 1033 Pine Avenue West,, Montreal, QC, Canada. [2]Department of Psychiatry, Mood Disorder Clinic, McGill University Health Center, McGill University, Montreal, QC, Canada. [3]Division of Neuroscience, San Raffaele Scientific Institute and Vita-Salute University, Milan, Italy. [4]Department of Psychology, Concordia University and Sainte-Justine Hospital Research Center, University of Montréal, Montréal, QC, Canada.

References

1. Ferrari AJ, Charlson FJ, Norman RE, Patten SB, Freedman G, Murray CJ, Vos T, Whiteford HA. Burden of depressive disorders by country, sex, age, and year: findings from the global burden of disease study 2010. PLoS Med. 2013; 10(11):e1001547.
2. Greden JF. The burden of disease for treatment-resistant depression. J Clin Psychiatry. 2001;62:26–31.
3. Kennedy N, Abbott R, Paykel E. Remission and recurrence of depression in the maintenance era: long-term outcome in a Cambridge cohort. Psychol Med. 2003;33(05):827–38.
4. Souery D, Papakostas GI, Trivedi MH. Treatment-resistant depression. J Clin Psychiatry. 2006;67:16.
5. Fava M. Diagnosis and definition of treatment-resistant depression. Biol Psychiatry. 2003;53(8):649–59.
6. Trivedi MH, Fava M, Wisniewski SR, Thase ME, Quitkin F, Warden D, Ritz L, Nierenberg AA, Lebowitz BD, Biggs MM. Medication augmentation after the failure of SSRIs for depression. N Engl J Med. 2006;354(12):1243–52.
7. Lam RW, Kennedy SH, Grigoriadis S, McIntyre RS, Milev R, Ramasubbu R, Parikh SV, Patten SB, Ravindran AV. Canadian network for mood and anxiety treatments (CANMAT) clinical guidelines for the management of major depressive disorder in adults.: III. Pharmacotherapy. J Affect Disord. 2009;117: S26–43.
8. Souery D, Amsterdam J, De Montigny C, Lecrubier Y, Montgomery S, Lipp O, Racagni G, Zohar J, Mendlewicz J. Treatment resistant depression: methodological overview and operational criteria. Eur Neuropsychopharmacol. 1999;9(1):83–91.
9. Berlim MT, Turecki G. Definition, assessment, and staging of treatment—resistant refractory major depression: a review of current concepts and methods. Can. J. Psychiatr. 2007;52(1):46–54.
10. Trivedi MH, Rush AJ, Wisniewski SR, Nierenberg AA, Warden D, Ritz L, Norquist G, Howland RH, Lebowitz B, McGrath PJ. Evaluation of outcomes with citalopram for depression using measurement-based care in STAR* D: implications for clinical practice. Am J Psychiatr. 2006;163(1):28–40.
11. Fornaro M, Giosuè P. Current nosology of treatment resistant depression: a controversy resistant to revision. Clinical Practice & Epidemiology in Mental Health. 2010;6(1)
12. Fornaro M, Giosuè P. Current nosology of treatment resistant depression: a controversy resistant to revision. 2010.
13. Souery D, Oswald P, Massat I, Bailer U, Bollen J, Demyttenaere K, Kasper S, Lecrubier Y, Montgomery S, Serretti A. Clinical factors associated with treatment resistance in major depressive disorder: results from a European multicenter study. J Clin Psychiatry. 2007;68(7):1062–70.
14. Balestri M, Calati R, Souery D, Kautzky A, Kasper S, Montgomery S, Zohar J, Mendlewicz J, Serretti A. Socio-demographic and clinical predictors of treatment resistant depression: a prospective European multicenter study. J Affect Disord. 2016;189:224–32.
15. Dudek D, Rybakowski JK, Siwek M, Pawłowski T, Lojko D, Roczeń R, Kiejna A. Risk factors of treatment resistance in major depression: association with bipolarity. J Affect Disord. 2010;126(1):268–71.
16. Bennabi D, Aouizerate B, El-Hage W, Doumy O, Moliere F, Courtet P, Nieto I, Bellivier F, Bubrovsky M, Vaiva G, et al. Risk factors for treatment resistance in unipolar depression: a systematic review. J Affect Disord. 2015;171:137–41.
17. Gobbi G, Ghabrash MF, Nuñez N, Tabaka J, Di Sante J, Saint-Laurent M, Vida S, Kolivakis T, Low N, Cervantes P, Comai S. Antidepressant combination versus antidepressants plus second-generation antipsychotic augmentation in treatment-resistant unipolar depression. Int Clin Psychopharmacol. 2018; 33(1):34–43.
18. Pacchiarotti I, Bond DJ, Baldessarini RJ, Nolen WA, Grunze H, Licht RW, Post RM, Berk M, Goodwin GM, Sachs GS. The International Society for Bipolar Disorders (ISBD) task force report on antidepressant use in bipolar disorders. Am J Psychiatr. 2013;170(11):1249–62.
19. Ghaemi SN, Boiman EE, Goodwin FK. Diagnosing bipolar disorder and the effect of antidepressants: a naturalistic study. J Clin Psychiatry. 2000;61(10)
20. Marchand WR. Recognizing and treating bipolar disorder. Hosp Physician. 2003;39(12):21–30.
21. Geller B, Luby J. Child and adolescent bipolar disorder: a review of the past 10 years. J Am Acad Child Adolesc Psychiatry. 1997;36(9):1168–76.
22. Akiskal HS, Walker P, Puzantian VR, King D, Rosenthal TL, Dranon M. Bipolar outcome in the course of depressive illness. Phenomenologic, familial, and pharmacologic predictors J Affect Disord. 1983;5(2):115–28.
23. Benazzi F. Symptoms of depression as possible markers of bipolar II disorder. Prog Neuro-Psychopharmacol Biol Psychiatry. 2006;30(3):471–7.
24. Perlis RH. A clinical risk stratification tool for predicting treatment resistance in major depressive disorder. Biol Psychiatry. 2013;74(1):7–14.
25. American Psychiatric Association: Diagnostic and statistical manual of mental disorders fourth edition text revision (DSM-IV-TR), vol. 4. Washington, DC; 2000.
26. First MB, Spitzer RL, Gibbon M, Williams JB. Structured clinical interview for DSM-IV-TR axis I disorders, research version, patient edition. In: SCID-I/P. 2002;
27. Fekadu WC, Poon KMBML, Cleare AJ. A multidimensional tool to quantify treatment resistance in depression: the Maudsley staging method. J. Clin. Psychiatry. 2009;70(2):177–84.
28. Young R, Biggs J, Ziegler V, Meyer D. A rating scale for mania: reliability, validity and sensitivity. Br J Psychiatry. 1978;133(5):429–35.
29. Zimmerman M, Martinez JH, Young D, Chelminski I, Dalrymple K. Severity classification on the Hamilton depression rating scale. J Affect Disord. 2013; 150(2):384–8.
30. Montgomery SA, Asberg M. A new depression scale designed to be sensitive to change. Br J Psychiatry. 1979;134(4):382–9.
31. Guy W. Clinical global impression scale. The ECDEU assessment manual for psychopharmacology-revised volume DHEW Publ no. ADM. 1976;76(338): 218–22.
32. Rush AJ, Trivedi MH, Ibrahim HM, Carmody TJ, Arnow B, Klein DN, Markowitz JC, Ninan PT, Kornstein S, Manber R. The 16-item quick inventory of depressive symptomatology (QIDS), clinician rating (QIDS-C), and self-report (QIDS-SR): a psychometric evaluation in patients with chronic major depression. Biol Psychiatry. 2003;54(5):573–83.
33. Hamilton M. A rating scale for depression. J Neurol Neurosurg Psychiatry. 1960;23(1):56–62.
34. Viera AJ, Garrett JM. Understanding interobserver agreement: the kappa statistic. Fam Med. 2005;37(5):360–3.
35. Cohen J. Weighted kappa: nominal scale agreement provision for scaled disagreement or partial credit. Psychol Bull. 1968;70(4):213.
36. Mitchell PB, Goodwin GM, Johnson GF, Hirschfeld R. Diagnostic guidelines for bipolar depression: a probabilistic approach. Bipolar Disord. 2008;10(1p2): 144–52.
37. Mitchell PB, Malhi GS. Bipolar depression: phenomenological overview and clinical characteristics. Bipolar Disord. 2004;6(6):530–9.
38. Vergunst FK, Fekadu A, Wooderson SC, Tunnard CS, Rane LJ, Markopoulou K, Cleare AJ. Longitudinal course of symptom severity and fluctuation in patients with treatment-resistant unipolar and bipolar depression. Psychiatry Res. 2013;207(3):143–9.

39. Benazzi F. Depression with DSM-IV atypical features: a marker for bipolar II disorder. Eur Arch Psychiatry Clin Neurosci. 2000;250(1):53–5.
40. Zaninotto L, Souery D, Calati R, Sentissi O, Kasper S, Akimova E, Zohar J, Montgomery S, Mendlewicz J, Serretti A. Treatment resistance in severe unipolar depression: no association with psychotic or melancholic features. Ann Clin Psychiatry. 2013;25(2):97–106.
41. Kornstein SG, Schneider RK. Clinical features of treatment-resistant depression. J Clin Psychiatry. 2001;62:18–25.
42. Friborg O, Martinsen EW, Martinussen M, Kaiser S, Øvergård KT, Rosenvinge JH. Comorbidity of personality disorders in mood disorders: a meta-analytic review of 122 studies from 1988 to 2010. J Affect Disord. 2014:152:1–11.
43. Vieta E, Colom F, Corbella B, Martínez-Arán A, Reinares M, Benabarre A, Gasto C. Clinical correlates of psychiatric comorbidity in bipolar I patients. Bipolar Disord. 2001;3(5):253–8.
44. Strawn JR, Adler CM, McNamara RK, Welge JA, Bitter SM, Mills NP, Barzman DH, Cerullo MA, Chang KD, Strakowski SM. Antidepressant tolerability in anxious and depressed youth at high risk for bipolar disorder: a prospective naturalistic treatment study. Bipolar Disord. 2014;16(5):523–30.
45. Angst J, Sellaro R, Stassen HH, Gamma A. Diagnostic conversion from depression to bipolar disorders: results of a long-term prospective study of hospital admissions. J Affect Disord. 2005;84(2):149–57.
46. Angst J. The bipolar spectrum. Bristish J Psychiatry. 2007;190:189–91.
47. Kessing L, Andersen P. Evidence for clinical progression of unipolar and bipolar disorders. Acta Psychiatr Scand. 2017;135(1):51–64.
48. Cassano GB, Rucci P, Frank E, Fagiolini A, Dell'Osso L, Shear MK, Kupfer DJ. The mood spectrum in unipolar and bipolar disorder: arguments for a unitary approach. Am J Psychiatry. 2004;161(7):1264-9.
49. Fagiolini A, Kupfer DJ. Is treatment-resistant depression a unique subtype of depression? Biol Psychiatry. 2003;53(8):640–8.
50. Schneider K. Die Schichtung des emotionalen Lebens und der Aufbau der Depressionszustände. Zeitschrift für die gesamte Neurologie und Psychiatrie. 1920;59(1):281–6.
51. Schneider K. Clinical psychopathology: Grune & Stratton; 1959.

2

Towards characterizing the regional cerebral perfusion in evaluating the severity of major depression disorder with SPECT/CT

Jinming Li[1,2†], Yuan Yang[3†], Yuankai Zhu[1], Liqiang Zhou[1], Yunfeng Han[1], Tao Yin[1], Zhaoting Cheng[1], Guopeng Zhang[1], Yanxia Shen[1] and Jing Chen[1*]

Abstract

Background: Major depressive disorder (MDD) is a common mental disorder worldwide, but now there is a lack of clinically effective assessment and management of MDD. In this study, we used technetium-99 m ethylcysteinate dimer ([^{99m}Tc]ECD) SPECT/CT to characterize the regional cerebral blood flow (rCBF) status of MDD patients, and to explore an objective image assessment model of MDD which is non- or minimally-invasive, convenient and accurate in a clinical setting.

Methods: The severity of MDD was assessed by three trained psychiatrists, based on scores obtained from HAMD and HAMA. [^{99m}Tc]ECD rCBF SPECT/CT was performed in 20 healthy controls and 74 unipolar MDD patients before receiving the treatment. The CT attenuation-corrected SPECT images data were automatically registered, analyzed simultaneously by 3D-SSP and eZIS.

Results: The mean score of HAMD and HAMA in the MDD patients was 25.49 ± 6.00, and 23.12 ± 5.83, respectively. There was a positive correlation between two scores. The MDD women had higher HAMD scores than MDD men. The decreased rCBF of MDD patients in frontal lobes (bilateral B11, B47 and right B4, B6, B10, B46), temporal lobe (right B21, B41, B42) and cingulated cortex (bilateral B24, B33), while their increased rCBF in occipital lobe (bilateral B17, B19 and left B18). Additionally, the depression severity was negatively correlated with decreased rCBF in left ventral anterior cingulate cortex B24, and was positively correlated with decreased rCBF in left inferior prefrontal gyrus B47 and increased rCBF in right associative visual cortex B19. The anxiety severity was negatively correlated with decreased rCBF in left subgenual cortex B25.

Conclusions: Although the mechanism underlying the correlation is not yet fully understood, our findings indicated that the rCBF SPECT/CT may provide an objective assessment for MDD severity. It might be used monitoring therapeutic efficacy in the management of MDD.

Keywords: Major depressive disorder, Cerebral blood flow, SPECT/CT, [^{99m}Tc]ECD

* Correspondence: lindaxcx@vip.163.com
†Equal contributors
[1]Department of Nuclear Medicine, Tongji Hospital, Tongji Medical College, Huazhong University of Science and Technology, Wuhan, Hubei Province 430030, China
Full list of author information is available at the end of the article

Background

Major depressive disorder (MDD) is a common mental disorder worldwide. It is characterized by a persistent low mood and a loss of interest or pleasure [1]. MDD is also a disabling condition that adversely affects the sufferers' whole lives. Moreover, MDD can lead to suicide. Over 800,000 people die by suicide every year, and most of them are suffering from MDD [2]. However, fewer than 10% of MDD sufferers have ever received effective treatments, and one of the most significant barriers is lack of effective assessment and management of MDD [2].

Today, the most widely used criterion for assessing MDD is the fourth edition of the Diagnostic and Statistical Manual of Mental Disorders (DSM-IV) published by American Psychiatric Association, and the 10th revision of International Statistical Classification of Diseases and Related Health Problems (ICD-10) list by the World Health Organization. DSM-IV is more popular among mental health professionals [3]. The Hamilton Rating Scale for Depression (HAMD) is a multiple-item scale for measuring the severity of depression. However, it has been criticized for its subjectivity [4]. There is a demand for objective assessment of MDD, which is non- or minimal-invasive, convenient and accurate in a clinical setting.

Since the late 1970s, functional neuroimaging, including single photon emission computed tomography (SPECT), positron emission tomography (PET), magnetic resonance imaging (MRI) and fusing imaging (SPECT/CT, PET/CT or PET/MRI) has been extensively used in MDD [5–9]. Regional cerebral blood flow (rCBF) SPECT is a nuclear medicine imaging method in routine clinical practice, and is also one of the earliest functional neuroimaging studies in MDD [10]. According to previous research, there is almost complete agreement that blood flow in the frontal lobe is reduced in MDD patients [9, 11–14], but the controversies still exist in the extent of the rCBF involvement [15–17]. It has been speculated that the various patterns of rCBF abnormalities in MDD patients may be related to the various clinical presentation of MDD [15–17].

In this study, the rCBF status of MDD patients was characterized with technetium-99 m ethylcysteinate dimer ([^{99m}Tc]ECD) SPECT/CT. The localization of abnormal rCBF was represented by Brodmann areas. In addition, we explore the relationship in MDD patients between the imaging features, clinical presentation and the severity of the symptoms. It is expected that the conventional nuclear medicine imaging could help add an objective image assessment model of MDD in current psychiatric practice that relies mainly on self-reporting of symptoms and clinical interviews.

Methods

Subjects

74 patients (21 men and 53 women) who fulfilled the DSM-IV criteria [1] for unipolar MDD were enrolled in this study, with age ranging from 20 to 72 years (mean 41.9 years old). All patients were outpatients from the department of psychiatry, Tongji Hospital of Tongji Medical College, Huazhong University of Science and Technology (HUST). The severity of MDD was assessed by three trained psychiatrists, based on scores obtained from HAMD and Hamilton Rating Scale for Anxiety (HAMA). 20 healthy controls (8 men and 12 women) were recruited through local advertisements, ranging from ages 22 to 59 (mean 38.0 years old). All MDD patients and healthy controls subjects were right handed, had never taken psychotropic medication, and had no central nervous system disorders and other medical disorders clearly affecting cerebral blood flow and cognitive function.

This study was approved by the local ethics committee at Tongji Hospital of Tongji Medical College, HUST (Permit Number: TJ-C20141220). All subjects received a detailed description of the study and gave written informed consent.

SPECT/CT

^{99}Mo-^{99m}Tc generator was provided by Beijing Atomic High-tech Co., Ltd., China. The ECD kit was purchased from Jiangsu Atom Medicine Research Institute Jiangyuan Pharmaceutical Factory, China. The radiochemical purity of ^{99m}Tc]ECD was over 95%.

[^{99m}Tc]ECD rCBF SPECT/CT was performed using a hybrid system (Discovery NM/670, General Electric) at the department of Nuclear Medicine, Tongji Hospital of Tongji Medical College, HUST, in 20 healthy controls and 74 unipolar MDD patients before receiving treatment. The hybrid system consists of a double-headed SPECT equipped with low-energy high-resolution collimators and a 16-detector row CT. The SPECT resolution is 9.9 mm. All subjects were administrated 740 MBq (20 mCi) [^{99m}Tc]ECD after resting 30 min with eyes closed in a dimly quiet room. Followed resting another 30 min, SPECT/CT fusing imaging were performed with a 20% window width centered at 140 KeV and a 128 × 128 matrix. Reconstructed images were displayed as CT images, SPECT images, and fusion images in the axial, coronal, and sagittal planes as well as maximum intensity projection images.

Image analysis

The images were interpreted by three nuclear medicine physicians. The abnormal rCBF was defined using a three-dimensional stereotactic surface projection (3D-SSP) technique, developed as part of a neurologic statistical image analysis (NEUROSTAT) program

(Department of Internal Medicine, University of Michigan, Ann Arbor, MI, USA). All CT attenuation-corrected SPECT data were automatically registered, analyzed and compared with a normalized database using 3D-SSP. A Z-score-based semi-quantitative analysis was used, and the Z-score of 1.5 was set as a cutoff point to identify the brain areas with abnormal rCBF. The localization of abnormal rCBF was presented by Brodmann areas (B). Besides, regions of interest (ROIs) were drawn on the transverse sections of the SPECT/CT fusion images by one operator over caudate nucleus, globus pallidus, hippocampus and cerebellum, which cannot be identified clearly by B. The mean counts of cerebellum were measured correcting for background counts, which mostly remains unchanged rCBF in all subjects according to our observational study. The fraction of mean counts in the targeted area ROI-to-cerebellum ROI was calculated as [^{99m}Tc]ECD uptake index (UI).

The same CT attenuation-corrected SPECT images data were also processed using statistical parametric mapping (SPM12; Functional Imaging Laboratory, University College London, London, UK) and easy Z score imaging system (eZIS; Fijifilm Ri Pharma Co., Kanazawa, Japan).

Statistical analysis

Data were processed using the IBM SPSS Statistics V19.0 (SPSS Inc., Chicago, IL, USA). Results were expressed as mean ± SD. A P value ($P<0.05$) is considered statistically significant. Student t-test was used to compare the difference in the HAMD score / HAMA score between groups, and to identify abnormal rCBF between healthy controls and MDD patients. Pearson correlation analysis and multiple linear regression analysis were used to infer causal relationships between regional cerebral Z-scores and HAMD scores / HAMA scores in MDD patients. The result of eZIS was visualized using xjView toolbox (http://www.alivelearn.net/xjview).

Results

The mean HAMD score and the mean HAMA score in the MDD patients were 25.49 ± 6.00 and 23.12 ± 5.83, respectively, and as for healthy controls, the mean scores were 2.70 ± 1.42 and 0.65 ± 0.88, respectively. There was a positive correlation between two scores for MDD patients ($r = 0.732$, $p = 0.000$) (Fig. 1).

It is still controversial whether there are correlations between the MDD severity and the patient characteristics. In this study, the HAMD score showed no correlations with the ages of MDD patients ($r = 0.134$, $p = 0.255$). The MDD women (26.66 ± 5.11) had higher HAMD scores than the MDD men (22.52 ± 7.08, $t = 2.801$, $p = 0.007$).

Compared with the normal controls data, 3D-SSP analysis showed that the MDD patients had decreased rCBF in frontal lobe (bilateral B4, B9, B10, B11, B47 and left B8 and right B6, B44, B46), parietal lobe (left B312), temporal lobe (right B21, B41, B42), cingulated cortex (bilateral B24, B32) and hypophysis. And it also showed in the MDD patients increased rCBF in parietal lobe (right B7), temporal lobe (right B28), occipital lobe (bilateral B17, B19 and left B18) and cingulated cortex (left

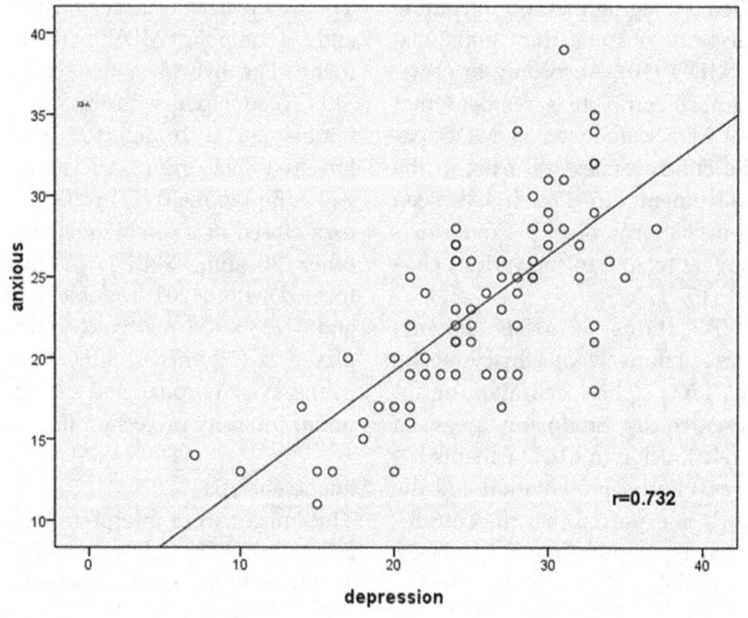

Fig. 1 The correlation between the score for HAMD and that for HAMA

B23 and right B31, B33). The detailed Z-scores were shown in Table 1. There was no statistically significant difference between MDD patients and normal controls for rCBF in hippocampus, caudate nucleus and globus pallidus (Table 2).

The HAMD score had a negative correlation with decreased rCBF in left ventral anterior cingulate cortex B24, a positive correlation with decreased CBF in left inferior prefrontal gyrus B47 and increased rCBF in right associative visual cortex B19 ($R = 0.400$, $F = 4.453$, $p = 0.006$). In addition, there was a negative correlation between the HAMA score and decreased rCBF in left subgenual cortex B25 ($r = -0.309$, $p = 0.007$).

Table 1 Z-scores of the increased/decreased rCBF areas in MDD patients from 3D-SSP

			Z-score		t value	p value
			MDD	CON		
INC:	B7	R	4.60 ± 1.78	3.74 ± 1.97	2.371	0.019
	B17	L	6.12 ± 1.22	4.80 ± 1.76	4.703	0.000
		R	5.47 ± 1.70	4.30 ± 1.45	3.685	0.000
	B18	L	6.35 ± 0.96	5.72 ± 0.99	3.323	0.001
	B19	L	6.70 ± 0.80	6.38 ± 0.80	2.033	0.044
		R	6.19 ± 1.08	5.41 ± 1.13	3.593	0.000
	B23	L	3.43 ± 1.92	2.67 ± 1.84	2.050	0.043
	B28	R	1.60 ± 2.83	0.00 ± 0.00	4.873	0.000
	B31	R	4.52 ± 1.96	3.59 ± 2.00	2.414	0.017
	B33	R	3.36 ± 2.53	2.49 ± 1.89	2.086	0.039
DEC:	B123	L	1.79 ± 2.28	2.77 ± 1.93	2.312	0.023
	B4	L	1.46 ± 1.99	2.39 ± 2.09	2.354	0.020
		R	6.39 ± 1.09	6.77 ± 0.37	2.658	0.009
	B6	R	2.17 ± 2.05	3.18 ± 1.82	2.590	0.011
	B8	L	−3.84 ± 1.97	−2.99 ± 1.75	2.276	0.025
	B9	L	1.72 ± 1.61	2.69 ± 1.17	3.653	0.000
		R	1.79 ± 1.67	2.74 ± 1.58	2.941	0.004
	B10	L	1.55 ± 1.70	2.73 ± 1.78	3.466	0.001
		R	1.33 ± 1.77	2.91 ± 1.58	4.723	0.000
	B11	L	2.50 ± 2.15	3.41 ± 1.86	2.357	0.021
		R	2.81 ± 2.16	3.74 ± 1.94	2.256	0.026
	B21	R	2.89 ± 1.88	3.70 ± 1.88	2.205	0.030
	B24	L	1.61 ± 1.84	2.26 ± 1.32	2.162	0.033
		R	3.60 ± 1.64	4.18 ± 0.91	2.436	0.016
	B32	L	1.72 ± 1.61	2.95 ± 1.31	4.398	0.000
		R	1.72 ± 1.66	3.31 ± 1.25	5.772	0.000
	B41	R	1.45 ± 1.86	2.30 ± 2.01	2.260	0.026
	B42	R	1.67 ± 1.91	2.46 ± 1.87	2.115	0.037
	B44	R	2.25 ± 1.92	3.22 ± 1.65	2.817	0.006
	B46	R	1.96 ± 1.99	3.02 ± 1.94	2.739	0.007
	B47	L	1.90 ± 1.88	2.92 ± 1.21	3.515	0.001
		R	2.46 ± 1.84	3.46 ± 1.29	3.392	0.001
	hypophysis		6.84 ± 0.45	7.00 ± 0.00	3.109	0.003

L left, *R* right, *DEC* the decreased rCBF areas, *INC* the increased rCBF areas, *rCBF* regional cerebral blood flow, *MDD* major depressive disorder, *CON* control

Table 2 Quantitative assessment of rCBF changes in caudate nucleus, globus pallidus and hippocampus from regions of interest method

		UI (mean ± SD)		t value	p value
		MDD group	Control group		
HIP	L	0.698 ± 0.103	0.718 ± 0.087	0.789	0.435
	R	0.677 ± 0.074	0.667 ± 0.088	0.527	0.600
CAU	L	0.850 ± 0.110	0.854 ± 0.117	0.141	0.888
	R	0.799 ± 0.102	0.800 ± 0.096	0.043	0.966
GLO	L	0.928 ± 0.110	0.967 ± 0.129	1.361	0.177
	R	0.910 ± 0.117	0.957 ± 0.099	1.657	0.101

MDD Major depressive disorder, *HIP* Hippocampal gyrus, *CAU* Caudate nucleus, *GLO* Globus pallidus, *UI* Uptake index, *rCBF* Regional cerebral blood flow

The differences of rCBF between MDD patients and normal controls were significant at the cluster lever ($P_{FWE\text{-}corr} < 0.05$) in the SPM and eZIP analysis. The results were listed in Table 3, and showed in Fig. 2 which was drawn from xjView toolbox and showed the decreased and increased rCBF foci in MDD patients.

According to 3D-SSP and eZIP analysis, the consistent results showed the decreased rCBF of MDD patients in frontal lobes (bilateral B11, B47 and right B4, B6, B10, B46), temporal lobe (right B21, B41, B42) and cingulated cortex (bilateral B24, B33), while their increased rCBF in occipital lobe (bilateral B17, B19 and left B18).

Discussion

MDD is a heterogeneous disorder with various clinical presentation and inconsistent response to treatment. But its pathogenesis is inadequately understood [6, 18]. The mechanism that underlies the altered rCBF in MDD patients is not fully elucidated, however, previous studies [19, 20] suggested that the depressive symptoms were associated with reduced parasympathetic and increased sympathetic tone resulting in a broad range of hemodynamic changes, including elevated systemic vascular resistance. In addition, activation of immune-inflammatory pathways in MDD may also contribute to the process. Our study showed that more severe MDD patients would experience more anxiety. It has been suggested to be caused partly by brain chemistry neurotransmitter imbalances [21]. Antidepressant medication and behavioral therapy can help MDD patients overcome both depression and anxiety. However, clinicians have observed when depression occurs together with anxiety, symptoms are more severe than when depression or anxiety occurs alone, furthermore, it may be

Table 3 Talairach Coordinates and Z-scores of areas with rCBF changes in MDD patients

Number of clusters	Co-ordinates			Region	Z-score
	X	Y	Z		($P_{FWE\text{-}corr}$ < 0.05)
INC: 2	**-32**	**-80**	**-10**	left occipital lobe (B17、B18、B19、B37)	5.91
	-8	-82	-8		5.43
	36	**-70**	**-14**	right occipital lobe (B17、B18、B19、B37)	4.87
DEC:4	**38**	**14**	**-24**	right temporal lobe (B22、B38、B41、B42), right insula and right frontal lobe (B11、B44、B45、B47)	6.07
	42	16	-12		5.30
	46	6	-24		5.09
	-32	**4**	**-4**	left insula, left frontal lobe (B11、B44、B45、B47), left temporal lobe (B22、B38、B41、B42) and [a]left anterior cingulate cortex (B24、B33)	5.30
	-38	-2	-2		5.07
	20	**22**	**0**	right frontal lobe (B4、B6、B10、B11、B44、B45、B46、B47), right temporal lobe (B21、B22、B38、B41、B42), right insula and [a]right anterior cingulate cortex (B24、B33)	4.50
	8	**22**	**-20**	right frontal lobe (B4、B6、B10、B46)	4.40

L Left, *R* Right, *DEC* The decreased rCBF areas, *INC* the increased rCBF areas, *rCBF* Regional cerebral blood flow, *PFWE-corr p*-value with FEW correction in %, FEW family-wise error

[a] only exist in $P < 0.001$

likely to develop treatment-resistant depression [22]. Additionally, our study also showed that the severity of depression had no correlations with age, and that women were found more likely than men to develop severe depression, the possible reasons may be as follows: women are more likely than men to show mood amplification; women have a greater propensity to be more passive than men; women may be exposed to more stressful life events than men [23].

To minimize the deviation errors caused by analysis software packages, 3D-SSP and eZIP image-processing programs were applied in the same CT attenuation-corrected SPECT images data of MDD patients and normal controls. According to previous studies [24, 25], the difference between 3D-SSP and eZIP lies in smoothing process after anatomic standardization. The smoothing process by eZIP is based on an SPM algorithm and effectively enhances the signal-noise ratio of images, which might overestimate cerebral hypoperfusion [24, 25]. So we apply corrections for multiple comparisons based on family-wise error (FEW), and $P_{FWE\text{-}corr} < 0.05$ is considered statistically significant in eZIP analysis. On the other hand, due to uninvolving such a smoothing process the preanalysis image reconstruction conditions might affect the results of 3D-SSP. Therefore, in 3D-SSP analysis all CT attenuation-corrected SPECT images data of MDD patients were compared with a normalized database and those of normal controls data simultaneously. Finally, the consistent results from 2 statistical image analysis methods were defined as the abnormal rCBF status of MDD patients. By 3D-SSP and eZIP analysis, we concluded that the decreased rCBF of MDD patients was in frontal lobes (bilateral B11, B47 and right B4, B6, B10, B46), temporal lobe (right B21, B41, B42) and cingulated cortex (bilateral B24, B33), while their increased rCBF was in occipital lobe (bilateral B17, B19 and left B18). Thus it can be seen that the rCBF abnormalities of MDD patients appear in bilateral cerebral hemisphere, and the hypoperfused regions showed right-hemisphere dominance while the area of hyperperfusion had a slight left-hemisphere dominance.

In the previous studies about brain structure [7, 26], metabolism [27] and perfusion [17], the medial prefrontal cortex (mPFC) and anterior cingulate cortex (ACC) in MDD patients have been found increased functional connectivity, which was related to one of possible pathophysiological mechanisms of depression——-dysfunction of default mode network (DMN) [21, 28]. The hypoperfused areas of frontal lobes and cingulated cortex in MDD patients of this study largely coincided with what have been reported in the past [9, 16, 29, 30]. Although there was no consensus in regard to the hypoperfusion of temporal lobe and the hyperperfusion of occipital lobe, some researchers [9] have mentioned the abnormal perfusion of these cerebral regions in patients with treatment-resistant depression, and other researchers [31] suggested that abnormal activation of the occipital lobes may be an initiating factor cognitive disorder in depressed patients. We found there was no significant difference in the cerebellar blood flow of MDD patients as compared with that of normal controls, which was inconsistent with the findings of Gardner et al[28], in which cerebellum resulted to be heavily implicated in a large cohort of patients with persistent depressive disorder (PDD). The discrepancy may be due to the various clinical presentations of MDD patients, and interindividual variability in the patterns of functional connections between brain regions also existed in the

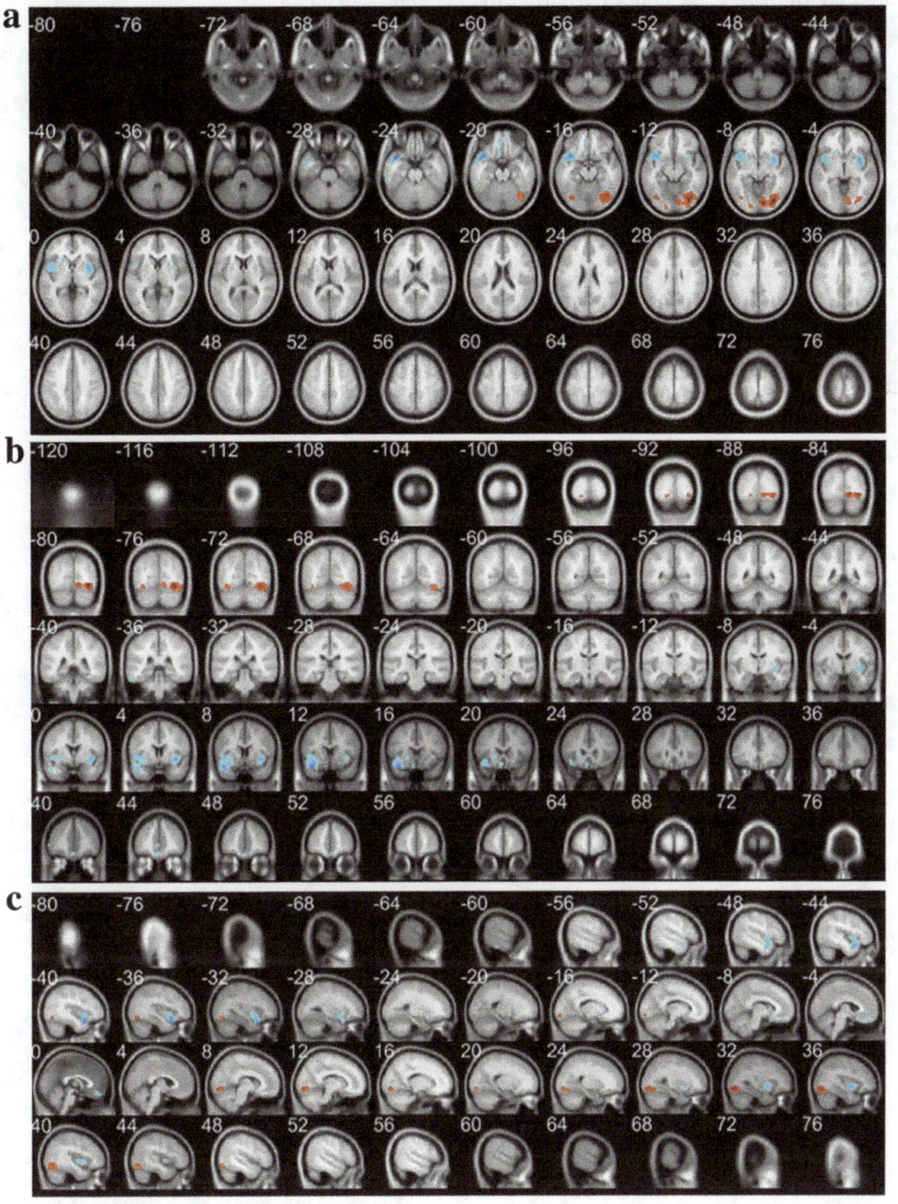

Fig. 2 The decreased (blue) and increased (red) rCBF foci in the reconstructed transverse slices (a), coronal slices (b) and sagittal slices (c) of MDD patients, which was analyzed by SPM and eZIP and viewed by xjView toolbox

specific MDD symptom clusters [17, 28]. The MDD patients involved in our study mostly have high HAMD scores and HAMA scores with the most common complaints——feeling down and insomnia, and this may be the reason why the different distribution of abnormal rCBF appeared in the MDD patients of this study.

In addition, our present study revealed that among these recruited MDD patients with relatively high HAMD and HAMA scores, the depression severity was negatively correlated with decreased rCBF in left ventral anterior cingulate cortex B24, and was positively correlated with decreased rCBF in left inferior prefrontal gyrus B47 and increased rCBF in right associative visual cortex B19. It also indicated that the anxiety severity was negatively correlated with decreased rCBF in left subgenual cortex B25. These results may be helpful in monitoring therapeutic efficacy of MDD, although a large-scale study is still necessary to verify the above characteristics of rCBF alteration in the progression of MDD and during follow-up after treatment. On the other hand, there were several additional limitations in this study including: our results weren't compared with the findings from MRI techniques, such as 3D-arterial spin labelling; the age range of the included healthy controls

(22–59 years) is smaller than that of MDD patients (20–72 years). Further studies are required to resolve these issues.

Conclusions

In conclusion, blood flow abnormalities were found in bilateral brain hemisphere of MDD patients with right-hemisphere dominant hypoperfused regions and a slight left- hemisphere dominance in the area of hyperperfusion. The depression severity was associated with decreased rCBF in B24 and B47 of left hemisphere, and increased rCBF of right B19. The rCBF SPECT/CT may provide an objective assessment for MDD severity. And it might be used monitoring therapeutic efficacy in the management of MDD.

Abbreviations

[^{99m}Tc]ECD: [^{99m}Tc]ethylcysteinate dimer; 3D-SSP: Three-dimensional stereotactic surface projection; ACC: Anterior cingulate cortex; B: Brodmann areas; CT: Computed tomography; DMN: Default mode network; DSM-IV: The fourth edition of the Diagnostic and Statistical Manual of Mental Disorders; eZIS: easy Z score imaging system; HAMA: Hamilton Rating Scale for Anxiety; HAMD: Hamilton Rating Scale for Depression; HUST: Huazhong University of Science and Technology; ICD-10: The 10th revision of International Statistical Classification of Diseases and Related Health Problems; MDD: Major depressive disorder; mPFC: Medial prefrontal cortex; MRI: Magnetic resonance imaging; PET: Positron emission tomography; rCBF: Regional cerebral blood flow; ROIs: Regions of interest; SPECT: Single photon emission computed tomography; UI: Uptake index

Acknowledgements

We thank Dr. Xiaofan Zhang and Dr. Wei Zou (Department of Neurology, Tongji Hospital, Tongji Medical College, HUST), Mr. Jian Hu and Mr. Jian Zhou (Department of Nuclear Medicine, Tongji Hospital, Tongji Medical College, HUST), for assistance in data collection.

Funding

Not applicable.

Authors' contributions

CJ and YY conceived and designed the experiments. LJM, YY and CJ were major contributors in writing the manuscript. YY and CJ analyzed and interpreted the MDD patient clinical data. LJM, ZYK, CJ, CZT and SYX analyzed and interpreted the imaging data. LJM, ZLQ, HYF, ZGP and YT contributed to acquisition imaging data. All authors read and approved the final manuscript.

Consent for publication

Not applicable.

Competing interests

The authors declare that they have no competing interests.

Author details

[1]Department of Nuclear Medicine, Tongji Hospital, Tongji Medical College, Huazhong University of Science and Technology, Wuhan, Hubei Province 430030, China. [2]Department of Nuclear Medicine, Renmin Hospital of Wuhan University, Wuhan, Hubei Province 430060, China. [3]Department of Neurology, Tongji Hospital, Tongji Medical College, Huazhong University of Science and Technology, Wuhan, Hubei Province 430030, China.

References

1. Belmaker RH, Agam G. Major depressive disorder. N Engl J Med. 2008;358(1): 55–68.
2. Alimohammadi AM, Mehrpisheh S, Memarian A. Epidemiology of Cases of Suicide due to Hanging who Referred to Forensic Center of Shahriar in 2011. International Journal of Medical Toxicology & Forensic Medicine. 2013; 3(4):121–125.
3. Andrews G, Slade T, Peters L. Classification in psychiatry: ICD-10 versus DSM-IV. Br J Psychiatry. 1999;174:3–5.
4. Maske UE, Buttery AK, Beesdo-Baum K, Riedel-Heller S, Hapke U, Prevalence BMA. Correlates of DSM-IV-TR major depressive disorder, self-reported diagnosed depression and current depressive symptoms among adults in Germany. J Affect Disord. 2016;190:167–77.
5. McGrath CL, Kelley ME, Holtzheimer PE, Dunlop BW, Craighead WE, Franco AR, Craddock RC, Mayberg HS. Toward a neuroimaging treatment selection biomarker for major depressive disorder. JAMA Psychiatry. 2013;70(8):821–9.
6. Zhang K, Zhu Y, Wu S, Liu H, Zhang W, Xu C, Zhang H, Hayashi T, Tian M. Molecular, functional, and structural imaging of major depressive disorder. Neurosci Bull. 2016;32(3):273–85.
7. Lener MS, Iosifescu DV. In pursuit of neuroimaging biomarkers to guide treatment selection in major depressive disorder: a review of the literature. Ann N Y Acad Sci. 2015;1344:50–65.
8. Kerestes R, Davey CG, Stephanou K, Whittle S, Harrison BJ. Functional brain imaging studies of youth depression: a systematic review. Neuroimage Clin. 2014;4:209–31.
9. Nagafusa Y, Okamoto N, Sakamoto K, Yamashita F, Kawaguchi A, Higuchi T, Matsuda H. Assessment of cerebral blood flow findings using 99mTc-ECD single-photon emission computed tomography in patients diagnosed with major depressive disorder. J Affect Disord. 2012;140(3):296–9.
10. Banas A, Lass P, Straniewska D. Single photon emission computed tomography (SPECT) for the diagnosis of depressive disorders, neurotic and eating disorders. Psychiatr Pol. 2005;39(3):497–507.
11. Hu S-Y, Shi G-Q, S-e W, Qiu J. Changes in regional cerebral blood flow with Chaihu-Shugan-San in the treatment of major depression. Pharmacognosy Magazine. 2014;10(40):503.
12. Brockmann H, Zobel A, Joe A, Biermann K, Scheef L, Schuhmacher A, von Widdern O, Metten M, Biersack HJ, Maier W, et al. The value of HMPAO SPECT in predicting treatment response to citalopram in patients with major depression. Psychiatry Res. 2009;173(2):107–12.
13. Oda K, Okubo Y, Ishida R, Murata Y, Ohta K, Matsuda T, Matsushima E, Ichimiya T, Suhara T, Shibuya H, et al. Regional cerebral blood flow in depressed patients with white matter magnetic resonance hyperintensity. Biol Psychiatry. 2003;53(2):150–6.
14. Navarro Vc GC, Lomeña F, Mateos JJ, Marcos T. Frontal cerebral perfusion dysfunction in elderly late-onset major depression assessed by 99MTC-HMPAO Spect. NeuroImage. 2001;14(1):202–5.
15. Watanabe M, Umezaki Y, Miura A, Shinohara Y, Yoshikawa T, Sakuma T, Shitano C, Katagiri A, Takenoshita M, Toriihara A, et al. Comparison of cerebral blood flow in oral somatic delusion in patients with and without a history of depression: a comparative case series. BMC Psychiatry. 2015;15(1):42.
16. Takahashi S, Ukai S, Tsuji T, Kose A, Shoyama M, Yamamoto M, Okumura M, Shinosaki K. Cerebral blood flow in the subgenual anterior cingulate cortex and modulation of the mood-regulatory networks in a successful rTMS treatment for major depressive disorder. Neurocase. 2013;19(3):262–7.
17. Périco CA-M, Skaf CR, Yamada A, Duran F, Buchpiguel CA, Castro CC, Soares JC, Busatto GF. Relationship between regional cerebral blood flow and separate symptom clusters of major depression: a single photon emission computed tomography study using statistical parametric mapping. Neurosci Lett. 2005;384(3):265–70.

18. GBoDS C. Global, regional, and national incidence, prevalence, and years lived with disability for 301 acute and chronic diseases and injuries in 188 countries, 1990-2013: a systematic analysis for the global burden of disease study 2013. Lancet. 2015;386(9995):743–800.
19. Ménard C, Hodes GE, Russo SJ. Pathogenesis of depression: insights from human and rodent studies. Neuroscience. 2016;321:138–62.
20. Matthews SC, Nelesen RA, Dimsdale JE. Depressive symptoms are associated with increased systemic vascular resistance to stress. Psychosom Med. 2005; 67(4):509–13.
21. Monteggia LM, Malenka RC, Depression DK. The best way forward. Nature. 2014;515(7526):200–1.
22. Chi KF, Korgaonkar M, Grieve SM. Imaging predictors of remission to anti-depressant medications in major depressive disorder. J Affect Disord. 2015; 186:134–44.
23. Parker G, Brotchie H. Gender differences in depression. Int Rev Psychiatry. 2010;22(5):429–36.
24. Onishi H, Matsutake Y, Matsutomo N, Kai Y, Amijima H. Effect of prefiltering cutoff frequency and scatter and attenuation corrections during normal database creation for statistical imaging analysis of the brain. J Nucl Med Technol. 2011;39(3):231–6.
25. Onishi H, Matsutake Y, Kawashima H, Matsutomo N, Amijima H. Comparative study of anatomical normalization errors in SPM and 3D-SSP using digital brain phantom. Ann Nucl Med. 2011;25(1):59–67.
26. Shad MU, Muddasani S, Rao U. Gray matter differences between healthy and depressed adolescents: a voxel-based morphometry study. J Child Adolesc Psychopharmacol. 2012;22(3):190–7.
27. Tomasi D, Wang GJ, Volkow ND. Energetic cost of brain functional connectivity. Proc Natl Acad Sci U S A. 2013;110(33):13642–7.
28. Finn ES, Shen X, Scheinost D, Rosenberg MD, Huang J, Chun MM, Papademetris X, Constable RT. Functional connectome fingerprinting: identifying individuals using patterns of brain connectivity. Nat Neurosci. 2015;18(11):1664–71.
29. Neuropsychological GGM. Neuroimaging evidence for the involvement of the frontal lobes in depression: 20 years on. J Psychopharmacol. 2016;30(11): 1090–4.
30. Gardner AÅD, Öberg J, Jacobsson H, Jonsson C, Larsson S, Pagani M. Towards mapping the brain connectome in depression: functional connectivity by perfusion SPECT. Psychiatry Res. 2014;223(2):171–7.
31. Li J. Xu C, Cao X, Gao Q, Wang Y, Wang Y, Peng J, Zhang K. Abnormal activation of the occipital lobes during emotion picture processing in major depressive disorder patients. Neural Regen Res. 2013;8(18):1693–701.

3

Predicting intentions to seek help for depression among undergraduates in Sri Lanka

Santushi D. Amarasuriya[1,2*], Anthony F. Jorm[2] and Nicola J. Reavley[2]

Abstract

Background: Studies have found that although there are high rates of depression among university students, their help-seeking practices are poor. It is important to identify students who are less likely to seek the necessary help, to encourage better help-seeking among them. This study, which was conducted among undergraduates in Sri Lanka, examined the associations between personal characteristics of the undergraduates and their intentions to seek help for depression.

Methods: This was a cross-sectional study in which 4461 undergraduates (Male: $n = 1358$, 30.4%, Female: $n = 3099$, 69.5%; Mean age = 22.18; $SD = 1.47$) indicated their intentions to seek help if personally affected by depression, which was described in a hypothetical vignette about a peer experiencing depression symptomatology. The predictors of the undergraduates' help-seeking intentions, including their sociodemographic characteristics, prior exposure to and recognition of the problem, and their stigma towards those with depression were examined using binary logistic regression analyses models.

Results: The undergraduates' ability to recognise the problem was one of the strongest predictors of their intentions to seek professional help. Those with higher levels of stigma were less likely to seek both professional and informal help. While females were less likely to consider professional help, they were more likely to consider the help of informal help-providers and to consider religious strategies. Medical undergraduates and those who had sought help for personal experiences of the problem were also more likely to consider informal help. However, all these associations resulted in small effect sizes, except for those between recognition of the problem and the undergraduates' intentions to seek professional help, where medium to very large effect sizes were observed in the case of some the associations examined.

Conclusions: Improvement of problem-recognition may be a key strategy for improving help-seeking among these undergraduates. Reduction of stigma may also be associated with better depression-related help-seeking of undergraduates. Females and medical undergraduates need to be educated about the importance of seeking appropriate types of help, and their informal social networks must be educated about how best to help them.

Keywords: Help-seeking, Helping-seeking intentions, Mental health literacy, Depression, Professional help, Informal help, Undergraduate, University student, Sri Lanka

* Correspondence: santushi@gmail.com; santushi@med.cmb.ac.lk
[1]Department of Medical Humanities, Faculty of Medicine, University of Colombo, PO Box 271, 25, Kynsey Road, Colombo 8, Sri Lanka
[2]Centre for Mental Health, Melbourne School of Population and Global Health, University of Melbourne, 207 Bouverie Street, Parkville, VIC 3010, Australia

Background

The high rates of depression found among university students [1, 2] highlight that many may require mental health support. While this indicates the need for examining the depression-related help-seeking practices of these students, it is also important to examine the predictors of such help-seeking and to identify those who are less likely to seek the necessary help.

In attempts to understand and predict help-seeking practices that university students might demonstrate if affected by a mental health problem, many studies have examined their help-seeking intentions, and likeliness and willingness to seek help for their problem [3–6]. The Theory of Planned Behaviour [7] provides strong support for the examination of help-seeking intentions as a predictor of actual help-seeking practices. In light of this, as part of a survey of depression-related literacy of undergraduates in Sri Lanka, Amarasuriya et al. [8] examined the intentions of these undergraduates to seek help if they were personally affected by depression. The condition was described using a vignette of an undergraduate who was exhibiting symptomatology of Major Depression as per the DSM-IV [9] and the participants were asked what they thought was wrong with the person in the vignette. Although only a low proportion of undergraduates were able to recognise the condition as being "depression", as discussed in Amarasuriya et al. [9], this may have been due to the lack of lay terminology for the condition in the local languages [10, 11]. The following help-seeking actions were nominated by approximately ≥5% of the undergraduates as those they would engage in if they were affected by this problem ($N = 4461$): *Professional help*: psychiatrist/related help (7.3%), doctor/medical treatment (7.7%), counsellor/counselling (6.5%); *Informal help*: help from friends (34.2%), parents (20.2%), family (4.8%), persons not specified (13.9); *Self-help strategies*: doing enjoyable/relaxing/physical activities or taking a break (16.1%), dealing with educational difficulties/focussing on education/ managing work (9.0%); using religious-oriented strategies (7. 2%) and understanding problem/self-initiated effort to get rid of problem (6.5%).

Although health pluralism is observed in Sri Lanka where, in addition to professional help, the population has endorsed a range of healers, such as alternative medicine practitioners [12, 13] and religious figures and practices [14, 15], the undergraduates in the Amarasuriya et al. study [9] mostly considered professional help and the help of their social network. However, it is noteworthy that when they were asked to rate the helpfulness of a list of potential help-providers, the clergy/religious priests were among those highly endorsed, indicating the presence of related treatment beliefs. However, these help-providers were not among those identified by the undergraduates in relation to their personal help-seeking intentions.

It is also noteworthy that although 9.3% of the undergraduates screened positive for Major Depression [8], which indicates that such students may require professional help, the findings as a whole show that the undergraduates are more likely to seek help from parents and friends than from professional sources, such as psychiatrists and counsellors [9]. This highlights the important roles the undergraduates' informal social network may play in assisting them, including as a gate-way to treatment [16]. Their importance is further emphasized when considering the shortage of professional mental health services in the country [17]. It would be useful to identify any factors which predict the different help-seeking intentions of these undergraduates in order to understand those who should be targeted when attempting to promote appropriate help-seeking in this group.

Among factors found in previous studies to influence the help-seeking intentions of university students and young people are their gender [6, 18–21], stage of study and age [6, 18], ability to recognise their mental health problems [22], personal experiences of the problem or experiences of it through their family [18, 20, 23–25], and their stigmatising attitudes [26, 27]. However, findings regarding the associations between the help-seeking intentions of these young persons and the aforementioned factors have been sometimes inconsistent. For example, although many studies have found that female university students and adolescents show better help-seeking intentions [6, 18–21], the ability to recognise the problem has only sometimes been found to be associated with higher intentions to seek help among these groups [6, 22]. Furthermore, while certain stigmatising attitudes held by these groups have been associated with their lesser intentions to seek professional help, other types of stigma have been inversely associated with such help-seeking intentions [26, 27]. There is a dearth of published research examining how such factors may affect mental health-related help-seeking of Sri Lankan university students and the Sri Lankan population in general. One study found that the perceptions of carers of mentally ill patients regarding the stigma held by others was associated with delayed help-seeking of the patients they cared for [28]. More research is needed to understand the factors which may affect the help-seeking practices of university students in Sri Lanka. Accordingly, the aim of the present study was to examine the personal characteristics of undergraduates in Sri Lanka which predict their intentions to seek help for depression.

Method

Study design, setting and participants

The methodology of this cross-sectional study, which was conducted from June to November 2013, has already been described in Amarasuriya et al. [9, 29]. The study population consisted of undergraduates enrolled in a Sri Lankan university.

The study sites included five of the six undergraduate faculties of the University of Colombo, namely the Faculties of Arts and Education, Law, Management and Finance, Medicine, and Science, as well as the School of Computing, which is an affiliated institute of the university. The sampling strategy, which involved clustered sampling, aimed to produce as large a sample as possible by approaching all those attending a lecture (the cluster) which was common for each year of study in the research sites. In the case of the Faculty of Arts in which students had varied subject combinations, lectures with the largest student cohorts were approached for data collection. Data was not collected in the Faculty of Education, as the second and third year students of this faculty attended lectures in the Faculty of Arts, and as only fourth year students had lectures exclusively at this faculty. The strategy of systematically approaching students from all faculties and years of study during the identified lectures was considered to reduce any bias in sampling.

Measures

Depression and depression literacy of the undergraduates was examined using a paper-based dual language questionnaire that was available in two versions, i.e., as English-Sinhala and English-Tamil versions. Participants could choose their preferred version. A vignette which described an undergraduate named 'Z', who exhibited symptoms of Major Depression as per the Diagnostic and Statistical Manual of Mental Disorders-IV, was provided as the problem trigger. The present paper examines the predictors of the undergraduates' personal help-seeking intentions. Therefore, it only describes the questionnaire items relevant to this aim. The complete depression literacy questionnaire, including the depression vignette that was used and details regarding its development, have been previously published [9, 29]. The questionnaire has been provided as Additional file 1 for the convenience of the reader.

Help-seeking intentions

The undergraduates' help-seeking intentions were elicited in relation to the depression vignette using the following open-ended question: "If you have this problem, what would you do?" Multiple responses were possible.

Problem recognition

This was examined using the following open-ended question: "What do you think is wrong with 'Z'?" Multiple responses were possible. Amarasuriya et al. [29] categorised these responses as follows: recognised as depression, recognised using other mental health-related labels (pertaining to the label categories "mental illness", "stress/pressure/mental suffering", "mental issue"), and not recognized (where responses were not relevant to either of the two previous response categories).

Screening positive for major depression

The Patient Health Questionnaire-9 (PHQ-9) is a self-administered measure which consists of nine items, based on the nine symptoms of Major Depression in the DSM-IV (Kroenke & Spitzer, 2002). This measure instructed respondents to rate the degree to which they were bothered by the symptoms presented in the measure during the previous two weeks, using a four point scale consisting of the following rating options: *Not at all, Several days, More than half the days, Nearly every day.* These rating options were scored from 0 to 3 respectively. Therefore, a maximum score of 27 could be obtained. If five of the nine symptoms were found to be present for *More than half the days* or *Nearly every day*, then a diagnosis of *Major Depression* was given. However, for these diagnoses to be given, either the symptom relating to depressed mood or anhedonia had to be present. If the symptom relating to suicidal thoughts was present at all, it was then considered within the symptom count for these diagnoses.

Stigmatizing attitudes

The questionnaire examined the undergraduates' stigmatising attitudes towards those with depression, by examining their negative attitudes towards 'Z' using the Personal Stigma Scale, and their willingness to interact with 'Z' using the Social Distance Scale.

The Personal Stigma Scale is a component of the Depression Stigma Scale [30]. This study used a version of this scale adapted for use among young persons between 12 and 25 years of age (Jorm & Wright, 2008). The scale consisted of seven statements and asked participants to indicate how much they agreed or disagreed with the statements, by using a five-point rating scale (scored from 1 to 5) consisting of the following rating options: *Strongly agree, Agree, Neither agree nor disagree, Disagree, Strongly disagree.* The items were reverse-scored so that higher scores indicated a higher level of personal stigma. A total score of 35 could be obtained.

The Social Distance Scale which was used is based on a social distance scale for adults [31], that was later adapted for use among a population of young persons between 12 and 25 years of age (Jorm & Wright, 2008). The scale consists of five items which ask participants to indicate their willingness to do the activities which are listed with 'Z', using a four-point rating scale (scored from 1 to 4), consisting of the following rating options: *Yes, definitely, Yes, probably, Probably not, Definitely not.* Higher scores on the scale indicate lesser willingness to interact with 'Z' and hence, greater desire for social distance from 'Z'. A total score of 20 could be obtained.

Amarasuriya et al. [32] found that the Personal Stigma scale consisted of two dimensions of stigma, i.e., the Weak-not-Sick and Dangerous-Undesirable dimensions (consisting of three items each), while the Social Distance scale consisted of one dimension (consisting of five items), which was labelled as Social Distance. This led to the construction of three subscales which reflected these three dimensions of stigma (see Amarasuriya et al. [32] for details regarding construction of the scales, factor loadings of scale items, reliabilities of scales and their limitations relating to low reliability estimates).

Exposure to problem and help-seeking

Three closed questions were used to examine the undergraduates' previous experiences of the problem and their related help-seeking practices. Participants were asked if anyone in their family or close circle of friends had experienced a problem like 'Z's (response options: *Yes, No, Don't know*), if they had ever had a problem like 'Z's (response options: *Yes, No, Don't know*), and in the case of responding as *'Yes'* or *'don't know'* to the latter, if they had dealt with the problem on their own, without getting help from others (response options: *Yes, Tried first but got help later, No*).

Demographic characteristics

The following variables were examined: faculty of study (open-ended question), gender, year of study, age, religion (response options: *Buddhist, Hindu, Islamic, Christian, Roman Catholic, Atheist, Other*) and residence (response options: *at home, hostel, rented place, home of friend/relative, other*).

Procedure

The questionnaires were distributed to the undergraduates during lectures. Participation was voluntary and anonymous. Implied consent procedures were used, where consent to participate was implied when a filled questionnaire was returned. The undergraduates took approximately 20 min to complete the questionnaire.

Statistical analysis

The aggregates for all types of professional and informal help that the undergraduates identified as those they would seek if personally affected by the problem were calculated. The category "person not specified" was excluded from the aggregate for informal help due to the ambiguity of this response. The aggregate for help-seeking intentions relating to self-help strategies was not calculated, as there were a range of differing responses, some of which may have been unhelpful when dealing with depression. The correlation between the aggregates for intentions to seek professional and informal help was also found using the phi correlation coefficient.

Binary logistic regression models were used to examine the predictors (IVs) of each of the aforementioned help-seeking intentions of the undergraduates (DVs) (i.e., professional help, informal help and self-help strategies). The following categorical variables were simultaneously entered into binary logistic regression models to examine the predictors of each of these types of help-providers/strategies of help-seeking, where the variable sub-categories which are italicised were the reference categories for each of the respective variables: gender (*male*, female); faculty of study (*Medicine*, Arts and Education, Law, Management and Finance, Science, School of Computing); year of study (*1st year*, 2nd year, 3rd year, 4th year, 5th year Medicine); age category (*18–20 years*, 21–23 years, 24 years and above); ability to recognise the problem in vignette (*not recognised*, recognised as depression, recognised using other mental health-related labels (pertaining to the label categories "mental illness", "stress/pressure/mental suffering", "mental issue"); if the respondents screened positive for Major Depression as per the PHQ-9 (*no*, yes); if the problem in the vignette had been experienced by family or friends (*no*, yes, don't know); if the problem was personally experienced (*no*, yes, don't know); and from those who responded as *yes* or *don't know* to the latter question, if they had sought help for the problem (*help not sought*, tried first but got help later, help sought; those who did not indicate personal experience of the problem were included in the analysis, but were dummy coded as a *not relevant* category). The stigma scale scores, which were continuous variables, were entered into the model in relation to the Weak-not-Sick, Dangerous-Undesirable and Social Distance scales that have been described in Amarasuriya et al. [32]. As simultaneous regression analysis models were used, this allowed for an examination of each of these variables as predictors of the undergraduates' help-seeking intentions while adjusting for all the other variables entered into the model. The analyses were also adjusted for the participants' religion, residence and language of response. Given the large number of predictors entered into each of the regression models, the $p < .01$ significance level was used to reduce the Type I error rate.

In order to examine the effect sizes of these associations, in instances in which the ORs were < 1, these were converted to 1/OR to place all effects in a common frame of reference [33]. ORs of 1.5 were considered as small effect sizes, 2.5 as medium effect sizes, 4 as a large effect sizes and 10 as very large effect sizes [34]. The results were interpreted in relation to these effect size estimates. As described in Mackinnon [35], the dichotomization of continuous scaled predictors for use in logistic regression analyses reduces the power of these scaled predictors. Therefore, as recommended by Mackinnon, in the case of the stigma scores which were continuous scaled predictors, Interquartile Odds Ratios (IQOR) which retain the full power of these predictors were calculated. This placed these variables within a common frame of reference with the other predictor variables when examining their effect sizes.

It must be noted that problem recognition as a predictor of intentions to seek help from professional help-providers has already been examined in Amarasuriya et al. [9]. The present analysis adjusted for a larger number of variables (stigma, exposure to problem and whether help was sought if problem was personally experienced), and also examined whether problem-recognition is a predictor of the undergraduates' intentions to seek help from informal help-providers or to engage in the self-help strategies identified.

Data was analysed using the Statistical Package for the Social Sciences, version 23.

Results

From a total of 4671 undergraduates who participated in the depression literacy survey, 4461 indicated their help-seeking intentions if personally affected by the problem described in the case vignette. Sample characteristics of those who indicated their help-seeking intentions are provided in Table 1. Interquartile ranges (IQR) for the stigma scale scores were as follows: Weak-not-Sick: IQR = 3, Dangerous-Undesirable: IQR = 2 and Social Distance: IQR = 4.

Overall, 23.5% undergraduates indicated that they would use some type of professional option of help, while 45.5% indicated intentions to use some type of informal help. A weak negative correlation was found between the aggregates of the undergraduates' intentions to seek professional and informal help (phi correlation coefficient = – 0.10, $p < .001$).

Subsequent to exclusion of cases due to missing values of the studied variables, the predictors of the help-seeking intentions of 3760 undergraduates were examined. The adjusted odds ratios (ORs) for the variables which were found to be significant predictors of the undergraduates' intentions to seek professional/formal help, to seek informal help and to engage in self-help/other strategies are presented in Tables 2, 3 and 4 respectively. The IQORs for instances in which significant associations were found between the stigma scale scores and the undergraduates' help-seeking intentions are also provided in these tables. The Nagelkerke's R^2, which is a generalization of the coefficient of determination in linear regression to logistic models and useful for comparing models within the same dataset is reported in relation to each of the analyses [36].

Following is a description of the significant effects found, including an interpretation of the effect sizes of the ORs/IQORs that were obtained.

Predictors of intending to seek professional/formal help

Those who recognized the problem as depression had higher odds of seeking psychiatric help, (OR = 12.85), while such problem recognition was also associated with higher odds of considering all types of professional help (OR = 3.53). These associations resulted in very large and medium effect sizes respectively. Recognition of the problem using a mental health-related label (excluding "depression") was associated with higher odds of considering the help of psychiatrists (OR = 4.16) and resulted in a large effect size.

All other significant associations found between the undergraduates' intentions to seek professional/formal help and the examined factors had small effect sizes. Relatedly, while those who recognised the problem as depression, or by using a mental health-related label had higher odds of considering the help of doctors and counsellors, those who used mental health-related labels had higher odds of considering professional help in general; those in the Faculty of Arts and Education (compared to medical undergraduates) had higher odds of intending to seek professional help in general; female undergraduates had lower odds of considering the help of psychiatrists and professional help in general; those who had been exposed to the problem through family and friends had lower odds of considering the help of doctors/to get medical assistance; and those with higher scores on the Weak-not-Sick scale had lower odds of intending to seek all types of professional help.

Predictors of intending to seek informal help

All significant associations which were observed resulted in small effect sizes. Relatedly, female undergraduates had higher odds of considering the help of their parents and informal help in general; those who had sought help for the problem or had sought help after trying to deal with it alone had higher odds of considering the help of both the aforementioned help-providers as well as their friends; those using mental health-related labels for the problem (excluding the label "depression") had higher odds of indicating intentions to seek help from their parents, while those in the third year had lower odds of intending to seek such help; those in the Faculties of Arts and Education, Management and Finance and the School of Computing (compared to Medical undergraduates) had lower odds of intending to seek help from their friends and of seeking informal help in general; Management and Finance undergraduates also had lower odds of intending to seek help from their parents and family; those with higher scores on the Dangerous-Undesirable and Social Distance scales had lower odds of considering informal help in general as well as the help of their friends, while those with higher scores on the Dangerous-Undesirable scale also had lower odds of indicating intentions to seek help from their parents.

Predictors of intending to engage in self-help/other strategies

A few of the examined associations resulted in medium to large effect sizes. Those who recognised the problem as "depression" had lower odds of indicating that they

Table 1 Demographic and other characteristics of undergraduates who indicated their personal help-seeking intentions ($n = 4461$)

Variables	n	%
Gender		
Male	1358	30.4
Female	3099	69.5
Faculty		
Medicine	581	13.0
Arts and Education	1146	25.7
Law	601	13.5
Management and Finance	993	22.3
Science	638	14.3
School of Computing	501	11.2
Year of Study		
1st year	1845	41.4
2nd year	1188	26.6
3rd year	802	18.0
4th year	516	11.6
5th year (Medicine)[a]	110	2.5
Age group (Mean = 22.18; *SD* = 1.47)		
18–20 years	486	10.9
21–23 years	3199	71.7
24 and above	771	17.3
Ethnicity		
Sinhala	4096	91.8
Tamil	176	3.9
Sri Lankan Moor	140	3.1
Other	45	1.0
Religion		
Buddhism	3889	87.2
Hinduism	145	3.3
Islam	144	3.2
Roman Catholicism	206	4.6
Other	71	1.6
Residence when going to University		
Home	1684	37.7
Hostel	1340	30.0
Rented place	1125	25.2
Home of friend or relative	258	5.8
Other	50	1.1
Screening positive for Major Depression[b] ($n = 4123$)		
No	3747	90.9
Yes	376	9.1
Exposure to problem through family/ friends		
No	1700	38.1
Yes	1651	37.0
Don't know	982	22.0
Personal experience of problem		
No	2409	54.0
Yes	1463	32.8
Don't know	308	6.9
If problem personally experienced (responding as 'Yes' or 'Don't know), if help sought ($n = 1771$)		
Help not sought	658	37.2
Tried first but got help later	683	38.6
Help sought	364	20.6

Notes
[a]Only the Faculty of Medicine has a 5th year of study
[b]Only responses which had ≤ 1 missing response on the PHQ-9 were considered valid for this variable
Percentages do not total to 100% due to missing values

would deal with their educational difficulties (OR = 0.20; Equivalent OR for estimating effect size of association = 5.0), while 5th year Medical undergraduates had lower odds of indicating their intentions to engage in enjoyable/relaxing/physical activities or of taking a break (OR = 0.22; Equivalent OR for estimating effect size of association = 4.54); Both these associations resulted in large effect sizes. Those who sought help for their problem had lower odds of intending to understand the problem/of engaging in self-initiated efforts to resolve the problem (OR = 0.26; Equivalent OR for estimating effect size of association = 3.85), while those from the Faculties of Arts and Education (compared to Medicine) had lower odds of indicating that they would deal with their educational difficulties (OR = 0.39; Equivalent OR for estimating effect size of association = 2.56); These latter two associations resulted in medium effect sizes.

All other significant associations which were observed resulted in small effect sizes. Relatedly, females had higher odds of intending to use religious-oriented strategies. Females and those with higher scores on the Weak-not-Sick Scale had higher odds of indicating that they would deal with their educational difficulties, while the odds of using this strategy were lower for those who screened positive for Major Depression and those who recognised the problem by using other mental health-related labels. While the odds of intending to engage in enjoyable/relaxing/physical activities or of taking a break was higher among those who recognised the problem as "depression" or used other mental health-related labels

Table 2 Predictors of intending to seek professional help examined using simultaneous binary logistic regression (n = 3760)

Predictor variable	Psychiatrist/ related help	Doctor/medical treatment	Counsellor/counselling	All types of professional help
	Adjusted OR (99% CI)	Adjusted OR (99% CI)	Adjusted OR (99% CI)	Adjusted OR (99% CI)
Gender (reference group: Male)				
Female	0.65^{**} (0.44, 0.96) [Equiv OR = 1.54]			0.72^{**} (0.57, 0.92) [Equiv OR = 1.39]
Faculty (reference group: Medicine)				
Arts and Education				1.87^{**} (1.16, 3.00)
Exposure to problem through family and friends (reference group: response: no)				
Response: Yes		0.64^{**} (0.42, 0.96) [Equiv OR = 1.56]		
Recognition of problem (reference group: not recognised)				
Recognised as depression	12.85^{***} (6.03, 27.41)	1.90^{**} (1.07, 3.40)	2.34^{***} (1.29, 4.23)	3.53^{***} (2.44, 5.12)
Recognised using mental health-related labels (excluding the label "depression")	4.16^{***} (2.19, 7.92)	1.87^{***} (1.21, 2.90)	1.70^{**} (1.06, 2.72)	2.30^{***} (1.74, 3.06)
Stigma Scale Scores				
Weak-not-Sick Scale	0.86^{***} (0.80, 0.92) [IQOR = 0.63] [Equiv OR = 1.59]	0.86^{***} (0.80, 0.92) [IQOR = 0.63] [Equiv OR = 1.59]	0.92^{**} (0.86, 1.00) [IQOR = 0.79] [Equiv OR = 1.26]	0.86^{***} (0.82, 0.90) [IQOR = 0.64] [Equiv OR = 1.56]
Nagelkerke R^2	0.16	0.08	0.05	0.12

$^{**}p < .01$; $^{***}p < .001$
Notes
Interquartile ORs abbreviated as IQOR
ORs < 1 were converted into 1/OR and have been presented as Equiv OR
Only adjusted ORs for the variables which were found to be significant predictors of the undergraduates' intentions to seek professional help have been provided

for this purpose, odds of considering such help was lower among those who sought help when they personally experienced the problem.

Discussion

This study attempts to identify some of the personal characteristics of the undergraduates which predict their help-seeking intentions. The findings indicate that while those who recognise the problem have greater intentions to seek professional assistance, those with various stigmatising attitudes show lesser intentions to seek both professional and informal help. The findings also indicate that those who have sought help for their personal experiences of the problem are more likely to consider the help of informal help-providers. There is some evidence that female undergraduates are less likely to seek professional assistance and more likely to seek help from informal help-providers and to engage in informal strategies of help. Medical undergraduates are also more likely to seek help from their informal social network. Some of the examined variables also predicted the undergraduates' intentions to engage in some of the self-help strategies, where these associations ranged from medium to large effect sizes. However, it must be noted that a majority of the examined associations resulted in small effect sizes.

While those who recognised the problem as "depression" were more likely to consider psychiatric help (very large effect size) as well as professional help in general (medium effect size), recognition using mental health-related labels was also associated with being more likely to seek psychiatric help (large effect size). The results highlight that problem recognition is a key predictor of the undergraduates' intentions to seek professional help. Recognition of the problem as "depression" was the strongest predictor of the undergraduates' intentions to seek any type of help. This study supports previous findings which have indicated that accurate use of psychiatric labels is associated with preference to seek professional help among young people [22]. While the present findings indicate that the undergraduates' ability to recognise depression is important to their help-seeking, they highlight that the low rates of depression recognition found in this population need attention [9]. However, as discussed in Amarasuriya et al., [9], the low rates of depression recognition found may be due to the lack of lay terminology for the condition in Sri Lanka. This highlights the challenges that may be faced in initiatives to improve the use of the depression label in this population. Therefore, as an initial step, the undergraduates should be helped to at least recognise the problem as being mental health-related, as this may also be related to improved help-seeking among them. Although depression recognition was associated with poorer intentions to deal with

Table 3 Predictors of intending to seek help from informal help-providers examined using simultaneous binary logistic regression ($n = 3760$)

Predictor variable	Friend	Parent	Family	All types of informal help
	Adjusted OR (99% CI)	Adjusted OR (99% CI)	Adjusted OR (99% CI)	Adjusted OR (99% CI)
Gender (reference group: Male)				
Female		2.22*** (1.68, 2.94)		1.51*** (1.23, 1.86)
Faculty (reference group: Medicine)				
Arts and Education	0.61** (0.41, 0.92) [Equiv OR = 1.64]			0.60** (0.41, 0.90) [Equiv OR = 1.67]
Management and Finance	0.65** (0.45, 0.96) [Equiv OR = 1.54]	0.59** (0.38, 0.93) [Equiv OR = 1.69]	0.46** (0.22, 0.97) [Equiv OR = 2.17]	0.61** (0.42, 0.89) [Equiv OR = 1.64]
Computer	0.62** (0.40, 0.94) [Equiv OR = 1.61]			0.66** (0.44, 0.98) [Equiv OR = 1.52]
Year of study (reference group: 1st year)				
3rd Year		0.70** (0.49, 0.98) [Equiv OR = 1.43]		
Whether those who personally experienced problem sought help (reference group: help not sought)				
Tried first but got help later	1.74*** (1.25, 2.43)	1.95*** (1.25, 3.05)		1.83*** (1.33, 2.52)
Help sought	1.91*** (1.28, 2.84)	1.76*** (1.05, 2.98)		1.94*** (1.32, 2.86)
Recognition of problem (reference group: not recognised)				
Recognised using mental health-related labels (excluding the label "depression")		1.33** (1.02, 1.74)		
Stigma Scale Scores				
Dangerous-Undesirable Scale	0.95** (0.90, 1.00) [IQOR = 0.90] [Equiv OR = 1.11]	0.93** (0.87, 0.99) [IQOR = 0.86] [Equiv OR = 1.16]		0.94** (0.89, 0.98) [IQOR = 0.87] [Equiv OR = 1.15]
Social Distance Scale	0.94*** (0.90, 0.97) [IQOR = 0.77] [Equiv OR = 1.30]			0.96** (0.93,1.00) [IQOR = 0.86] [Equiv OR = 1.16]
Nagelkerke R^2	0.04	0.10	0.05	0.06

**$p < .01$; ***$p < .001$

Notes

Interquartile ORs abbreviated as IQOR

ORs < 1 were converted into 1/OR and have been presented as Equiv OR

Only adjusted ORs for the variables which were found to be significant predictors of the undergraduates' intentions to seek informal help have been provided

educational difficulties and resulted in a large effect size, the results also indicate that recognition was associated with higher intentions to engage in enjoyable/relaxing activities (small effect size), which have been found to be effective self-help strategies for dealing with depression [37].

Many of the other significant associations that were observed between the examined variables and the help-seeking intentions of the undergraduates resulted in small effect sizes, except for a few concerning the undergraduates' intentions to engage in self-help strategies that resulted in medium to large effect sizes. However, it would be useful to consider how all these associations may influence the help-seeking practices of this population. The findings indicate that stigmatising attitudes of the undergraduates towards those who are depressed may be negatively associated with their personal help-seeking. While stigma that the problem is a "weakness" and not a "sickness" seems to be associated with lesser acknowledgement of the need for professional help, other stigmatising attitudes, such as the perception that those with depression are "dangerous" and "undesirable" and the desire for social distance from such individuals, may also be negatively associated with these undergraduates' attempts to seek help from their informal help-providers. The findings indicate that the examined dimensions of stigma could have a consistently negative effect on the help-seeking of these undergraduates. The current findings together with recent findings from Sri Lanka, that perceived stigma of carers of mentally ill patients may result in help-seeking delays of these patients [28], highlight how the different dimensions of mental health-related stigma might have detrimental effects on the help-seeking practices of the Sri Lankan population.

The findings indicate that females may be less likely than males to seek professional help if personally affected by the problem. This finding does not align with the findings of many previous studies among university students in other countries, which have found instead that males are more reluctant to seek professional help

Table 4 Predictors of intending to engage in self-help/other strategies examined using simultaneous binary logistic regression (n = 3760)

Predictor variable	Enjoyable/relaxing/physical activities or taking break	Using religious-oriented strategies	Dealing with educational difficulties	Understand problem/self-initiated effort to resolve it
	Adjusted OR (99% CI)	Adjusted OR (99% CI)	Adjusted OR (99% CI)	Adjusted OR (99% CI)
Gender (reference group: Male)				
Female		1.73** (1.11, 2.70)	1.72*** (1.17, 2.52)	
Faculty (reference group: Medicine)				
Arts and Education			0.39** (0.19, 0.79) [Equiv OR = 2.56]	
Year of study (reference group: 1st year)				
5th Year (Medicine)	0.22** (0.05, 0.96) [Equiv OR = 4.54]			
Whether those who personally experienced the problem sought help (reference group: help not sought)				
Help sought	0.55** (0.33, 0.90) [Equiv OR = 1.82]			0.26** (0.09, 0.76) [Equiv OR = 3.85]
Screening positive for Major Depression (reference group: No)				
Yes			0.55** (0.30, 1.00) [Equiv OR = 1.82]	
Recognition of problem (reference group: not recognised)				
Recognised as depression	1.78*** (1.20, 2.63)		0.20*** (0.10, 0.39) [Equiv OR = 5.00]	
Recognised using mental health-related labels (excluding the label "depression")	1.44** (1.07, 1.92)		0.47*** (0.34, 0.66) [Equiv OR = 2.13]	
Stigma Scale Scores				
Weak-not-Sick Scale			1.10** (1.02, 1.18) [IQOR = 1.33]	
Nagelkerke R^2	0.06	0.06	0.09	0.04

**$p < .01$; ***$p < .001$

Notes

Interquartile ORs abbreviated as IQOR

ORs < 1 were converted into 1/OR and have been presented as Equiv OR

Only adjusted ORs for the variables which were found to be significant predictors of the undergraduates' intentions to seek self-help strategies have been provided

for their problems [6, 18–21], where this may be associated with their identification with traditional masculinity roles [38–40]. However, in Asian cultures in which there may be greater reliance on family and friends when dealing with mental health problems, females may be more influenced by such cultural influences in their help-seeking practices [41, 42]. The findings also provide evidence of the female undergraduates' greater reliance on social support, such as from their parents, and their greater endorsement of informal strategies of help, such as religious-oriented activities, when dealing with the problem. These findings may be highlighting a greater tendency for female undergraduates to first activate such socially-sanctioned informal pathways of help when attempting to deal with their mental health problems. Alternatively, such greater endorsement of informal help by females may be reflecting their greater preference for emotional support and person-centred and social-network-related help when attempting to deal with the problem [43–45].

While the medical undergraduates seem to be more likely to consider informal help for the problem than their non-medical counterparts, they do not show any difference in their inclination to seek professional help, despite their medical training. In fact, intentions to seek professional help were lower among the medical students as compared to those in the Arts and Education Faculties. Many previous studies have shown that professional help-seeking among medical students is low [46–48] and that they prefer to seek help from informal sources [47, 49–51]. A further analysis of the help-seeking intentions of medical vs. non-medical undergraduates is presented in Amarasuriya et al. [52]. Other noteworthy findings were that those in the Medical Faculty were more likely to focus on dealing with education-related difficulties than those in the Arts Faculty, and that those in the 5th year of Medicine were less likely to consider engaging in relaxing and enjoyable activities and that these associations resulted in medium to large effect sizes. Both these findings may be reflective of the academic and time-related pressures on those undertaking medical training.

Data was not obtained regarding the types of help sought by those who reported previous experiences of the problem and related help-seeking. However, the results indicate that previous experiences of seeking help for the problem are associated with being less likely to try to understand the problem and/or engage in self-initiated efforts to deal with the problem (medium effect size). Therefore, those who have sought help for previous personal experiences of the problem seem to be less inclined to personally deal with the problem. There were also no significant associations found between such previous help-seeking and the undergraduates' intentions to seek professional help. However, the findings did indicate that those who had sought help previously were more likely to indicate that they would seek informal help for the problem, such as from parents and friends. Such findings could be indicating that these undergraduates' past help-seeking experiences with these informal help-providers were positive. This would be encouraging, given the inclination of the undergraduates to seek such informal help for their problems [9]. However, such an association is only speculative at present.

Other findings relating to students who indicated that they had experienced or were experiencing the problem were nevertheless discouraging. For example, those who screened positive for Major Depression did not differ from those screening negative with regard to their intentions to seek help from both the formal and informal help-providers. Furthermore, while those who had personally experienced the problem were less likely to consider self-help strategies, such as engagement in relaxing and enjoyable activities, those who were exposed to the problem through their family or friends were less likely to consider the help of doctors. These findings concur with the findings of many previous studies which have found that the personal experience of depression or other mental health problems, or experiences of these through family members, could be negatively associated with help-seeking among university students [20, 23–25]. Such findings are concerning, as they indicate that those who are most likely to be in need of help may not seek it. Therefore, it is important to address factors which may act as barriers and impede the help-seeking of these groups and improve contact between suitable help-providers and the affected groups. As seen in many previous studies, such experiences of seeking help may in turn improve the subsequent help-seeking practices of these university students [21, 41].

The undergraduates could benefit from the support of both professional help-providers, in receiving the necessary treatment and interventions for their depression, and their informal social networks, with regard to provision of care, emotional support and encouragement/support to seek professional help. However, overall, the help-seeking pattern of the undergraduates indicates that those who seek professional help have a lesser tendency to seek help from their informal help-providers, while those who seek help from their informal help-providers have a lesser tendency to seek help from professional help-providers. Therefore, it may be necessary to educate these undergraduates about the importance of reaching out to these different sources of help and support. Furthermore, given the evidence that those who seek help from informal help-providers are less inclined to seek professional help, it is also important to educate the social networks of these undergraduates about the need for professional help for depression, as they may play pivotal roles as gate-way providers to treatment [16].

The findings need to be considered in light of the limitations of the study. The depression vignette is limited in its ability to capture the different factors which could influence the help-seeking intentions of the undergraduates in real-life. Furthermore, the methodology of open-ended questions was dependent on the undergraduates' motivation to provide descriptive and comprehensive responses relating to their help-seeking intentions. However, such methodology could be considered to reflect the cognitive mechanisms that the undergraduates would undergo in deciding how to deal with the problem, and therefore to be a suitable strategy to examine their help-seeking intentions. It is also necessary to note that many of the predictors of the undergraduates' help-seeking intentions were associated with small effect sizes [33]. Furthermore, the predictors which were examined only accounted for a small percentage of variance in the undergraduates' help-seeking intentions, indicating that there were other factors influencing these variables that had not been considered in the study. The use of qualitative methodology in the future, such as in-depth interviews, would help in gaining a more comprehensive understanding of the help-seeking practices of the undergraduates and the factors which influence these practices. Although data was collected only from one University in Sri Lanka, the large sample size, including undergraduates from diverse disciplines and all years of study, indicate that the findings are useful in identifying the personal characteristics which predict intentions to seek help for depression among undergraduates in Sri Lanka.

Conclusions

The findings indicate that among the personal characteristics of the undergraduates that were examined, their ability to recognize the problem is a key predictor of their inclination to seek help. Reduction of their stigma may also be associated with such an outcome. There is also some evidence indicating that both female and medical undergraduates are inclined to seek informal help and that their intentions to seek professional help need to be improved. Such findings emphasise the importance of educating these groups about the need to seek help for their depression, as well as educating the informal help-providers that they approach about how best to assist these undergraduates.

Abbreviations
IQOR: Interquartile odds ratio; IQR: Interquartile range

Acknowledgements
The authors thank the academic and administrative staff of the University of Colombo for their ready co-operation during data collection. We also convey our grateful thanks to the undergraduates of the University of Colombo who voluntarily participated in this study.

Funding
No funding was received for this project other than for printing the paper-based questionnaires and for data entry obtained through a NHMRC Australia Fellowship awarded to AFJ.

Authors' contributions
SDA was the primary investigator and designed the study, managed data collection and analysis under the guidance of AFJ and NJR. SDA prepared the initial manuscript which was reviewed critically for important intellectual content by AFJ and NJR, who provided necessary inputs where necessary. All authors read and approved the final manuscript.

Authors' information
SDA is a senior lecturer at the Department of Medical Humanities of the Faculty of Medicine, University of Colombo and an Honorary Fellow at the Centre for Mental Health at the Melbourne School of Population and Global Health at the University of Melbourne. This work is related to her PhD project which was supervised by AFJ, a Professorial Fellow and the Head of the Population Mental Health Group at the Centre for Mental Health at the Melbourne School of Population and Global Health, University of Melbourne, and NJR, an Associate Professor in this Centre.

Consent for publication
Not applicable. The identity of the participants remained anonymous throughout the study.

Competing interests
The authors declare that they have no competing interests.

References

1. Ibrahim AK, Kelly SJ, Adams CE, Glazebrook C. A systematic review of studies of depression prevalence in university students. J Psychiatr Res. 2013;47(3):391–400. https://doi.org/10.1016/j.jpsychires.2012.11.015.
2. Peltzer K, Pengpid S. Depressive symptoms and social demographic, stress and health risk behaviour among university students in 26 low-, middle- and high-income countries. Int J Psychiatry Clin Pract. 2015;19(4):259–65. https://doi.org/10.3109/13651501.2015.1082598.
3. Hickie IB, Davenport TA, Luscombe GM, Rong Y, Hickie ML, Bell MI. The assessment of depression awareness and help-seeking behaviour: experiences with the international depression literacy survey. BMC Psychiatry. 2007;7(48) https://doi.org/10.1186/1471-244X-7-48.
4. Rong Y, Luscombe GM, Davenport TA, Huang Y, Glozier N, Hickie IB. Recognition and treatment of depression: a comparison of Australian and Chinese medical students. Soc Psychiatry Psychiatr Epidemiol. 2009;44(8): 636–42. https://doi.org/10.1007/s00127-008-0471-5
5. Smith CL, Shochet IM. The impact of mental health literacy on help-seeking intentions: results of a pilot study with first year psychology students. Int J Men Health Promot. 2011;13(2):14–20. https://doi.org/10.1080/14623730.2011.9715652
6. Reavley NJ, McCann TV, Jorm AF. Mental health literacy in higher education students. Early Interv Psychiatry. 2012;6(1):45–52. https://doi.org/10.1111/j.1751-7893.2011.00314.x.
7. Ajzen I. The theory of planned behavior. Organ Behav Hum Decis Process. 1991;50(2):179–211. https://doi.org/10.1016/0749-5978(91)90020-T.
8. Amarasuriya SD, Jorm AF, Reavley NJ. Prevalence of depression and its correlates among undergraduates in Sri Lanka. Asian J Psychiatry. 2015;15: 32–7. https://doi.org/10.1016/j.ajp.2015.04.012.
9. Amarasuriya SD, Jorm AF, Reavley NJ. Depression literacy of undergraduates in a non-western developing context: the case of Sri Lanka. BMC Res Notes. 2015;8(593) https://doi.org/10.1186/s13104-015-1589-7.
10. Abeyasinghe DRR, Tennakoon S, Rajapakse TN. The development and validation of the Peradeniya depression scale (PDS)—a culturally relevant tool for screening of depression in Sri Lanka. J Affect Disord. 2012;142(1–3): 143–9. https://doi.org/10.1016/j.jad.2012.04.019.
11. de Silva VA, Ekanayake S, Hanwella R. Validity of the Sinhala version of the Centre for Epidemiological Studies Depression Scale (CES-D) in out-patients. Ceylon Med J. 2014;59(1):8–12. https://doi.org/10.4038/cmj.v59i1.6732.
12. Sumathipala A, Siribaddana S, Hewege S, Sumathipala K, Prince M, Mann A. Understanding the explanatory model of the patient on their medically unexplained symptoms and its implication on treatment development research: a Sri Lanka study. BMC Psychiatry. 2008;8:54. https://doi.org/10.1186/1471-244X-8-54.
13. Ediriweera HW, Fernando SM, Pai NB. Mental health literacy survey among Sri Lankan carers of patients with schizophrenia and depression. Asian J Psychiatry. 2012;5(3):246–50. https://doi.org/10.1016/j.ajp.2012.02.016.
14. Hollifield M, Hewage C, Gunawardena CN, Kodituwakku P, Bopagoda K, Weerarathnege K. Symptoms and coping in Sri Lanka 20–21 months after the 2004 tsunami. Br J Psychiatry. 2008;192(1):39–44. https://doi.org/10.1192/bjp.bp.107.038422.
15. Somasundaram D, Thivakaran T, Bhugra D. Possession states in northern Sri Lanka. Psychopathology. 2008;41(4):245–53. https://doi.org/10.1159/000125558.
16. Stiffman AR, Pescosolido B, Cabassa LJ. Building a model to understand youth service access: the gateway provider model. Ment Health Serv Res 2004;6(4):189–198. https://doi.org/10.1023/B:MHSR.0000044745.09952.33.
17. Bruckner TA, Scheffler RM, Shen G, Yoon J, Chisholm D, Morris J et al. The mental health workforce gap in low- and middle-income countries: a needs-based approach. Bull World Health Organ 2011;89(3):184–194. https://doi.org/10.2471/BLT.10.082784.
18. Stigma HMJ. Help seeking related to depression: a study of nursing students. J Psychosoc Nurs Ment Health Serv. 2004;42(2):42–51.
19. Seyfi F, Poudel KC, Junko Y, Keiko O, Masamine J. Intention to seek professional psychological help among college students in Turkey: influence of help-seeking attitudes. BMC Res Notes. 2013;6:519. https://doi.org/10.1186/1756-0500-6-519.
20. Zochil ML, Thorsteinsson EB. Exploring poor sleep, mental health, and help-seeking intention in university students. Aust J Psychol. 2017; https://doi.org/10.1111/ajpy.12160.
21. Erkan S, Ozbay Y, Cihangir-Cankaya Z. Terzi Ş. The prediction of university students' willingness to seek counseling. Educ Sci: Theory Pract. 2012;12(1):35–42.
22. Yap MBH, Reavley NJ, Jorm AF. The associations between psychiatric label use and young people's help-seeking preferences: results from an Australian national survey. Epidemiol Psychiatr Sci. 2014;23(1):51–9. https://doi.org/10.1017/S2045796013000073.
23. Chan W, Batterham P, Christensen H, Galletly C. Suicide literacy, suicide stigma and help-seeking intentions in Australian medical students. Australas Psychiatry. 2014;22(2):132–9. https://doi.org/10.1177/1039856214522528.
24. Wilson CJ, Rickwood D, Deane FP. Depressive symptoms and help-seeking intentions in young people. Clin Psychol. 2007;11(3):98–107. https://doi.org/10.1080/13284200701870954.
25. Kenny R, Dooley B, Fitzgerald A. How psychological resources mediate and perceived social support moderates the relationship between depressive symptoms and help-seeking intentions in college students. Br J Guid Counc 2016;44(4):402–413. https://doi.org/10.1080/03069885.2016.1190445.
26. Yap MBH, Wright A, Jorm AF. The influence of stigma on young people's help-seeking intentions and beliefs about the helpfulness of various sources of help. Soc Psychiatry Psychiatr Epidemiol. 2011;46(12):1257–65. https://doi.org/10.1007/s00127-010-0300-5.

27. Lally J, O'Conghaile A, Quigley S, Bainbridge E, McDonald C. Stigma of mental illness and help-seeking intention in university students. Psychiatrist. 2013;37(8):253. https://doi.org/10.1192/pb.bp.112.041483.
28. Fernando SM, Deane FP, McLeod HJ. The delaying effect of stigma on mental health help-seeking in Sri Lanka. Asia-Pac Psychiatry. 2017;(1). https://doi.org/10.1111/appy.12255.
29. Amarasuriya SD, Jorm AF, Quantifying RNJ. Predicting depression literacy of undergraduates: a cross sectional study in Sri Lanka. BMC Psychiatry. 2015; 15(269) https://doi.org/10.1186/s12888-015-0658-8.
30. Griffiths KM, Christensen H, Jorm AF, Evans K, Groves C. Effect of web-based depression literacy and cognitive-behavioural therapy interventions on stigmatising attitudes to depression: randomised controlled trial. Br J Psychiatry. 2004;185(4):342–9. https://doi.org/10.1192/bjp.185.4.342.
31. Link BG, Phelan JC, Bresnahan M, Stueve A, Pescosolido BA. Public conceptions of mental illness: labels, causes, dangerousness, and social distance. Am J Pub Health 1999;89(9):1328–1333. https://doi.org/10.2105/AJPH.89.9.1328.
32. Amarasuriya SD, Jorm AF, Reavley NJ, Mackinnon AJ. Stigmatising attitudes of undergraduates towards their peers with depression: a cross-sectional study in Sri Lanka. BMC Psychiatry. 2015;15(129). https://doi.org/10.1186/s12888-015-0523-9.
33. Chen H, Cohen P, Chen S. How big is a big odds ratio? Interpreting the magnitudes of odds ratios in epidemiological studies. Commun Stat- Simul Comput. 2010;39(4):860–4. https://doi.org/10.1080/03610911003650383.
34. Rosenthal JA. Qualitative descriptors of strength of association and effect size. J Soc Serv Res. 1996;21(4):37–59. https://doi.org/10.1300/J079v21n04_02.
35. Mackinnon A. The inter-quartile odds ratio: a suggestion for the presentation of results from continous predictors in logistic regression. Int J Methods Psychiatr Res. 1992;2:233–5.
36. Nagelkerke NJD. A note on a general definition of the coefficient of determination. Biometrika. 1991;(3):691. https://doi.org/10.2307/2337038.
37. Morgan AJ, Jorm AF. Self-help interventions for depressive disorders and depressive symptoms: a systematic review. Ann General Psychiatry. 2008;7: 13. https://doi.org/10.1186/1744-859x-7-13.
38. Yousaf O, Popat A, Hunter MS. An investigation of masculinity attitudes, gender, and attitudes toward psychological help-seeking. Psychol Men & Masc. 2015;16(2):234–7. https://doi.org/10.1037/a0036241.
39. Pattyn E, Verhaeghe M, B P. The gender gap in mental health service use. Soc Psychiatry Psychiatr Epidemiol. 2015;50(7):1089–95. https://doi.org/10.1007/s00127-015-1038-x.
40. Addis ME, Mahalik JR. Men, masculinity, and the contexts of help seeking. Am Psychol. 2003;58(1):5–14. https://doi.org/10.1037/0003-066X.58.1.5.
41. Chang H. Help-seeking for stressful events among chinese college students in Taiwan: roles of gender, prior history of counseling, and help-seeking attitudes. J Coll Stud Dev 2008;49(1):41–51. https://doi.org/10.1353/csd.2008.0003.
42. Nam SK, Chu HJ, Lee MK, Lee JH, Kim N, Lee SM. A meta-analysis of gender differences in attitudes toward seeking professional psychological help. J Am Coll Heal. 2010;59(2):110–6. https://doi.org/10.1080/07448481.2010.483714.
43. Ashton WA, Fuehrer A. Effects of gender and gender role identification of participant and type of social support resource on support seeking. Sex Roles. 1993;28(7/8):461–76. https://doi.org/10.1007/BF00289608.
44. Flaherty J, Richman J. Gender differences in the perception and utilization of social support: theoretical perspectives and an empirical test. Soc Sci Med. 1989;28(12):1221–8. https://doi.org/10.1016/0277-9536(89)90340-7.
45. Ptacek JT, Smith RE, Gender ZJ. Appraisal, and coping: a longitudinal analysis. J Pers. 1992;60(4):747–70. https://doi.org/10.1111/1467-6494.ep9212283735.
46. Gold JA, Johnson B, Leydon G, Rohrbaugh RM, Wilkins KM. Mental health self-care in medical students: a comprehensive look at help-seeking. Acad Psychiatry. 2015;39(1):37–46. https://doi.org/10.1007/s40596-014-0202-z.
47. Dyrbye LN, Eacker A, Durning SJ, Brazeau C, Moutier C, Massie FS et al. The impact of stigma and personal experiences on the help-seeking behaviors of medical students with burnout. Acad Med 2015;90(7):961–969. https://doi.org/10.1097/ACM.0000000000000655.
48. Dahlin ME, Burnout RB. Psychiatric morbidity among medical students entering clinical training: a three year prospective questionnaire and interview-based study. BMC Med Educ. 2007;7(6) https://doi.org/10.1186/1472-6920-7-6.
49. Thistlethwaite J, Quirk F, Evans R. Medical students seeking medical help: a qualitative study. Med Teach. 2010;32(2):164–6. https://doi.org/10.3109/01421590903434177
50. Brimstone R, Thistlethwaite JE, Quirk F. Behaviour of medical students in seeking mental and physical health care: exploration and comparison with psychology students. Med Educ. 2007;41(1):74–83. https://doi.org/10.1111/j.1365-2929.2006.02649.x.
51. Chew-Graham CA, Rogers A, Yassin N. I wouldn't want it on my CV or their records': medical students' experiences of help-seeking for mental health problems. Med Educ. 2003;37(10):873–80. https://doi.org/10.1046/j.1365-2923.2003.01627.x.
52. Amarasuriya SD, Jorm AF, Perceptions RNJ. Intentions relating to seeking help for depression among medical undergraduates in Sri Lanka: a cross-sectional comparison with non-medical undergraduates. BMC Med Educ. 2015;15(162) https://doi.org/10.1186/s12909-015-0453-8.

4

Differential mitochondrial DNA copy number in three mood states of bipolar disorder

Dong Wang[1,4], Zongchang Li[1,2], Weiqing Liu[3], Jun Zhou[1,4], Xiaoqian Ma[1,4], Jinsong Tang[1,4,5,6,7*] and Xiaogang Chen[1,4,5,6,7*]

Abstract

Background: Accumulating evidences indicated that mitochondrial abnormalities were associated with bipolar disorder. As a sensitive index of mitochondrial function and biogenesis, Mitochondrial DNA copy number (mtDNAcn) may be involved in the pathophysiology of bipolar disorder.

Methods: Leukocyte relative mtDNAcn was measured by quantitative polymerase chain reaction in subjects with BD ($n = 131$) in manic, depressive, and euthymic symptoms. Thirty-four healthy individuals were used as comparison control. BD clinical symptomatology was evaluated by Young Mania Rating Scale (YMRS), Hamilton Depression Scale (HAM-D), Clinical Global Impression-Bipolar Disorder-Severity of Illness Scale (CGI-BD-S), and the Positive and Negative Syndrome Scale (PANSS).

Results: Compared to healthy controls, BD patients with manic and depressive symptoms presented significantly decreased mtDNAcn levels (p-value = 0.009 and 0.041, respectively). No significant differences were detected in mtDNAcn between euthymic patients and healthy controls. The mtDNAcn was negatively correlated with the number of relapses in manic patients ($\beta = -0.341$, $p = 0.044$).

Conclusions: Our study described the first evidence of (1) a significant decline of mtDNAcn in manic BD patients, (2) a similar decreased level of mtDNAcn between manic and depressed BD patients, (3) a negative correlation of mtDNAcn with number of relapses in patients suffering from manic states. Alterations of mtDNAcn in manic and depressed patients, which may reflect disturbances of energy metabolism, supported the role of mitochondrial abnormalities in the pathophysiology of BD.

Keywords: Bipolar disorder, Mitochondrial DNA copy number, Mania, Depression

Background

Bipolar disorder (BD) is a chronic and several psychiatric illness, characterized by recurrent episodes of mania and depression, and interspersed with remission period. Although many systems and pathways have been involved in the pathophysiology of BD together containing signal transduction pathways, various neurotransmitter abnormalities, mitochondrial and metabolic dysfunctions and so on [1]; the definitive mechanisms of BD remains to be fully elucidated.

Mitochondria serve as key organelles in eukaryotic cells, well known for synthesizing adenosine triphosphate (ATP) from glucose by oxidative phosphorylation for energy production. Especially, the energy source of neurons relies primarily on mitochondrial oxidative phosphorylation. Additionally, mitochondria also play a vital role in calcium signaling, cell resilience, apoptosis, the regulation of reactive oxygen species (ROS) and DNA damage [2–4]. Mitochondrial DNA (mtDNA) is a double-stranded DNA molecule with no introns and histones. Without protection of histones and due to limited DNA repair capacity, these mtDNA is very prone to oxidative or genotoxic injury. As a result, mitochondria may increase their own copy number to compensate for

* Correspondence: Tangjinsong@csu.edu.cn; Chenxiaogang@csu.edu.cn
[1]Department of Psychiatry, the Second Xiangya Hospital, Central South University, Changsha, Hunan, China

the defects or impairment. Excessive oxidative stresses in pathological conditions may induce structural and functional changes of mitochondrial [5]. Postmortem, brain imaging, genetic and peripheral cells studies all support that mitochondrial dysfunction is associated with BD [6–10]. Using magnetic resonance spectroscopy, some studies showed lower level of phosphocreatine, N-acetyl-aspartate and inorganic phosphate and inorganic phosphate, which are supposed to reflect impaired mitochondrial function in several brain regions of living BD patients [6, 7]. There were lines of evidences revealing abnormal mitochondrial morphology in neurons of postmortem brain and peripheral cells of BD patients [8, 9]. Additionally, many SNPs across the genome of mitochondria were associated with BD [10, 11]. These observed changes maybe indicate an important role of mitochondria in the pathogenesis of BD.

Mitochondrial DNA copy number (mtDNAcn) that reflects the mitochondrial function and biogenesis could be measured per cell [12]. Abnormal mtDNAcn has been suggested to associate with various psychiatric disorders [13–15]. With regard to BD, few studies were conducted to address the possible role of mtDNAcn in BD. Vawter et al. firstly found the alteration of mtDNAcn in a post-mortem study [16], but other three post-mortem studies got negative results [17–19]. In peripheral blood leukocytes, Chang et al. revealed that euthymic BD patients had a lower mtDNAcn than control group [20]; While de Sousa et al. found no significant differences in mtDNA content between depressed BD patients and health controls [21]. Furthermore, the mtDNA content still did not have a significant decrease after lithium carbonate treatment.

Mitochondrial dysfunction may be a cause of BD symptoms. Given the heterogeneity of the disease itself and the inconsistent results from studies, it is necessary to find more evidence to interpret the effect of mitochondrial dysfunction in BD. Human leukocytes have been proved to reflect virtually the plasma oxidative damage to DNA [22]. Heretofore, no studies have assessed the mtDNA content in leukocytes of patients suffering mania or different states of BD. In this study, mtDNAcn was measured in BD patients with three different states and healthy individuals to identify how mtDNA content is altered in different mood states. We hypothesized that mtDNAcn variation may associate with BD, and would differentiate mood states as well as bipolar euthymia from healthy controls.

Methods

Participants

The study was approved by the ethics committee of the Second Xiangya Hospital of Central South University. All subjects voluntarily participated in the research and signed the informed consent. These procedures were performed in accordance with Declaration of the Helsinki. Acute BD patients were recruited from the inpatient and outpatient departments of the Second Xiangya Hospital in Hunan Province of China. The Euthymic patients of BD were primarily recruited from the outpatient clinic.

BD type I is defined by a pattern of depressive episodes and manic episodes. Subjects with BD type I were diagnosed by two or more trained psychiatrists using the Structured Clinical Interview for DSM- IV Axis I Disorders (SCID-IV) and its researcher version with psychotic screen (SCID-I/P). The exclusion criteria for BD patients included electroconvulsive therapy within past 3 months; substance abuse; other mental illness; neurological diseases; serious medical conditions; positive pregnancy test or lactation. Meanwhile, healthy volunteers were recruited by advertisements from local communities. Healthy controls with substance use, history of mental or neurological disorders, serious medical disorders, positive pregnancy test or lactation were excluded from the study (see Additional file 1).

Assessment

One hundred thirty-one subjects with BD type I and 34 healthy volunteers were enrolled in the study. There were 55 patients meeting the Diagnostic and Statistical Manual of Mental Disorders Fourth Edition (DSM-IV) criteria suffering from manic episodes, 47 patients in depressive episodes and 29 patients in euthymic states. Young Mania Rating Scale (YMRS), Hamilton Depression Scale (HAM-D), Clinical Global Impression-Bipolar Disorder-Severity of Illness Scale (CGI-BD-S) were used to assess the symptom severity respectively. Euthymic BD patients were clinically stable for more than 6 months and the index score for CGI-BD-S ≤ 2. When all patients were recruited in the study, the psychiatric assessment and blood collection would be completed in next 24 h.

Assays

Blood samples (3 ml) were collected in EDTA tubes from the 165 participants and kept at – 80 °C. Genomic DNA was extracted from 200 μl blood samples following the manufacturer's protocol using QIAamp DNA Mini Kit (Qiagen, Hilden, Germany). The quantity and purity of the DNA were measured by Nanodrop 2000 spectrophotometer.

The detailed methods and procedures were described in our previous research [13]. In brief, the mtDNAcn was evaluated by the ratio of the amount of mtDNAcn (ND1) to a reference nuclear single copy gene (hemoglobin subunit beta HBB) copy number. The primers for ND1 were as follow: F (5-CCCTAAAACCCGCCACATCT-3) and R (5-GAGCGATGGTGAGAGCTAAGGT-3). The primers for (HBB) were F (5-GTGCACCTGACTCCTGAGGAGA-3) and R (5-CCTTGATACCA ACCTGCCCAG-3).

The assays were conducted by using LightCycler® 480 SYBR Green I Master on a Roche LightCycler® 480 machine (Roche, Manheim, Germany). The double-standard curves method of relative quantification PCR was employed, which is an improved, simple, accurate method [23]. The quantitative assay was based on amplification using conditions, primer sequences according to Xing et al. [24]. PCR cycling condition of ND1 gene was 95 °C 10 min for 1 cycle, 30 cycles of 95 °C for 15 s, 60 °C for 1 m. The cycling condition of HBB gene was 95 °C 10 min, 40 cycles of 95 °C 15 s, 56 °C for 1 m. Each sample was run in triplicate using 10 ng DNA templates in a 10 ul reaction volume and randomly assigned to 96-well plates. The ND1 and HBB genes PCR reactions were performed on separate plates with the same samples located at the same positions., The measures of mtDNAcn for each sample were obtained by the ratio of ND1 copy number to HBB copy number from standard curves. The ratio was normalized to a calibrator DNA in order to standardize between different independent assays. The calibrator DNA sample was from a health control individual and used for comparison with results of different runs. The calibrator DNA sample was diluted 1:4 to build a five-point standard curve between 0.0195 and 20 ng/ul. The amplification efficiencies of the standards were between 92.3 and 108.2%. A negative control and a calibrator DNA were enrolled in each run. The inter-assay coefficient of variation (CV) was 0.15–3.5%, and the intra-assay CV was 1.13–4.37%.

Statistical analysis

Statistical analysis was conducted using Minitab 16 (Minitab Inc., Pennsylvania) and SPSS 23.0 (SPSS Inc., Chicago, IL) for windows. Dichotomous categorical variables in groups were compared using Chi-square test. Continuous variables with normal distribution were analyzed using T test or one-way analysis of variance analysis (ANOVA) test. The mtDNAcn in four groups were skewed distributed, and then adapted into normal distribution using Box-Cox transformation in Minitab software [25]. The Box-Cox (1964) transformation model in Minitab could select the best mathematical function to obtain a normal distribution of the transformed data [26]. The primary outcome analysis was conducted using ANOVA test. When significance was shown in ANOVA, Generalized linear model and Bonferroni post hoc test were performed to examine the intergroup differences of mtDNAcn, after adjusting sexuality, age, years of education, body mass index (BMI). Effect sizes were calculated using Cohen's eta squared η^2 in ANOVA test and R^2 in multiple regression analyses [27]. Cohen J suggested effect sizesη^2 of < 0.01 were small, 0.06 medium, and ≥ 0.14 large. For each BD group, multiple regression analyses were used to explore the association between mtDNAcn and other variables. Descriptive statistics were shown as the mean ± standard deviation or median (interquartile range), and significance level was set at $P < 0.05$ (two-tailed).

Results

Demographic and clinical data of the sample

Table 1 lists demographic, clinical and medication information, and the mtDNAcn median (range) of the study sample. BD patients and healthy controls did not differ in terms of age, gender, BMI, months of education (all $P > 0.05$). Second generation antipsychotic drugs were prescribed for BD patients in the research, and their doses were converted to CPZ equivalents available [28]. As showed, there were no significant differences in using CPZ equivalents, anticonvulsants, benzodiazepines and Lithium (all $P > 0.05$). Manic subjects demonstrated more severe symptoms than depressive and euthymic subjects on Young Mania Rating Scale; and depressed group showed significantly higher HDRS scores than manic and euthymic groups. To identify effect of illness history on mtDNAcn, the detailed information about duration of illness and number of previous episodes were recorded. Both Length of illness and number of previous episodes were similar in three groups ($P > 0.05$).

MtDNA copy number in subjects with BD patients and controls

After transformation, the mean mtDNAcn of four groups were 0.5 ± 0.40 (manic group), 0.57 ± 0.44 (depressed group), 0.86 ± 0.49 (euthymic group), 0.73 ± 0.45 (healthy control). The results of ANOVA showed a significant difference ($F = 4.78$, df = 3161, $P = 0.003, \eta^2 = 0.085$). After controlling for age, gender, BMI, years of schooling as covariates, there remained a significant difference ($F = 2.54$, df = 6158, $P = 0.023, \eta^2 = 0.087$). Besides, we found on the model, these covariates did not associate with mtDNAcn (all $P > 0.05$). The Bonferroni post hoc test revealed that, comparing with healthy group, depressed and manic groups showed a significantly lower level of mtDNAcn respectively, ($P = 0.041, \eta^2 = 0.068$, $s = 0.083$; $P = 0.009, \eta^2 = 0.049$, $s = 0.081$) (Fig. 1). No differences were detected in the mtDNAcn between manic group and depressed group ($P > 0.05$). The euthymic patients had a similar level of mtDNAcn with healthy volunteers ($P > 0.05$) (Table 2). Although the mtDNAcn of BD euthymic group were increased in comparison with manic and depressed BD group, the differences did not reach a significant level (euthymic vs. manic $P = 0.056$, euthymic vs. depressive $P = 0.11$).

Association of mtDNAcn with clinical characteristics within bipolar subjects

Multiple regression analysis was conducted in each group to confirm the relationship between mtDNAcn and clinical information (Table 2). For the manic group, the mtDNAcn was negatively correlated with the

Table 1 Demographic, clinical and medication information of bipolar patients and healthy controls

	Bipolar patients			Health control	Statistic		
	Manic $N=55$	Depression $N=47$	Euthymic $N=29$	$N=34$			
Age, mean (SD)	26.67 (7.15)	26.94 (8.91)	23.76 (3.94)	24.50 (3.82)	ANOVA, F = 2.05, $P=0.108$		
Sex							
Male	26	23	9	19			
Female	23	24	20	15	df = 3, $X^2=4.13$, $P=0.25$		
Years of education, mean (SD)	12.55 (2.80)	12.38 (3.47)	12.24 (2.52)	13.56 (2.78)	ANOVA, F = 1.41, $P=0.13$		
BMI, mean(SD)	21.63 (1.89)	21.45 (1.78)	21.93 (1.69)	21.5 (1.40)	ANOVA, F = 1.63, $P=0.18$		
Medication information							
Antipsychotics	51/55	37/47	23/29		df = 2, $X^2=4.69$, $P=0.09$		
Anticonvulsants	24/55	21/47	18/29		df = 2, $X^2=2.92$, $P=0.23$		
CPZ equivalents, mean(SD)	241.58 (93.43)	224.55 (79.90)	227.31 (64.16)		ANOVA, F = 0.519, $P=0.67$		
Benzodiazepines	15/55	17/47	5/29		df = 2, $X^2=3.22$, $P=0.20$		
Lithium	22/55	19/47	12/29		df = 2, $X^2=4.72$, $P=0.094$		
Clinical characteristics					Man vs Eut	Dep vs Eut	Man vs Dep
Duration of illness, months, mean (SD)	70.91(59.24)	67.70 (61.91)	47.45 (34.66)		$P=0.140$	$P=0.361$	$P=1$
YMRS, mean(SD)	33.78 (6.08)	8.19 (7.31)	2.78 (2.24)		$P<0.001$	$P<0.001$	$P<0.001$
HDRS, mean(SD)	6.90 (8.24)	27.89 (6.61)	2.63 (3.18)		$P<0.001$	$P<0.001$	$P<0.001$
Number of Previous Episodes, mean (SD)	3.55 (1.74)	3.60 (1.70)	2.90 (2.28)		$P=0.713$	$P=0.654$	$P=1$
MtDNAcn, Median (range)	1.59 (1.31,2.07)	1.83 (1.22,2.31)	2.05 (1.5,2.96)	2.38 (1.77,3.24)			

Abbreviations: *BMI* body mass index, *SD* standard deviation, *YMRS* young mania rating scale. *HDRS* hamilton depression rating scale, *ANOVA* one-way analysis of variance, *Man* manic, *Dep* depression, *Eut* euthymic

number of relapses ($\beta=-0.341$, $t=-2.61$, $P=0.044$, $s=0.039$) (Fig. 2), while no similar findings happened in depressed group ($\beta=0.319$, $t=1.19$, $P=0.964$, $s=0.044$). The other clinical characteristics or variables had no significant association with mtDNAcn in BD patients (all $P>0.05$).

Discussion

To our knowledge, this is the first study to examine mtDNA content across the depressed, manic and euthymic states in BD patients. This current research has three main findings. (1) The acute BD patients had markedly lower mtDNA amount than healthy controls,

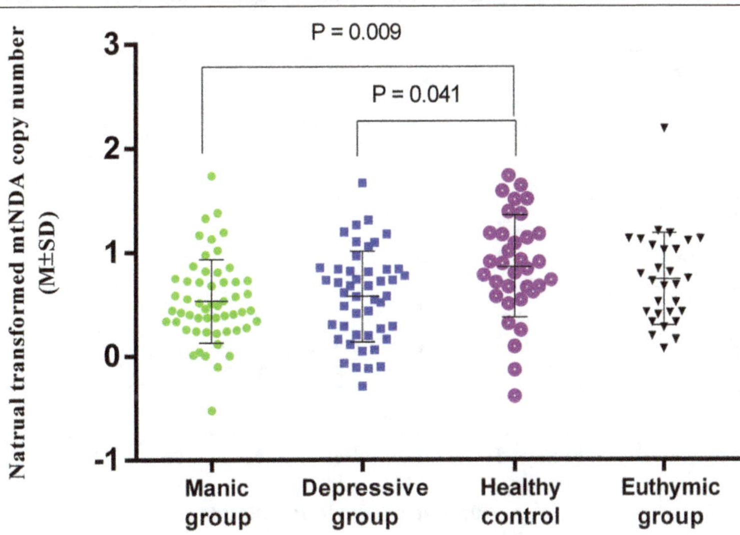

Fig. 1 MtDNA copy number in manic, depressive, euthymic BD patients and healthy controls

Table 2 Effect sizes for healthy control versus patients groups and for multiple regression analyses in each patients group

	Manic group		Depressive group		Euthymic group	
	ES(SE)	*P*	ES	*P*	ES	*P*
healthy control	0.068 [c](0.081)	0.009[a]*	0.049[c](0.083)	0.041[a]*	0.008[c](0.091)	1[a]
Clinical characteristics						
Duration of illness	0.002[d](0.001)	0.825 [b]	0.003[d](0.001)	0.743[b]	0.009[d](0.004)	0.77[b]
YMRS/HDRS	0.040[d](0.012)	0.262[b]	0.100[d](0.016)	0.796[b]	0.259[d](0.076)	0.212[b]
Number of Previous Episodes	0.116[d](0.039)	0.044[b]*	0.102[d](0.044)	0.964[b]	0.006[d](0.065)	0.679[b]
CGI-BD-S	0.009[d](0.067)	0.632[b]	0.02[d](0.088)	0.724[b]	0.072[d](0.081)	0.536[b]

ES effect size, *SE* standard error, *YMRS* young mania rating scale, *HDRS* hamilton depression rating scale, *CGI-BD-S* clinical global impression-bipolar disorder-severity of illness scale, [a]adjusted *p*-values of one way ANOVA test; [b]adjusted p-values of multiple regression analyses; [c]Cohen's eta squared η^2 in ANOVA test; [d]R^2 in multiple regression analyses; *$P < 0.05$

after controlling covariates; there were no differences in mtDNAcn between manic patients and depressed patients. (2) The euthymic group showed a comparable content of mtDNA with healthy control group. (3) The mtDNAcn was inversely correlated with the number of relapses in BD subjects during manic episodes.

Change of mtDNAcn is an important sensitive index of mitochondrial dysfunction and oxidative stress [29]. Our findings indicated that there may be explicit mitochondrial impairments during episodes of BD. In the current study, we firstly reported decreased mtDNA amount in peripheral leukocytes of BD patients undergoing manic episodes. Our data suggested, manic group may display a similar level of mtDNA with depressive group. In contrast, there was nearly normal level of mtDNA in euthymic patients. Hence, we speculate that, leukocyte mtDNA content may change with mood states in BD. Nicod et al. suggested the mtDNA content of patients changed with time during 8-week treatment in major depression [30]. Acute patients could recover after treatment, and gradually transit to euthymic states. According to the findings and clinical observations above, the mtDNAcn of acute patients in peripheral blood might be gradually restored to some extent as time goes on.

The results of prior data on mtDNAcn in peripheral leukocytes and brain tissues of mood disorder were not consistent. Compatible with our result, de Sousa et al. showed a slight decreased mtDNAcn in depressive patients with BD type I, although the differences just failed to be significant ($P = 0.05$), due to a small sample ($N = 7$) [21]. Chang et al. described that mtDNAcn was still significantly lower in the BD euthymic patients [20]. One plausible explanation is that mtDNAcn was negatively correlated with age in BD [21], and their subjects were older than ours. Accumulated evidences demonstrate BD may be an accelerated aging disease [31]. Aging was also reported to be associated with the downregulation of mtDNA-associated genes and a decline level of mtDNAcn [32]. Therefor accelerated aging in BD may affect the levels of mtDNA. According to threshold hypothesis of mtDNAcn control [12], low mtDNAcn triggers the upregulation of mtDNA replication and high mtDNAcn triggers the machinery to degradate mtDNA. Taken together, low threshold and accelerated aging may

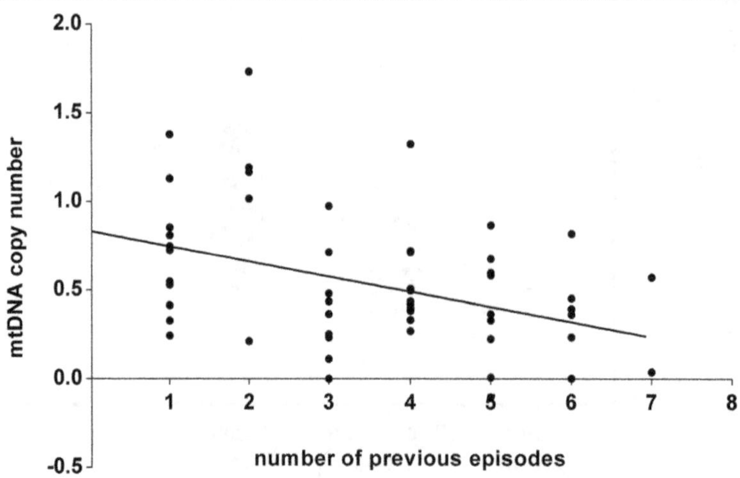

Fig. 2 Correlation between number of previous episodes and mtDNA copy number ($\beta = -0.341$, $t = -2.61$, $p = 0.044$) within manic BD patients

induce the decrease of mtDNAcn. Regarding mtDNAcn in postmortem brains, three out of four studies reported a negative result in BD [16–19]. It was not clear about what kinds of mood states that those subjects suffered from. Thus, the comparison cannot be made with ours. Additional, another innegligible factor is using different tissues or cells in studies, which may confound the results. .

MtDNA polymerase gamma (POLG) is the only one polymerase responsible for the mtDNA replication. POLG is prone to oxidative damage,and its deleterious variants were suggested as a risk for BD [33]. Munkholm et al. revealed downregulation of POLG expression in BD across mania, hypomania, depression or mixed states in peripheral leukocyte [34]. We suppose that POLG downregulation in acute phases of BD may be another important point of resulting in decrease of mtDNAcn.

There are also several evidences for abnormal mtDNA amounts in major depression [35–38]. A large sample multicenter study reported patients with major depression showed increased mtDNA level than controls in saliva and blood [37]. Two studies found a lower peripheral mtDNA level in both depressive and euthymic states [35, 38]. Nicod et al. suggested mtDNA content of patients changed with time in major depression [30].Overall it is not consistent about changes of mtDNA content in major depression and bipolar depression. However all studies indicate the importance of mtDNA in mood disorder. Future research is warranted to explore the relationship in different states of mood disorders.

The relationship observed between mtDNAcn and the number of episodes in manic patients deserves attention. In the current study, we found that mtDNA content was negatively correlated with the number of episodes in BD patients. BD patients often experience recurrent episodes or relapses which appear to cause chronicity of this illness and vulnerability for high stress response [39]. The subjects suffering manic episode are at a high stress level [40]. The "sensitivity" state of oxidative stress may accelerate illness course, and cause cell deficits as well as rapid decline of mitochondrial function.. However, similar findings were not found in the depressive subjects of this study. Hence, the results should be interpreted cautiously, due to the heterogeneity and complexity of BD.

Although antipsychotic agents and mood stabilizers were reported to exert some effect on mitochondrial function [4, 41–43]. de Sousa and our previous studies showed that six or eight weeks lithium or risperidone treatment have no significant effect on mtDNAcn in subjects with psychiatric disorders [13, 21]. Accordingly, we suppose the mtDNAcn of the acute patients would make no significant changes after short–term treatment. Whereas our euthymic patients were medically stabilized for more than 6 months, and may have enough time to recover from various damage in cell.

There are several limitations to be considered. Since we didn't have more clinical data, including smoking status, glucose intolerance, and serum lipid, the possible influence of these variables cannot be completely excluded. Although using peripheral blood is more convenient and less invasive to quantify mtDNAcn, these finding cannot be extrapolated mechanically to other tissues. In addition, only mtDNAcn was measured in this cross-sectional data, it does not indicate any information about causal relationship between oxidative stress, mtDNA variations, and BD. More biological parameters and longitudinal studies regarding mitochondria involved in the pathophysiology of BD are warranted in future.

Conclusion

This study provides novel observations that Leukocyte mtDNA content was significantly decreased in BD patients suffering manic and depressive episodes, as compared with healthy controls. Our results also showed mtDNAcn was negatively correlated with the number of relapses in manic BD patients. Mitochondrial abnormalities in acute patients might involve in the pathophysiology of BD. The findings maybe promote a further understanding on the role of mitochondria in BD. Although our data indicated the mtDNAcn might change with mood states, the underlying mechanisms are complex and still unclear. More effort for a better explanation of the processes engaged in BD is required in further investigation.

Abbreviations

ANCOVA: One-way analysis of covariance; ANOVA: one-way analysis of variance; ATP: adenosine triphosphate; BD: Bipolar disorder; BMI: Body Mass Index; CGI-BD-S: Clinical Global Impression-Bipolar Disorder-Severity of Illness Scale; CPZ: chlorpromazine; Dep: Depression; DSM-IV: Diagnostic and Statistical Manual of Mental Disorders Fourth Edition; Eut: Euthymic; HAM-D: Hamilton Depression Scale; Man: Manic; mtDNAcn: mitochondrial DNA; mtDNAcn: Mitochondrial DNA copy number; POLG: polymerase gamma; ROS: reactive oxygen species; SCID-IV: Structured Clinical Interview for DSM-IV Axis I Disorders; SD: Standard Deviation; YMRS: Young Mania Rating Scale

Funding

This work was supported by the social development program of Wuxi [CSE31N1724 to D.W]; National Natural Science Foundation of China [81471361 to X.C, 81371480 to J.T], Human Provincial Innovation Foundation for Postgraduate [12700–150140005 to Z.L]. The funders had no role in study design, data collection and analysis, decision to publish or preparation of the manuscript.

Authors' contributions
XC, JT, designed the study. DW, ZL, JZ, XM performed the data collection and WL, DW performed data analyses. DW was responsible for manuscript writing. All authors have read and approved the final manuscript.

Competing interests
The authors declare that they have no competing interests.

Author details
[1]Department of Psychiatry, the Second Xiangya Hospital, Central South University, Changsha, Hunan, China. [2]Laboratory of Medical Genetics, School of Life Sciences, Central South University, Changsha, Hunan, China. [3]Department of Psychiatry, First Affiliated Hospital of Kunming Medical University, Kunming, Yunnan, China. [4]Mental Health Institute, the Second Xiangya Hospital, Central South University, Changsha, Hunan, China. [5]National Clinical Research Center on Mental Disorders, Changsha, Hunan, China. [6]National Technology Institute on Mental Disorders, Changsha, Hunan, China. [7]Hunan Key Laboratory of Psychiatry and Mental Health, Changsha, Hunan, China.

References
1. Sigitova E, Fisar Z, Hroudova J, Cikankova T, Raboch J. Biological hypotheses and biomarkers of bipolar disorder. Psychiatry Clin Neurosci. 2017;71(2):77–103.
2. Bolisetty S, Jaimes EA. Mitochondria and reactive oxygen species: physiology and pathophysiology. Int J Mol Sci. 2013;14(3):6306–44.
3. Niizuma K, Yoshioka H, Chen H, Kim GS, Jung JE, Katsu M, Okami N, Chan PH. Mitochondrial and apoptotic neuronal death signaling pathways in cerebral ischemia. Biochim Biophys Acta. 2010;1802(1):92–9.
4. Scaini G, Rezin GT, Carvalho AF, Streck EL, Berk M, Quevedo J. Mitochondrial dysfunction in bipolar disorder: evidence, pathophysiology and translational implications. Neurosci Biobehav Rev. 2016;68:694–713.
5. Clay HB, Sillivan S, Konradi C. Mitochondrial dysfunction and pathology in bipolar disorder and schizophrenia. Int J Dev Neurosci. 2011;29(3):311–24.
6. Bertolino A, Frye M, Callicott JH, Mattay VS, Rakow R, Shelton-Repella J, Post R, Weinberger DR. Neuronal pathology in the hippocampal area of patients with bipolar disorder: a study with proton magnetic resonance spectroscopic imaging. Biol Psychiatry. 2003;53(10):906–13.
7. Sikoglu EM, Jensen JE, Vitaliano G, Liso NAA, Renshaw PF, Frazier JA, Moore CM. Bioenergetic measurements in children with bipolar disorder: a pilot 31P magnetic resonance spectroscopy study. PLoS One. 2013;8(1):e54536.
8. Cataldo AM, McPhie DL, Lange NT, Punzell S, Elmiligy S, Ye NZ, Froimowitz MP, Hassinger LC, Menesale EB, Sargent LW, et al. Abnormalities in mitochondrial structure in cells from patients with bipolar disorder. Am J Pathol. 2010;177(2):575–85.
9. Kvajo M, Dhilla A, Swor DE, Karayiorgou M, Gogos JA. Evidence implicating the candidate schizophrenia/bipolar disorder susceptibility gene G72 in mitochondrial function. Mol Psychiatry. 2008;13(7):685–96.
10. Ueno H, Nishigaki Y, Kong QP, Fuku N, Kojima S, Iwata N, Ozaki N, Tanaka M. Analysis of mitochondrial DNA variants in Japanese patients with schizophrenia. Mitochondrion. 2009;9(6):385–93.
11. Muller DJ, Zai CC, Shinkai T, Strauss J, Kennedy JL. Association between the DAOA/G72 gene and bipolar disorder and meta-analyses in bipolar disorder and schizophrenia. Bipolar Disord. 2011;13(2):198–207.
12. Clay MLL, Deng JJ, Bai Y. Number matters: control of mammalian mitochondrial DNA copy number. J Genet Genomics. 2009;36(3):125–31.
13. Li Z, Hu M, Zong X, He Y, Wang D, Dai L, Dong M, Zhou J, Cao H, Lv L, et al. Association of telomere length and mitochondrial DNA copy number with risperidone treatment response in first-episode antipsychotic-naive schizophrenia. Sci Rep. 2015;5:18553.
14. Bersani FS, Morley C, Lindqvist D, Epel ES, Picard M, Yehuda R, Flory J, Bierer LM, Makotkine I, Abu-Amara D, et al. Mitochondrial DNA copy number is reduced in male combat veterans with PTSD. Prog Neuro-Psychopharmacol Biol Psychiatry. 2016;64:10–7.
15. Yoo HJ, Park M, Kim SA. Difference in mitochondrial DNA copy number in peripheral blood cells between probands with autism spectrum disorders and their unaffected siblings. World J Biol Psychiatry. 2017; 18(2):151–6.
16. Vawter MP, Tomita H, Meng F, Bolstad B, Li J, Evans S, Choudary P, Atz M, Shao L, Neal C, et al. Mitochondrial-related gene expression changes are sensitive to agonal-pH state: implications for brain disorders. Mol Psychiatry. 2006;11(7):615. 663-679
17. Torrell H, Montana E, Abasolo N, Roig B, Gaviria AM, Vilella E, Martorell L. Mitochondrial DNA (mtDNA) in brain samples from patients with major psychiatric disorders: gene expression profiles, mtDNA content and presence of the mtDNA common deletion. Am J Med Genet B Neuropsychiatr Genet. 2013;162B(2):213–23.
18. Sabunciyan S, Kirches E, Krause G, Bogerts B, Mawrin C, Llenos IC, Weis S. Quantification of total mitochondrial DNA and mitochondrial common deletion in the frontal cortex of patients with schizophrenia and bipolar disorder. J Neural Transn (Vienna). 2007;114(5):665–74.
19. Kakiuchi C, Ishiwata M, Kametani M, Nelson C, Iwamoto K, Kato T. Quantitative analysis of mitochondrial DNA deletions in the brains of patients with bipolar disorder and schizophrenia. Int J Neuropsychopharmacol. 2005;8(4):515–22.
20. Chang CC, Jou SH, Lin TT, Liu CS. Mitochondrial DNA variation and increased oxidative damage in euthymic patients with bipolar disorder. Psychiatry Clin Neurosci. 2014;68(7):551–7.
21. de Sousa RT, Uno M, Zanetti MV, Shinjo SM, Busatto GF, Gattaz WF, Marie SK, Machado-Vieira R. Leukocyte mitochondrial DNA copy number in bipolar disorder. Prog Neuro-Psychopharmacol Biol Psychiatry. 2014;48:32–5.
22. Liu CS, Tsai CS, Kuo CL, Chen HW, Lii CK, Ma YS, Wei YH. Oxidative stress-related alteration of the copy number of mitochondrial DNA in human leukocytes. Free Radic Res. 2003;37(12):1307–17.
23. Zhang C, Xu S, Huang X. A novel and convenient relative quantitative method of fluorescence real time RT–PCR assay based on slope of standard curve. Prog Biochem Biophys. 2005;32(9):883–8. (http://europepmc.org/abstract/cba/596524)
24. Xing J, Chen M, Wood CG, Lin J, Spitz MR, Ma J, Amos CI, Shields PG, Benowitz NL, Gu J. Mitochondrial DNA content: its genetic heritability and association with renal cell carcinoma. J Natl Cancer Inst. 2008;100(15):1104.
25. Box GEP, Cox DR. An analysis of transformations. J R Stat Soc Ser B Methodol. 1964;26(2):211–52. http://www.jstor.org/stable/2984418.
26. Sakia RM. The box-cox transformation technique: a review. J R Stat Soc. 1992;41(2):169–78. (http://www.jstor.org/stable/2348250)
27. Cohen J. Statistical power analysis for the behavioral sciences. 2nd ed. Hillsdale, NJ: L. Erlbaum Associates; 1988.
28. Woods SW. Chlorpromazine equivalent doses for the newer atypical antipsychotics. J Clin Psychiatry. 2003;64(6):663–7.
29. Malik AN, Czajka A. Is mitochondrial DNA content a potential biomarker of mitochondrial dysfunction? Mitochondrion. 2013;13(5):481–92.
30. Nicod J, Wagner S, Vonberg F, Bhomra A, Schlicht KF, Tadic A, Mott R, Lieb K, Flint J. The amount of mitochondrial DNA in blood reflects the course of a depressive episode. Biol Psychiatry. 2016;80(6):e41.
31. Rizzo LB, Costa LG, Mansur RB, Swardfager W, Belangero SI, Grassi-Oliveira R, McIntyre RS, Bauer ME, Brietzke E. The theory of bipolar disorder as an illness of accelerated aging: implications for clinical care and research. Neurosci Biobehav Rev. 2014;42:157–69.
32. Hartmann N, Reichwald K, Wittig I, Drose S, Schmeisser S, Luck C, Hahn C, Graf M, Gausmann U, Terzibasi E, et al. Mitochondrial DNA copy number and function decrease with age in the short-lived fish Nothobranchius furzeri. Aging Cell. 2011;10(5):824–31.
33. Kasahara T, Ishiwata M, Kakiuchi C, Fuke S, Iwata N, Ozaki N, Kunugi H, Minabe Y, Nakamura K, Iwata Y, et al. Enrichment of deleterious variants of mitochondrial DNA polymerase gene (POLG1) in bipolar disorder. Psychiatry Clin Neurosci. 2017;71(8):518–29.
34. Munkholm K, Peijs L, Vinberg M, Kessing LV. A composite peripheral blood gene expression measure as a potential diagnostic biomarker in bipolar disorder. Transl Psychiatry. 2015;5:e614.
35. Chang CC, Jou SH, Lin TT, Lai TJ, Liu CS. Mitochondria DNA change and oxidative damage in clinically stable patients with major depressive disorder. PLoS One. 2015;10(5):e0125855.

36. He Y, Tang J, Li Z, Li H, Liao Y, Tang Y, Tan L, Chen J, Xia K, Chen X. Leukocyte mitochondrial DNA copy number in blood is not associated with major depressive disorder in young adults. PLoS One. 2014;9(5):e96869.
37. Cai N, Chang S, Li Y, Li Q, Hu J, Liang J, Song L, Kretzschmar W, Gan X, Nicod J, et al. Molecular signatures of major depression. Curr Biol. 2015; 25(9):1146–56.
38. Kageyama Y, Kasahara T, Kato M, Sakai S, Deguchi Y, Tani M, Kuroda K, Hattori K, Yoshida S, Goto Y, et al. The relationship between circulating mitochondrial DNA and inflammatory cytokines in patients with major depression. J Affect Disord. 2018;233:15–20.
39. Pfaffenseller B, Fries GR, Wollenhaupt-Aguiar B, Colpo GD, Stertz L, Panizzutti B, Magalhaes PV, Kapczinski F. Neurotrophins, inflammation and oxidative stress as illness activity biomarkers in bipolar disorder. Expert Rev Neurother. 2013;13(7):827–42.
40. Kapczinski F, Dal-Pizzol F, Teixeira AL, Magalhaes PV, Kauer-Sant'Anna M, Klamt F, Pasquali MA, Quevedo J, Gama CS, Post R. A systemic toxicity index developed to assess peripheral changes in mood episodes. Mol Psychiatry. 2010;15(8):784–6.
41. Inuwa IM, Peet M, Williams MA. QSAR modeling and transmission electron microscopy stereology of altered mitochondrial ultrastructure of white blood cells in patients diagnosed as schizophrenic and treated with antipsychotic drugs. Biotech Histochem. 2005;80(3–4):133–7.
42. Bachmann RF, Wang Y, Yuan P, Zhou R, Li X, Alesci S, Du J, Manji HK. Common effects of lithium and valproate on mitochondrial functions: protection against methamphetamine-induced mitochondrial damage. Int J Neuropsychopharmacol. 2009;12(6):805–22.
43. Eftekhari A, Azarmi Y, Parvizpur A, Eghbal MA. Involvement of oxidative stress and mitochondrial/lysosomal cross-talk in olanzapine cytotoxicity in freshly isolated rat hepatocytes. Xenobiotica. 2016;46(4):369–78.

5

Prevalence, patterns and predictors of depression treatment among community-dwelling older adults with stroke in the United States

Sandipan Bhattacharjee[1*], Majed Al Yami[2], Sawsan Kurdi[2] and David Rhys Axon[1]

Abstract

Background: Depression is one of the most common psychiatric conditions among stroke survivors and is associated with several negative health outcomes. However, little is known about the depression treatment patterns among stroke survivors. The objective of this study was to examine national-level prevalence, patterns and predictors of depression treatment among community-dwelling stroke survivors.

Methods: This study adopted a retrospective, cross-sectional study design using multiple years of Medical Expenditure Panel Survey (MEPS) (2002–2012) data. The study population consisted of older adults (age ≥ 50 years) who (i) were stroke survivors (ICD-9-CM codes of 430–438), (ii) did not die during the calendar year, and (iii) had co-occurring depression (ICD-9-CM code of 296.xx, or 311.xx). Depression treatment, identified by antidepressant medication and/or psychotherapy use, was the dependent variable of this study. Multinomial logistic regression analysis was conducted to examine the association of individual level factors with depression treatment among stroke survivors with co-occurring depression.

Results: The final study sample consisted 370 (unweighted) community-dwelling older adults with self-reported stroke and depression. The prevalence of co-occurring depression among stroke survivors was 22.03% [95% Confidence Interval (CI) 19.7–24.4%]. An overwhelming majority (87.6%) of stroke survivors with co-occurring depression reported some form of depression treatment. Antidepressants only and combination therapy was reported by 74.8% (95% CI, 71.6–78.0%] and 12.8% (95% CI, 10.5–15.1%) by stroke survivors with co-occurring depression respectively. Approximately, 61% of stroke survivors with co-occurring depression reported using SSRIs, followed by SNRIs (15.2%), miscellaneous antidepressants (12.1%), TCAs (9.8%), phenylpiperazine antidepressants (5.2%), and tetracyclic antidepressants (4%). Sertraline (15.8, 95% CI, 12.7–19.0%) had the highest reported use among individual antidepressants.

Conclusions: Vast majority (nearly 90%) of the study sample received some form of depression treatment and several individual level factors (such as age, education) were associated with the report of depression treatment use. Future longitudinal studies are warranted to assess the comparative treatment benefits of antidepressants, psychotherapy and their combination. Healthcare providers should carefully assess the risks and benefits of antidepressant (such as SSRIs or TCAs) use in this vulnerable population prior to their use.

Keywords: Stroke, Depression, Antidepressants, Psychotherapy

* Correspondence: bhattacharjee@pharmacy.arizona.edu
[1]Department of Pharmacy Practice and Science, College of Pharmacy, The University of Arizona, 1295 North Martin Avenue, Tucson, AZ 85721, USA
Full list of author information is available at the end of the article

Background

Stroke is a common and costly disease, which is a major burden on patients' lives and the health system economy. On average, every 40 s, someone in the United States (US) has either a new or recurrent stroke, with an annual incidence of 795,000 [1]. Other than being the fifth leading cause of mortality, stroke is the leading cause of long-term adult disability in the US [1]. Due to advances in awareness, risk factor control, and the aging population, stroke survivors' prevalence has been increasing [1]. However, recovery after stroke takes time, and usually stroke survivors live with some degree of functional disability and depression is a common sequelae after stroke [2]. A pooled estimate indicates that depressive symptoms are present in one third of all stroke survivors at any time during the follow-up [3]. Another study reported that pooled prevalence of minor and major depression in community based setting after stroke are 9 and 14%, respectively [4].

Co-occurring depression among stroke survivors is associated with poor rehabilitation outcome [5], compromised quality of life [6], social isolation, poor medications adherence [7], and higher rate of mortality [8]. Given the array of negative outcomes associated with co-occurring depression among stroke survivors, it is critical to treat depression in this vulnerable population, which in turn may improve patients' health outcomes and quality of life. In general, depression can be treated by using antidepressants, psychotherapy, or both. Existing randomized controlled trials (RCTs) have demonstrated the benefits of these depression treatment modalities in reducing depression burden among stroke survivors [9–14]. Moreover, in a Cochrane review of 12 clinical trials, the use of antidepressant treatment in older adults(age range of 60–78), was associated with an improvement in rates of depression (OR 0.47, 95% CI 0.22–0.98) [15]. A recent systematic review and meta-analysis of RCTs investigating the effectiveness of antidepressants in post-stroke depression found a standardized mean effect size of − 0.96 (95% CI = − 1.41, − 0.51) between antidepressants versus placebo, indicating a significant advantage of antidepressants over placebo ($p < 0.0001$) [16]. Furthermore, Mitchell et al. found that a combination of antidepressant and behavioral therapy was more effective in reducing depression compared to antidepressants alone [11].

Despite the evidence of the efficacy of depression treatment modalities (antidepressants only, psychotherapy only, and antidepressant and psychotherapy combination) ,, to the best of our knowledge, no study to date has been conducted to examine the national-level prevalence, patterns and predictors of depression treatment among community-dwelling stroke survivors with co-occurring depression in the United States (US). Examining the current treatment patterns can help to understand whether the demonstration of depression treatment efficaciousness among stroke survivors from RCTs have helped in adoption of depression treatment into real-world clinical practice. Moreover, determining the predictors of depression treatment among stroke survivors can provide insights into factors where there is/are need of intervention(s) to improve depression care. Hence, this study is a first of its kind to examine national-level prevalence, patterns and predictors of depression treatment among community-dwelling stroke survivors in the US.

Methods

Study design

We adopted a retrospective, cross-sectional study design using pooled data from Medical Expenditure Panel Survey (MEPS) (2002–2012). Respondents of the MEPS are followed for two years. In order to eliminate the chances of including the same respondent between consecutive years, we used alternate years of data (2002, 2004, 2006, 2008, 2010, and 2012) [17]. It is recommended that multiple years of MEPS data be used to achieve adequate sample size [18].

Data source

MEPS is a nationwide survey of US citizens, their healthcare providers and employers which records healthcare cost, use and insurance coverage [19], collected by the Agency for Healthcare Research and Quality (AHRQ). MEPS uses the sampling framework of the National Health Interview Survey (NHIS) and contains information about medical and mental health conditions, as well as services and treatments such as prescription drugs and counseling therapies. The survey oversamples minority groups and disabled people in order to achieve nationally representative estimates. The survey consists of a household component (MEPS-HC) and an insurance component (MEPS-IC). The MEPS-HC uses a nationally representative sample panel of households selected annually whereby household respondents provide information about their medical conditions. This information is then converted into International Classification of Diseases, 9th Edition, Clinical Modification (ICD-9-CM) codes and clinical classification codes by professional coders. Data in each panel are collected for two calendar years. Information from MEPS-HC was used to obtain data of self-reported medical conditions and socio-demographic data. The MEPS-IC is conducted by the U.S. Census Bureau and contains information on establishment characteristics, whether an establishment offers health insurance, and details on health plans. Household respondents medical conditions have been found to typically correlate with medical care provider data. It has been demonstrated that

MEPS participant reported conditions are consistent with those provided by their medical providers for chronic conditions (such as diabetes, mental health, hypertension) with a median sensitivity of 70% [20]. The MEPS Medical Conditions file was used to identify the comorbidities, the Prescription Use file was used to identify the medication use, and Outpatient and Office-based Provider Visits files were used to identify psychotherapy use [19].

Study population

The study population consisted of older adults (age ≥ 50 years) who (i) were stroke survivors, (ii) did not die during the calendar year, and (iii) had co-occurring depression. Stroke was identified by using International Classification of Diseases, Ninth Revision, Clinical Modification (ICD-9-CM) code of 430.xx-438.xx [21]. These ICD-9-CM codes are used by the American Heart Association to report stroke statistics [22] and have also shown high sensitivity (≥ 82%), specificity (≥ 95%), and positive predictive value (≥ 81%) to identify overall diagnosis of acute or preexisting stroke [23]. Co-occurring depression was identified by using ICD-9-CM code of 296.xx, or 311.xx [24]. As MEPS publically available medical conditions file provides only three digit ICD-9-CM codes, there is a possibility of including some individuals with bipolar disorder with the use of ICD-9-CM code of 296.xx. However, it has been observed that most of the individuals with an ICD-9-CM code of 296.xx have major depressive disorder and overwhelming majority (> 90%) of them have an ICD-9-CM code of 311 that corresponds to unspecified depression [25]. Moreover, existing studies using MEPS data have used ICD-9-CM codes of 296.xx and 311.xx to identify depression [26, 27].

Dependent variable

Depression treatment constituted the dependent variable. Depression treatment was identified by antidepressant medication and/or psychotherapy use. Antidepressant use was ascertained from the prescription drug files. Multum Lexicon therapeutic class code (second level) of "249" was used to identify antidepressant use. The third level of Multum Lexicon therapeutic class codes were used to identify the subclasses of antidepressants. Antidepressants were classified into the following categories: (i) Selective serotonin reuptake inhibitors (SSRIs); (ii) Serotonin–norepinephrine reuptake inhibitors (SNRIs); (iii) Tricyclic antidepressants (TCAs); (iv) Monoamine oxidase inhibitor (MAO inhibitors); (v) phenylpiperazine antidepressants; (vi) Tetracyclic antidepressants; and (vii) Miscellaneous antidepressants. An additional file is provided showing detailed Multum Lexicon codes used to identify these subclasses of antidepressants [see Additional file 1: Table S1]. National Drug Codes (NDCs) were used to identify individual antidepressants. Psychotherapy use was obtained from the provider visits of outpatient and office-based files. Stroke survivors with co-occurring depression, who reported at least one visit for psychotherapy or mental health counseling services, were included in the group of psychotherapy receipt [28].

We defined depression treatment in two different ways. In the first measure, depression treatment was categorized as (i) receipt of antidepressants and/or psychotherapy; and (ii) no depression treatment. For the second measure, the depression treatment was classified into four groups: (i) antidepressant use alone; (ii) psychotherapy alone; (iii) antidepressant with psychotherapy; and (iv) no depression treatment. As the sample size of stroke survivors with co-occurring depression, who used psychotherapy alone (Unweighted $N = 13$) was very small, they were not included in the final study sample.

Independent variables

This study was conceptualized using Ronal M. Andersen's Behavioral Model of Health Services Use framework to investigate the association between predisposing, enabling, need, external environmental, and personal health practices factors with depression treatment [29]. The predisposing factors included age (50–64 years, 65 years and older), gender (male; female), and race/ethnicity (white and others). Enabling factors included education (less than high school; up to high school; and higher than high school), marital status (married and others), type of insurance (public; private; and uninsured), and poverty status [poor or near poor (< 200% of federal poverty level); middle income or high income (≥ 200% of federal poverty level)]. Need factors included chronic diseases (e.g. arthritis, osteoporosis, diabetes, thyroid disorder, heart disease, hypertension, asthma, gastro esophageal reflux disorder, depression, anxiety and other neurological conditions), limitations of activities of daily living (ADLs) (yes/no), limitations of instrumental activities of daily living (IADLs) (yes/no), activities limitations in work or housework (yes/no), functional activities limitations (yes/no), perceived physical health status (excellent/very good; good; and fair/poor), perceived mental health status (excellent/very good; good; and fair/poor), and pain (quite or extreme pain; moderate or little pain; and no pain). If a survey respondent required help or supervision on any of the ADLs (eating, dressing, bathing, toileting, getting in and out of bed, and mobility inside own residence) for at least another three months from the date of data collection (during any of the multiple interviews in a year), then they were considered to have ADL limitations. IADL limitations were defined similarly based on whether they required help or supervision with using the telephone, paying bills, taking medications, preparing light meals, doing laundry, or going shopping. MEPS participants were considered to have functional limitations if they had difficulties performing specific physical actions, or had problems with cognition, vision and hearing. The series of questions asked to evaluate difficulties with physical actions for at least three more months were: difficulty lifting 10 pounds, difficulty walking up 10 steps, difficulty walking 3 blocks, difficulty walking a mile, difficulty standing 20 min, difficulty bending or stooping, difficulty reaching over head, difficulty using fingers to grasp. Cognitive limitations were identified with a "yes" response to any of the following questions: (i) experienced confusion or memory loss, (ii) had problems making decisions, or (iii) required supervision for their own safety. Vision or hearing problems were identified by asking the respondent whether they had difficulty seeing or hearing respectively. Activities limitation was identified based on whether MEPS participants had any limitation in work, housework, or school. Perceived physical and mental health status were collected during any of the interview rounds by asking MEPS respondents to rate their physical and mental health status into any of the following categories: excellent, very good, good, fair, and poor. Personal health practices consisted of body mass index (BMI) categories (under or normal; and overweight or obese), and smoking status (current smoker; and others). External environmental factors consisted of region (Mid-West; Northeast; West; and South), and metropolitan status (metropolitan; and non-metropolitan).

Pain

Antidepressants are prescribed at certain times to alleviate pain associated with different chronic conditions [30] and hence can influence depression treatment patterns among stroke survivors with co-occurring depression. In order to minimize the effect of pain on depression treatment among stroke survivors with co-occurring depression, we adjusted pain as one of the variables in the multivariate regression models. MEPS respondents were asked if - *"During past 4 weeks, pain interfered with normal work outside the home and housework"*, which was used to construct the pain variable [31]. The pain variable was self-reported by MEPS respondents on a 5-point scale: (i) not at all; (ii) a little bit; (iii) moderately; (iv) quite a bit; and (v) extremely. We categorized pain into three categories for this study: (i) quite a bit/extreme pain; (ii) a little bit or moderate pain; and (iii) no pain.

Statistical analysis

Univariate analyses were conducted using chi-square tests to ascertain the statistically significant differences among different depression treatment groups (antidepressant use alone, antidepressant and psychotherapy combination and no depression treatment) in the study population. Multinomial logistic regression was conducted to assess the factors (predisposing, enabling, need, personal health choices, and external environmental factors) associated with depression treatment among stroke survivors with co-occurring depression. The levels of the depression treatment (dependent variable) consisted of: (i) antidepressant use alone; (ii) antidepressant and psychotherapy (combination therapy); and (iii) no depression treatment (which served as the reference group for the multinomial logistic regression). Sensitivity analyses was conducted by using logistic regression with any form of depression treatment (antidepressant and/or psychotherapy) compared to no depression treatment as dependent variable adjusting for predisposing, enabling, need, personal health practices, and external environmental factors. National estimates were obtained by adjusting for the complex survey design of MEPS. SAS version 9.4 (SAS institute Inc., Cary, NC, USA) was used to carry out all the analyses.

Results

The final study sample consisted 370 (unweighted) community-dwelling older adults with self-reported stroke and depression who were alive during the calendar year (2002, 2004, 2006, 2008, 2010, and 2012). The prevalence of co-occurring depression among stroke survivors was 22.03% [95% Confidence Interval (CI) 19.7–24.4%]. An overwhelming majority (87.6%) of stroke survivors with co-occurring depression reported some form of depression treatment. Antidepressants only and combination therapy was reported by 74.8% (95% CI, 71.6–78.0%] and 12.8% (95% CI, 10.5–15.1%) respectively by stroke survivors with co-occurring depression. Only 12.4% (95% CI, 9.9–14.8%) of stroke survivors with co-occurring depression reported that they did not receive any form of depression treatment.

Table 1 shows the overall distribution of predisposing, enabling, need, personal health practices and external environmental factors among stroke survivors with co-occurring depression as well as the distribution of these factors in different depression treatment groups. Overall, majority of stroke survivors with co-occurring depression were 65 years and older (60.4%), females (62.4%), whites (77.3%), reported fair or poor perceived physical health status (62.5%), experienced some form of pain (87.9%), reported functional disability (89.8%), had some chronic diseases (66.2%), and resided in metropolitan area (78%). From Table 1, it can be observed that there were subgroup differences in terms of age, race/ethnicity, education, poverty status, insurance, perceived mental health status, pain, ADL disability, chronic disease group, BMI status and region. For example, a

Table 1 Descriptive Statistics of Stroke Survivors with Co-occurring Depression Medical Expenditure Panel Survey (2002–2012)

	All (*N* = 370)	No Dep Tx (*N* = 55)	AD only (*N* = 268)	AD & Psych (*N* = 47)	Sig
	Wt.%	Wt.%	Wt.%	Wt.%	
		12.4	74.8	12.8	
Predisposing Factors					
Age					
50–64 years	39.6	42.8	34.8	64.9	***
65,+ years	60.4	57.2	65.2	35.1	
Gender					
Female	62.4	65.3	62.1	61.9	
Men	37.6	34.7	37.9	38.1	
Race/Ethnicity					
White	77.3	67.4	78.1	82.3	*
Other	22.7	32.6	21.9	17.7	
Enabling Factors					
Marital Status					
Married	49.4	41.5	51.4	45.2	
Other	50.6	58.5	48.6	54.8	
Education					
LT HS	25.7	39.7	24.5	17.3	***
HS	33.2	32.6	31.0	47.6	
> HS	41.0	27.7	44.5	35.1	
Poverty Status					
Poor	15.9	26.2	14.0	17.6	**
Near Poor	24.3	32.0	23.4	22.2	
Middle Income	33.2	29.9	33.8	33.0	
High Income	26.6	11.9	28.9	27.2	
Insurance					
Public	47.2	59.3	42.8	61.1	***
Others	52.8	40.7	57.2	38.9	
Need Factors					
Perceived Physical Health Status					
Ex/vgood	12.4	12.0	13.2	8.8	
Good	25.1	28.5	23.1	33.6	
Fair/poor	62.5	59.5	63.8	57.6	
Perceived Mental Health Status					
Ex/vgood	22.9	36.1	23.0	9.2	*
Good	38.0	28.2	39.2	39.8	
Fair/poor	39.2	35.7	37.7	50.9	
Pain					
Quite/Extreme	46.4	51.7	44.3	53.6	***
Little/Moderate	41.5	28.4	45.4	31.3	
No Pain	12.1	19.8	10.3	15.0	
ADL Disability					
Yes	31.2	32.9	33.1	18.3	*

Table 1 Descriptive Statistics of Stroke Survivors with Co-occurring Depression Medical Expenditure Panel Survey (2002–2012) *(Continued)*

	All (*N* = 370)	No Dep Tx (*N* = 55)	AD only (*N* = 268)	AD & Psych (*N* = 47)	Sig
	Wt.%	Wt.%	Wt.%	Wt.%	
		12.4	74.8	12.8	
No	68.8	67.1	66.9	81.7	
IADL Disability					
Yes	51.7	47.0	52.9	49.6	
No	48.3	53.0	47.1	50.4	
Functional Disability					
Yes	89.8	94.4	89.7	85.9	
No	10.2	5.6	10.3	14.1	
Activities Disability					
Yes	80.2	75.7	80.6	82.4	
No	19.8	24.3	19.4	17.6	
Chronic Disease Groups					
None	33.8	26.0	34.8	35.8	**
One	30.2	32.5	29.3	33.3	
Two	24.5	20.8	26.8	14.7	
Three or more	11.4	20.7	9.0	16.3	
Personal Health Practices Factors					
BMI Status					
Und/normal	58.8	77.5	58.4	43.6	***
Overwt/Obese	41.2	22.5	41.6	56.4	
Smoking Status					
Current smoker	16.3	8.1	17.4	17.6	
Other	83.7	91.9	82.6	82.4	
External Environmental Factors					
Area of Residence					
Metropolitan	78.0	84.9	78.2	70.3	
Non-Metropolitan	22.0	15.1	21.8	29.7	
Region					
Northeast	18.9	19.9	15.5	37.6	***
Mid-west	21.9	8.5	25.0	16.4	
South	37.7	48.1	38.8	21.8	
West	21.5	23.5	20.7	24.2	

Based on 370 older adults (age ≥ 50 years) with self-reported stroke and depression who were alive during the calendar year (2002, 2004, 2006, 2008, 2010, and 2012)

Abbreviations- No Dep Tx No Depression Treatment, *AD only* Antidepressants only, *AD & Psych* Antidepressants with Psychotherapy, *LT HS* Less than High School, *HS* High School, *Wt%* Weighted percentage, *Sig* Significant difference, *Ex/vgood* Excellent or Very Good, *ADL* Activity of Daily Living, *IADL* Instrumental Activity of Daily Living, *Und/normal* Underweight or Normal, *Overwt/Obese* Overweight or Obese, *BMI* Body Mass Index

Asterisks represent statistical significance between the different depression treatment groups [No Depression Treatment (Unweighted N = 55); Antidepressants only (Unweighted N = 268); and Antidepressants with Psychotherapy (Unweighted N = 47)] based on chi-square tests

****p* < 0.001; ** 0.001 ≤ *p* < 0.01; *0.01 ≤ *p* < 0.05*

greater proportion (64.9%) of stroke survivors with co-occurring depression who received combination therapy were in the age range of 50–64 years, whereas the majority (65.2%) of stroke survivors with co-occurring depression receiving antidepressants only were 65 years or older.

Table 2 provides the nationally representative patterns of depression treatment among stroke survivors with co-occurring depression. Approximately, 61% of stroke survivors with co-occurring depression reported using SSRIs, followed by SNRIs (15.2%), miscellaneous antidepressants (12.1%), TCAs (9.8%), phenylpiperazine antidepressants

Table 2 Dep Tx Patterns among Stroke Survivors with Co-occurring Depression Medical Expenditure Panel Survey (2002–2012)

	Wt.%
Any form of Dep Tx	87.6
SSRI	60.9
SNRI	15.2
TCA	9.8
PPAZ	5.2
Tetra Cyc	4.0
Misc ADP	12.1

Based on 370 older adults (age ≥ 50 years) with self-reported stroke and depression who were alive during the calendar year (2002, 2004, 2006, 2008, 2010, and 2012)
Abbreviations - Dep Tx Depression Treatment, *SSRI* Selective Serotonin Reuptake Inhibitor, *SNRI* Serotonin–Norepinephrine Reuptake Inhibitor, *TCA* Tricyclic Antidepressants, *PPAZ* Phenylpiperazine Antidepressants, *Tetra Cyc* Tetracyclic Antidepressants, *Misc ADP* Miscellaneous Antidepressants, *Wt%* Weighted percentage (nationally representative)
Total number of individual antidepressant classes may not add up to 100% due to intra-class polypharmacy
Denominator for Wt.% calculations for individual types of antidepressant classes was the total analytic sample (Unweighted N = 370)

(5.2%), and tetracyclic antidepressants (4%). Sertraline (15.8, 95% CI, 12.7–19.0%) had the highest reported use among individual antidepressants (data not presented in table). Other individual antidepressant use in the study population that should be noted include citalopram (13.9, 95% CI, 11.1–16.7%), paroxetine (12.5, 95% CI, 9.9–15.1%), escitalopram (11.4, 95% CI, 8.1% - 14.6), duloxetine (8.9, 95% CI, 6.2–11.6%), fluoxetine (8.8, 95% CI, 6.8–10.8%), bupropion (8.6, 95% CI, 7.2–10.1%), venlafaxine (7.1, 95% CI, 4.3–9.9%), trazodone (6.6, 95% CI, 4.8–8.4%), amitriptyline (5.5, 95% CI, 3.5–7.5%) and mirtazapine (4.7, 95% CI, 1.9% - 7.4).

Table 3 summarizes the findings from the multinomial logistic regression analysis. Several individual-level factors were associated with depression treatment. For example, among stroke survivors with co-occurring depression, those who were 65 years and older were nearly six times more likely [Adjusted Odds Ratio (AOR): 5.80, 95% CI 2.48–13.5] to report use of antidepressants only compared to those who were 50–64 years old. Stroke survivors with co-occurring depression who had less than high school education were 92% (AOR: 0.08, 95% CI 0.02–0.37) less likely to report the use combination therapy compared to those with higher than high school education. Details of the multinomial logistic regression are presented in Table 3 Sensitivity analyses with depression treatment (yes/no) showed similar findings (Table 4).

Discussion

The current study estimated the national level prevalence of co-occurring depression among community-dwelling older adults with stroke in the US to be 22.03%. To the best of our knowledge, this is the first study to date to estimate the national-level prevalence of co-occurring depression among community-dwelling stroke survivors in the US. Data from existing studies showed that the prevalence of depression among individuals with stroke varied widely across the world based on the region and method used, ranging from 11 to 79% [32–43], with epidemiological studies showing the co-occurrence of depression in 30% of stroke cases [44]. A recent study by McCarthy et al. (2016) using data from the greater Cincinnati/Northern Kentucky stroke study in the US found that 37% of stoke survivors were at risk for depression at 3-months post-stroke [45]. Another recent study by Fei et al. (2016) using data from the Prevent Recurrent All-Inner city Stroke through Education (PRAISE) study of 556 individuals in New York City in the US found that 31% of stroke survivors had post stroke depression [46]. Prevalence of depression observed in our study was slightly lower compared to the available estimates from the recent US studies [45, 46], that can be explained by the fact that these are self-reported by MEPS respondents, which are often associated with stigma of reporting mental illnesses, as well as the possibility of under-diagnosis of depression. Another possible explanation can be that some stroke survivors may not recently report depressive symptoms as they may have been successfully treated and are currently in remission. However, depression can be episodic, so regular depression screening is recommended.

The current study also provides the first national-level estimate of the receipt of depression treatment among community-dwelling stroke survivors with co-occurring depression. Among individual antidepressant classes, the current study found that SSRIs were reported as the mostly used antidepressants, which is not surprising as SSRIs have been found to be effective among stroke survivors in reducing dependency, disability, neurological impairment, anxiety as well as depression [47]. Moreover, in a population-based nested case control study, SSRIs were not found to be associated with recurrent stroke risk [48]. However, this study [48] found that TCAs, were associated with 41% higher likelihood of stroke recurrence. According to the current study findings, TCAs were reported to be used by approximately 10% of the study sample, and given the risk of recurrent stroke, close monitoring should be in place for individuals on TCAs. Another advantage of using SSRIs among stroke survivors with depression is the potential benefit of decreasing platelet aggregation and adhesion. However, this benefit has been examined and observed among individuals with different conditions such as myocardial infarction, depression, and ischemic heart disease (with depression) but not among stroke survivors [49–51]. It should however be kept in mind that SSRIs do have significant side effects as demonstrated by a

Table 3 Multinomial Logistic Regression among Stroke Survivors with Co-occurring Depression in terms of Depression Treatment Medical Expenditure Panel Survey (2002–2012)

	AD Only (*N* = 268)			AD & Psych (*N* = 47)		
	AOR	95% CI	Sig	AOR	95% CI	Sig
Predisposing Factors						
Age						
65,+ yrs. vs 50–64 yrs	5.80	[2.48,13.5]	***	1.16	[0.42,3.18]	
Gender						
Female vs Men	0.69	[0.33,1.42]		0.53	[0.21,1.31]	
Race/Ethnicity						
Other vs White	1.60	[0.77,3.32]		1.45	[0.58,3.61]	
Enabling Factors						
Marital Status						
Other vs Married	1.02	[0.45,2.31]		1.17	[0.32,4.27]	
Education						
LT HS vs > HS	0.07	[0.02,0.27]	***	0.08	[0.02,0.37]	**
HS vs > HS	0.24	[0.08,0.75]	*	0.57	[0.13,2.53]	
Insurance						
Public vs others	0.75	[0.22,2.54]		3.54	[0.65,19.2]	
Poverty Status						
Mid Inc./High Inc. vs Poor/Near Poor	1.60	[0.66,3.87]		3.90	[1.19,12.8]	*
Need Factors						
Pain						
Quite/Extreme vs No pain	1.09	[0.32,3.67]		1.02	[0.22,4.68]	
Little/Moderate vs No pain	1.97	[0.54,7.20]		1.11	[0.23,5.33]	
Perceived Physical Health Status						
Good vs Ex/vgood	0.49	[0.08,2.93]		0.72	[0.09,5.82]	
Fair/poor vs Ex/vgood	0.72	[0.22,2.41]		0.19	[0.06,0.60]	**
Perceived Mental Health Status						
Good vs MH Ex/vgood	4.55	[2.26,9.15]	***	11.04	[3.33,36.6]	***
Fair/poor vs MH Ex/vgood	3.60	[1.40,9.27]	**	19.19	[5.41,68.1]	***
ADL Disability						
Yes vs No	2.05	[0.72,5.86]		0.39	[0.11,1.34]	
IADL Disability						
Yes vs No	1.57	[0.52,4.78]		2.20	[0.64,7.50]	
Functional Disability						
Yes vs No	0.19	[0.04,0.83]	*	0.31	[0.06,1.65]	
Activities Disability						
Yes vs No	3.63	[0.89,14.8]		3.73	[0.71,19.6]	
Chronic Disease Groups						
One vs None	0.54	[0.17,1.69]		1.55	[0.41,5.86]	
Two vs None	0.91	[0.27,3.06]		1.33	[0.36,4.89]	
Three or more vs None	0.19	[0.07,0.48]	***	0.62	[0.06,5.92]	
CVD						
Yes vs No	0.02	[0.00,1.34]		0.08	[0.00,4.72]	

Table 3 Multinomial Logistic Regression among Stroke Survivors with Co-occurring Depression in terms of Depression Treatment Medical Expenditure Panel Survey (2002–2012) *(Continued)*

	AD Only (*N* = 268)			AD & Psych (*N* = 47)		
	AOR	95% CI	Sig	AOR	95% CI	Sig
Anxiety						
Yes vs No	0.79	[0.31,1.99]		1.09	[0.40,2.93]	
Hyperlipidemia						
Yes vs No	1.35	[0.69,2.66]		2.73	[0.94,7.96]	
Personal Health Practices Factors						
BMI Status						
Overwt/Obese vs Und/normal	5.18	[1.93,13.8]	**	9.35	[2.98,29.3]	***
Smoking Status						
Curr smoker vs Other	6.40	[1.51,27.0]	*	6.04	[1.42,25.6]	*
External Environmental Factors						
Metropolitan Status						
Non-Metropolitan vs Metropolitan	1.53	[0.67,3.46]		3.42	[1.13,10.2]	*
Region						
Mid-west vs Northeast	4.05	[1.28,12.7]	*	0.64	[0.17,2.40]	
South vs Northeast	0.83	[0.30,2.27]		0.20	[0.06,0.63]	**
West vs Northeast	0.53	[0.12,2.37]		0.36	[0.05,2.51]	

Based on 370 older adults (age ≥ 50 years) with self-reported stroke and depression who were alive during the calendar year (2002, 2004, 2006, 2008, 2010, and 2012)
Abbreviations -No Dep Tx No Depression Treatment, *AD only* Antidepressants only, *AD & Psych* Antidepressants with Psychotherapy, *LT HS* Less than High School, *HS* High School, *Wt%* Weighted percentage, *Sig* Significant difference, *Ex/vgood* Excellent or Very Good, *ADL* Activity of Daily Living, *IADL* Instrumental Activity of Daily Living, *Und/normal* Underweight or Normal, *Overwt/Obese* Overweight or Obese, *BMI* Body Mass Index, *AOR* Adjusted odds ratio, *Mid Inc./High Inc.* Middle Income or High Income
Asterisks represent statistical significance group differences by type of treatment compared to the reference group based on multinomial logistic regression. The reference group for the dependent variable in the multinomial logistic regression was "No Depression Treatment" ($N = 55$)
*$***p < 0.001$; ** $0.001 \leq p < 0.01$; *$0.01 \leq p < 0.05$*

study among post-menopausal women using the Women's Health Initiative (WHI) data [52]. This study using the WHI data observed that even though the absolute event risks are low, SSRIs are associated with higher risk of death, and hemorrhagic and fatal stroke [52]. Hence, the benefits to risk profile should always be assessed before using these medications. It is noteworthy to mention that currently there are three ongoing trials (FOCUS, AFFINITY, and EFFECTS) examining the effect of fluoxetine 20 mg daily for six months on different outcomes (such as modified Rankin scale, diagnosis of depression and adherence to medication) among stroke survivors [53]. Furthermore, there is an ongoing real-world study funded by the Patient Centered Outcomes Research Institute (PCORI) assessing the effectiveness of antidepressants among stroke survivors [54]. Findings from these studies have the potential to provide further evidence of antidepressant safety and effectiveness among stroke survivors.

Sertraline was the most frequently used individual antidepressant in this study sample. An open-label study [55] among stroke survivors with depression found that symptoms of depression and anxiety had consistent decline along with improvement in cognitive and functional performances with sertraline treatment and hence findings from this study are unsurprising. Approximately 14% of the current study sample reported using citalopram, which can be explained in the light of fewer side effects observed with citalopram in stroke survivors with depression [56], as well as the chances of significantly improving dexterity [57] after stroke. However, use of some individual antidepressants such as trazodone, mirtazapine and venlafaxine warrants constant monitoring as they have been observed to be associated high risks of several adverse events [58]. This study observed psychotherapy with antidepressant use in only 12.8% of stroke survivors with co-occurring depression. Even though specific data of the prevalence of psychotherapy use among stroke survivors is not available, but an existing study among depressed Medicare beneficiaries during 1992–1999 found psychotherapy use among a quarter of these patients [59]. However, the lower use of psychotherapy observed in the current study can be explained by the decline of outpatient psychotherapy in general population [60] as well as concerns about psychotherapy effectiveness among stroke survivors [61]. Selection of

Table 4 Logistic Regression among Stroke Survivors with Co-occurring Depression in terms of Depression Treatment Medical Expenditure Panel Survey (2002–2012)

	AOR	95% CI	Sig
Predisposing Factors			
Age			
65,+ yrs. vs 50–64 yrs	4.65	[2.10,10.2]	***
Gender			
Female vs Men	0.71	[0.36,1.41]	
Race + Ethnicity			
Other vs White	1.54	[0.78,3.05]	
Enabling Factors			
Marital Status			
Other vs Married	1.02	[0.46,2.26]	
Education			
LT HS vs > HS	0.08	[0.02,0.26]	***
HS vs > HS	0.29	[0.10,0.80]	*
Insurance			
Public vs others	0.89	[0.28,2.81]	
Poverty Status			
Mid Inc./High Inc. vs Poor/Near Poor	1.87	[0.87,4.01]	
Need Factors			
Pain			
Quite/Extreme vs No pain	1.20	[0.39,3.67]	
Little/Moderate vs No pain	1.99	[0.60,6.65]	
Perceived Physical Health Status			
Good vs Ex/vgood	0.56	[0.10,3.02]	
Fair/poor vs Ex/vgood	0.65	[0.21,2.01]	
Perceived Mental Health Status			
Good vs Ex/vgood	4.55	[2.37,8.72]	***
Fair/poor vs Ex/vgood	4.05	[1.69,9.73]	**
ADL Disability			
Yes vs No	1.68	[0.64,4.37]	
IADL Disability			
Yes vs No	1.62	[0.58,4.49]	
Functional Disability			
Yes vs No	0.20	[0.05,0.84]	*
Activities Disability			
Yes vs No	3.60	[0.97,13.2]	
Chronic Disease Groups			
One vs None	0.64	[0.22,1.86]	
Two vs None	1.00	[0.34,2.98]	
Three or more vs None	0.21	[0.08,0.52]	***
CVD			
Yes vs No	0.02	[0.00,1.12]	
Anxiety			
Yes vs No	0.88	[0.38,2.01]	
Hyperlipidemia			
Yes vs No	1.55	[0.82,2.93]	
Personal Health Practices Factors			
BMI Status			
Overwt/Obese vs Und/normal	5.71	[2.27,14.3]	***
Smoking Status			
Curr smoker vs Other	6.30	[1.65,240]	**
External Environmental Factors			
Metropolitan Status			
Non-Metropolitan vs Metropolitan	1.64	[0.77,3.49]	
Region			
Mid-west vs Northeast	2.80	[0.86,9.14]	
South vs Northeast	0.60	[0.22,1.66]	
West vs Northeast	0.41	[0.10,1.78]	

Based on 370 older adults (age ≥ 50 years) with self-reported stroke and depression who were alive during the calendar year (2002, 2004, 2006, 2008, 2010, and 2012)

Abbreviations- yrs. years, *LT HS* Less than High School, *HS* High School, *Wt%* Weighted percentage, *Sig* Significant difference, *Ex/vgood* Excellent or Very Good, *ADL* Activity of Daily Living, *IADL* Instrumental Activity of Daily Living, *Und/normal* Underweight or Normal, *Overwt/Obese* Overweight or Obese, *BMI* Body Mass Index, *AOR* Adjusted odds ratio, *Mid Inc./High Inc.* Middle Income or High Income

Asterisks represent statistical significance group differences by type of treatment (any form of depression treatment and no depression treatment) compared to the reference group based on binomial logistic regression. The reference group for the dependent variable in the binomial logistic regression was "No Depression Treatment"

***$p < 0.001$; ** $0.001 \le p < 0.01$; *$0.01 \le p < 0.05$

pharmacologic versus non-pharmacologic treatment modality is complicated and depends on several factors. For example, the choice of antidepressant treatment is generally influenced by the presence of multimorbidity, polypharmacy, and predisposition to antidepressant adverse effects [62]. In this context, non-pharmacologic treatment options (such as cognitive behavioral therapy) may present a favorable alternative. However, non-pharmacologic interventions are expensive, time consuming and usually show delayed response [62]. Thus, from a healthcare practice and policy perspective, it may be prudent to carefully weigh these different factors along with patient preferences, which has the potential to improve adherence and outcomes associated with these depression treatment modalities.

In certain cases, no depression treatment option is adopted among stroke survivors with co-occurring depression. In our study, not reporting any form of depression treatment among stroke survivors with co-occurring depression can be due to several reasons such as patient and/or physician preference, suboptimal detection of depression, depression therapy discontinuation due to adverse effects, non-adherence to depression therapy, or the possibility of improvement or remission of depressive symptoms. Future studies are warranted to understand the factors associated with no depression treatment in this vulnerable population.

In terms of predisposing factors, the current study showed that older adults (age ≥ 65 years) in the study sample were more likely to receive antidepressant therapy compared to those within 50–64 years of age. This finding can be partially explained by the overall increase in antidepressant use among older adults in the US from 3% in 1988–1994 [63] to 13.7% during 2007–2010 [64]. Moreover, a study of veterans who survived stroke with an average age of 69.4 years found it was clinically beneficial when patients were dispensed an antidepressant medication [65]. However, caution should be taken with the use of antidepressants in older adults, as with increasing age the chances of developing serotonin syndrome, falls and fractures risk, and mortality increases [58].

With respect to enabling factors, it was observed that stroke survivors with co-occurring depression with lower levels of education had less likelihood of receiving antidepressant therapy or combination therapy. This may be because lower levels of education are consistently associated with limited health literacy [66] and this may lead to less preventative care seeking behavior [67]. Appropriate interventions are required to improve health literacy as individuals with low literacy usually experience 1.5 to 3 times higher chances of poor health outcomes [68]. The current study also observed that stroke survivors with co-occurring depression who belonged to high or middle income status were more likely to receive combination therapy compared to individuals with lower incomes. This finding is not surprising as existing literature suggests that adults from low-income households have several barriers (lack of transport, childcare, health insurance, and difficult working hours) to accessing mental health services such as psychotherapy [69].

In terms of need factors, good and fair/poor perceived mental health status was associated with increased likelihood of antidepressant and combination therapy use. This study finding is consistent with an existing study by Olfson et al. (2006) [70], where longer-term antidepressant use was observed to be associated with perceived fair or poor mental health status, which can be partially attributed to greater motivation from these individuals or their caregivers. In the current study it was observed that having functional disability was associated with lower likelihood of antidepressant use. This finding is counterintuitive as existing double-blind randomized study demonstrated that antidepressant treatment was associated with improved recovery from disability among stroke survivors [71]. Future studies should explore the factors associated with the lower chances of antidepressant use among those with functional disability. Having three or more chronic diseases was associated with lower likelihood of receiving antidepressant treatment. Multiple factors could explain this finding such as competing demands from other disease conditions [72], risk of adverse events (such as falls) with polypharmacy including antidepressants [73] and drug interactions [74, 75].

In the domain of Personal Health Practices factors, both BMI and smoking status were significantly associated with higher likelihood of receiving antidepressant and combination therapy. The positive association of overweight or obese individuals with depression treatment can be explained by the fact that overweight adults are at an increased risk of depression [76], and that maybe the reason they are reporting higher depression treatment. However, caution should be taken while choosing antidepressants among overweight or obese individuals as some antidepressants (such as SSRIs) have been shown to be associated with abdominal obesity [77]. The present study finding suggests that current smokers had significantly higher likelihood of reporting antidepressants and combination therapy, which is not unexpected as adult smokers with depression smoke heavily [78] and may have higher need to treat depression to reduce smoking. Some antidepressants (such as bupropion) are used for smoking cessation and have been found to be effective in long-term smoking cessation [79], but in the present study population only 15% of current smoker reported using bupropion.

In terms of the external environmental factors, it was surprising to observe that stroke survivors with co-occurring depression who resided in rural areas were more likely to report combination therapy use compared to those residing in metropolitan areas. This finding is inconsistent with existing literature [80, 81], and reason is unclear as there was no significant differences among the study sample residing in metropolitan and rural areas in terms of perceived mental health status, functional disability, and chronic diseases. Future research is warranted to explore the reasons for this difference in metropolitan status. Another interesting finding from this study is that stroke survivors with co-occurring depression residing in Southern region were less likely to report combination therapy use. This is surprising because Southern region is the stroke belt of US and also as per the Darthmouth Atlas of Medicare Prescription Drug use, newer antidepressants use was concentrated in the Southern region [82].

Use of a nationally representative sample of community-dwelling older adults with stroke and co-occurring depression and use of a broad set of individual-level variables including pain, are some of the strengths of this study.

However, limitations of this study need to be kept in mind while interpreting the findings. MEPS uses self-reported data that are subject to potential recall bias. However, in order to minimize recall bias, interviews are conducted at regular intervals of 4–5 months by MEPS [20]. Sequence of stroke and depression (whether stroke preceded depression or vice-versa) cannot be obtained from the Medical Conditions file. Severity of stroke and depression is unavailable in MEPS data. It cannot be ascertained from MEPS whether psychotherapy was used specifically for depression or for other conditions (such as anxiety). This is also true for antidepressant use (whether it is specific for depression or it was for other conditions such as anxiety, sleep or appetite stimulation). Inability of establishing cause-effect relationship remains one of the inherent drawbacks of studies utilizing secondary data and hence limitations such as the exact reason for using any pharmacologic or non-pharmacologic option remains elusive. MEPS publically available data provide three digit ICD-9-CM codes that can lead to misclassification bias, however, stroke and depression ICD-9-CM codes used in this study have been validated and used in previous studies utilizing MEPS data. One of the other limitations of this study was that we were not able to segregate stroke subtypes (ischemic and hemorrhagic) as individuals with co-occurring hemorrhagic stroke and depression ($n = 3$) was extremely small. And finally, given the range of years of data (2002–2012) used in this study, it may not represent the current status of depression treatment among stroke survivors in the US.

Conclusions

Despite the limitations, this is the first study to date to provide national level estimates of depression treatment among community-dwelling older adults with stroke and co-occurring depression. Nearly 90% of the study sample received some form of depression treatment, with SSRIs reported as the most widely used class of antidepressant, and sertraline being the most reported individual antidepressant agent. Use of depression treatment was associated with several individual-level factors such as age, education, poverty status, perceived mental health status, functional disability, presence of other chronic conditions, BMI, smoking, metropolitan status, and region. Future longitudinal studies are warranted to assess the comparative treatment benefits of antidepressants (classes as well as individual antidepressants), psychotherapy and their combination that can add to the current knowledgebase and eventually improve different domains of quality of care (such as effectiveness, safety and patient centeredness). Future studies should also assess the incremental healthcare expenditures among stroke survivors due to the presence of depression and also if depression treatment reduces healthcare expenditure in this vulnerable population.

Abbreviations

ADL: Activity of Daily Living; AHRQ: Agency for Healthcare Research and Quality; AOR: Adjusted Odds Ratio; BMI: Body mass index; CI: Confidence Intervals; IADL: Instrumental Activity of Daily; ICD-9-CM: International Classification of Diseases, 9th Edition, Clinical Modification; MAOI: Mono-Amine Oxidase Inhibitors; MEPS: Medical Expenditure Panel Survey; MEPS-HC: Medical Expenditure Panel Survey-Household Component; MEPS-IC: Medical Expenditure Panel Survey-Insurance Component; NDC: National Drug Code; NHIS: National Health interview Survey; OR: Odds Ratio; PPAZ: Phenylpiperazine Antidepressants]; RCT: Randomized Controlled Trial; SNRI: Serotonin–Norepinephrine Reuptake Inhibitor; SSRI: Selective Serotonin Reuptake Inhibitor; TCA: Tricyclic Antidepressants; US: United States; WHI: Women's Health Initiative

Acknowledgements

A part of this research was presented as poster at the International Society for Pharmacoeconomics and Outcomes Research 22nd Annual International Meeting (May 20-24, 2017; Boston, MA, USA). The authors would like to thank Ms. Zufan Yegezu for her help with formatting of this manuscript.

Funding

This research did not receive any grant from funding agencies in the public, commercial, or not-for-profit sectors.

Authors' contributions

SB conceptualized the study, conducted analysis, drafted manuscript, and incorporated suggestion from co-authors in successive iterations. MAY and SK conducted literature review, drafted manuscript, and provided input on successive versions of the manuscript. DRA drafted manuscript, interpreted findings and provided input on successive versions of the manuscript. All authors read and approved the final manuscript.

Competing interests

The views and opinions expressed in this article are those of the authors and do not necessarily reflect the official policy or position of The University of Arizona or any other affiliated organizations. The author(s) declare that they have no competing interests.

Author details

[1]Department of Pharmacy Practice and Science, College of Pharmacy, The University of Arizona, 1295 North Martin Avenue, Tucson, AZ 85721, USA. [2]Health Outcomes & PharmacoEconomic Research (HOPE) Center, College of Pharmacy, The University of Arizona, Tucson, AZ, USA.

References

1. Mozaffarian D, Benjamin EJ, Go AS, Arnett DK, Blaha MJ, Cushman M, Das SR, de Ferranti S, Despres JP, Fullerton HJ, et al. Heart disease and stroke Statistics-2016 update: a report from the American Heart Association. Circulation. 2016;133(4):e38–60.

2. Hadidi N, Treat-Jacobson DJ, Lindquist R. Poststroke depression and functional outcome: a critical review of literature. Heart & lung : the journal of critical care. 2009;38(2):151–62.
3. de Man-van Ginkel JM, Hafsteinsdottir TB, Lindeman E, Ettema RG, Grobbee DE, Schuurmans MJ. In-hospital risk prediction for post-stroke depression: development and validation of the post-stroke depression prediction scale. Stroke. 2013;44(9):2441–5.
4. Robinson RG, Jorge RE. Post-stroke depression: a review. Am J Psychiatry. 2016;173(3):221–31.
5. Sinyor D, Amato P, Kaloupek DG, Becker R, Goldenberg M, Coopersmith H. Post-stroke depression: relationships to functional impairment, coping strategies, and rehabilitation outcome. Stroke. 1986;17(6):1102–7.
6. Guajardo VD, Terroni L, Sobreiro Mde F, Zerbini MI, Tinone G, Scaff M, Iosifescu DV, de Lucia MC, Fraguas R. The influence of depressive symptoms on quality of life after stroke: a prospective study. Journal of stroke and cerebrovascular diseases : the official journal of National Stroke Association. 2015;24(1):201–9.
7. Boden-Albala B, Litwak E, Elkind MS, Rundek T, Sacco RL. Social isolation and outcomes post stroke. Neurology. 2005;64(11):1888–92.
8. Morris PL, Robinson RG, Andrzejewski P, Samuels J, Price TR. Association of depression with 10-year poststroke mortality. Am J Psychiatry. 1993; 150(1):124–9.
9. Lipsey JR, Robinson RG, Pearlson GD, Rao K, Price TR. Nortriptyline treatment of post-stroke depression: a double-blind study. Lancet (London, England). 1984;1(8372):297–300.
10. Andersen G, Vestergaard K, Lauritzen L. Effective treatment of poststroke depression with the selective serotonin reuptake inhibitor citalopram. Stroke. 1994;25(6):1099–104.
11. Mitchell PH, Veith RC, Becker KJ, Buzaitis A, Cain KC, Fruin M, Tirschwell D, Teri L. Brief psychosocial-behavioral intervention with antidepressant reduces poststroke depression significantly more than usual care with antidepressant: living well with stroke: randomized, controlled trial. Stroke. 2009;40(9):3073–8.
12. Williams LS, Kroenke K, Bakas T, Plue LD, Brizendine E, Tu W, Hendrie H. Care management of poststroke depression: a randomized, controlled trial. Stroke. 2007;38(3):998–1003.
13. Rampello L, Alvano A, Chiechio S, Raffaele R, Vecchio I, Malaguarnera M. An evaluation of efficacy and safety of reboxetine in elderly patients affected by "retarded" post-stroke depression. A random, placebo-controlled study. Arch Gerontol Geriatr. 2005;40(3):275–85.
14. Fruehwald S, Gatterbauer E, Rehak P, Baumhackl U. Early fluoxetine treatment of post-stroke depression–a three-month double-blind placebo-controlled study with an open-label long-term follow up. J Neurol. 2003;250(3):347–51.
15. Hackett ML, Anderson CS, House A, Xia J. Interventions for treating depression after stroke. Cochrane Database Syst Rev. 2008;(4):CD003437. https://doi.org/10.1002/14651858.CD003437.pub3. Review. PubMed PMID: 18843644.
16. Xu XM, Zou DZ, Shen LY, Liu Y, Zhou XY, Pu JC, Dong MX, Wei YD. Efficacy and feasibility of antidepressant treatment in patients with post-stroke depression. Medicine (Baltimore). 2016;95(45):e5349.
17. Medical Expenditure Panel Survey. MEPS-HC Sample Design and Data Collection Process [http://meps.ahrq.gov/mepsweb/survey_comp/hc_data_collection.jsp]. Accessed 12 July 2017.
18. Sommers J. An Examination of State Estimates Using Multiple Years of Data from the Medical ExpenditurePanel Survey, Household Component [http://meps.ahrq.gov/mepsweb/data_files/publications/workingpapers/wp_06004.pdf]. Accessed 12 July 2017.
19. Medical Expenditure Panel Survey. MEPS Survey Background [http://meps.ahrq.gov/mepsweb/about_meps/survey_back.jsp]. Accessed 12 July 2017.
20. Machlin S, Cohen J, Elixhauser A, Beauregard K, Steiner C. Sensitivity of household reported medical conditions in the medical expenditure panel survey. Med Care. 2009;47(6):618–25.
21. Ma JWE, Siegel RL, Jemal A. Temporal trends in mortality in the United States, 1969-2013. JAMA. 2015;314(16):1731–9.
22. Benjamin EJ, Blaha MJ, Chiuve SE, Cushman M, Das SR, Deo R, de Ferranti SD, Floyd J, Fornage M, Gillespie C, et al. Heart disease and stroke Statistics-2017 update: a report from the American Heart Association. Circulation. 2017;135(10):e146–603.
23. McCormick N, Bhole V, Lacaille D, Avina-Zubieta JA. Validity of diagnostic codes for acute stroke in administrative databases: a systematic review. PLoS One. 2015;10(8):e01358e34.
24. Atkins EVSU, Bhattacharya R. Variations of depression treatment among women with hypertension. Healthcare for Women International. 2015;36(6):20.
25. Harman JS, Kelleher KJ, Reynolds CF, Pincus HA. Out-of-pocket healthcare expenditures of older Americans with depression. J Am Geriatr Soc. 2004; 52(5):809–13.
26. Bhattacharjee S, Oh YM, Reiman EM, Burke WJ. Prevalence, patterns, and predictors of depression treatment among community-dwelling elderly individuals with dementia in the United States. Am J Geriatr Psychiatry. 2017;25(7):803–13.
27. Nagar S, Sherer JT, Chen H, Aparasu RR. Extent of functional impairment in children and adolescents with depression. Curr Med Res Opin. 2010;26(9): 2057–64.
28. Harman JSEM, Fortney JC, Kallas H. The influence of comorbid chronic medical conditions on the adequacy of depression care for older Americans. J Am Geriatr Soc. 2005;53(12):6.
29. Andersen RM. Revisiting the behavioral model and access to medical care: does it matter? J Health Soc Behav. 1995;36(1):1–10.
30. DI Verdu B, Buclin T, Stiefel F, Berney A. Antidepressants for the treatment of chronic pain. Drugs. 2008;68(18):22.
31. MEPS HC-155 2012 Full Year Consolidated Data File. September 2014.MEPS Data Documentation: Pain definition 2012 [http://meps.ahrq.gov/mepsweb/data_stats/download_data/pufs/h155/h155doc.pdf]. Accessed 14 July 2017.
32. Gordon WA, Hibbard MR. Poststroke depression: an examination of the literature. Arch Phys Med Rehabil. 1997;78(6):658–63.
33. Desmaele S, Putman K, De Wit L, Dejaeger E, Gantenbein AR, Schupp W, Steurbaut S, Dupont AG, De Paepe K. A comparative study of medication use after stroke in four countries. Clin Neurol Neurosurg. 2016;148:96–104.
34. Santos EB, Rodrigues RA, Pontes-Neto OM. Prevalence and predictors of post stroke depression among elderly stroke survivors. Arq Neuropsiquiatr. 2016;74(8):621–5.
35. Tsai CS, Wu CL, Hung TH, Chou SY, Su JA. Incidence and risk factors of poststroke depression in patients with acute ischemic stroke: a 1-year prospective study in Taiwan. Biom J. 2016;39(3):195–200.
36. Mutai H, Furukawa T, Nakanishi K, Hanihara T. Longitudinal functional changes, depression, and health-related quality of life among stroke survivors living at home after inpatient rehabilitation. Psychogeriatrics. 2016; 16(3):185–90.
37. Ayis SA, Ayerbe L, Crichton SL, Rudd AG, Wolfe CD. The natural history of depression and trajectories of symptoms long term after stroke: the prospective South London stroke register. J Affect Disord. 2016;194:65–71.
38. Kowalska J, Bojko E, Szczepanska-Gieracha J, Rymaszewska J, Rozek-Piechura K. Occurrence of depressive symptoms among older adults after a stroke in the nursing home facility. Rehabil Nurs. 2016;41(2):112–9.
39. Alghwiri AA. The correlation between depression, balance, and physical functioning post stroke. Journal of stroke and cerebrovascular diseases : the official journal of National Stroke Association. 2016;25(2):475–9.
40. Gyagenda JO, Ddumba E, Odokonyero R, Kaddumukasa M, Sajatovic M, Smyth K, Katabira E. Post-stroke depression among stroke survivors attending two hospitals in Kampala Uganda. Afr Health Sci. 2015;15(4):1220–31.
41. Schottke H, Giabbiconi CM. Post-stroke depression and post-stroke anxiety: prevalence and predictors. Int Psychogeriatr. 2015;27(11):1805–12.
42. Barker-Collo SL. Depression and anxiety 3 months post stroke: prevalence and correlates. Arch Clin Neuropsychol. 2007;22(4):519–31.
43. Broomfield NM, Quinn TJ, Abdul-Rahim AH, Walters MR, Evans JJ. Depression and anxiety symptoms post-stroke/TIA: prevalence and associations in cross-sectional data from a regional stroke registry. BMC Neurol. 2014;14:198.
44. Paolucci S. Epidemiology and treatment of post-stroke depression. Neuropsychiatr Dis Treat. 2008;4(1):145–54.
45. McCarthy MJ, Sucharew HJ, Alwell K, Moomaw CJ, Woo D, Flaherty ML, Khatri P, Ferioli S, Adeoye O, Kleindorfer DO, et al. Age, subjective stress, and depression after ischemic stroke. J Behav Med. 2016;39(1):55–64.
46. Fei K, Benn EK, Negron R, Arniella G, Tuhrim S, Horowitz CR. Prevalence of depression among stroke survivors: racial-ethnic differences. Stroke. 2016; 47(2):512–5.
47. Mead GE, Hsieh CF, Lee R, Kutlubaev M, Claxton A, Hankey GJ, Hackett M. Selective serotonin reuptake inhibitors for stroke recovery: a systematic review and meta-analysis. Stroke. 2013;44(3):844–50.
48. Wang MT, Chu CL, Yeh CB, Chang LC, Malone DC, Liou JT. Antidepressant use and risk of recurrent stroke: a population-based nested case-control study. The Journal of clinical psychiatry. 2015;76(7):e877–85.

49. Halperin D, Reber G. Influence of antidepressants on hemostasis. Dialogues Clin Neurosci. 2007;9(1):47–59.
50. Schins A, Hamulyak K, Scharpe S, Lousberg R, Van Melle J, Crijns H, Honig A. Whole blood serotonin and platelet activation in depressed post-myocardial infarction patients. Life Sci. 2004;76(6):637–50.
51. Laghrissi-Thode F, Wagner WR, Pollock BG, Johnson PC, Finkel MS. Elevated platelet factor 4 and beta-thromboglobulin plasma levels in depressed patients with ischemic heart disease. Biol Psychiatry. 1997;42(4):290–5.
52. Smoller JW, Allison M, Cochrane BB, Curb JD, Perlis RH, Robinson JG, Rosal MC, Wenger NK, Wassertheil-Smoller S. Antidepressant use and risk of incident cardiovascular morbidity and mortality among postmenopausal women in the Women's Health Initiative study. Arch Intern Med. 2009; 169(22):2128–39.
53. Mead G, Hackett ML, Lundstrom E, Murray V, Hankey GJ, Dennis M. The FOCUS, AFFINITY and EFFECTS trials studying the effect(s) of fluoxetine in patients with a recent stroke: a study protocol for three multicentre randomised controlled trials. Trials. 2015;16:369.
54. Xian Y, O'Brien EC, Fonarow GC, Olson DM, Schwamm LH, Hannah D, Lindholm B, Maisch L, Lytle BL, Greiner MA, et al. Patient-centered research into outcomes stroke patients prefer and effectiveness research: implementing the patient-driven research paradigm to aid decision making in stroke care. Am Heart J. 2015;170(1):36–45. 45 e31-11
55. Spalletta G, Caltagirone C. Sertraline treatment of post-stroke major depression: an open study in patients with moderate to severe symptoms. Funct Neurol. 2003;18(4):227–32.
56. Tan S, Huang X, Ding L, Hong H. Efficacy and safety of citalopram in treating post-stroke depression: a meta-analysis. Eur Neurol. 2015;74(3–4): 188–201.
57. Zittel S, Weiller C, Liepert J. Citalopram improves dexterity in chronic stroke patients. Neurorehabil Neural Repair. 2008;22(3):311–4.
58. Coupland C, Dhiman P, Morriss R, Arthur A, Barton G, Hippisley-Cox J. Antidepressant use and risk of adverse outcomes in older people: population based cohort study. BMJ. 2011;343:d4551.
59. Wei W, Sambamoorthi U, Olfson M, Walkup JT, Crystal S. Use of psychotherapy for depression in older adults. Am J Psychiatry. 2005;162(4): 711–7.
60. Olfson M, Marcus SC. National trends in outpatient psychotherapy. Am J Psychiatry. 2010;167(12):1456–63.
61. Lincoln NB, Flannaghan T. Cognitive behavioral psychotherapy for depression following stroke: a randomized controlled trial. Stroke. 2003; 34(1):111–5.
62. Lokk J, Delbari A. Management of depression in elderly stroke patients. Neuropsychiatr Dis Treat. 2010;6:539–49.
63. National Center for Health S: Health, United States. Health, United States, 2013: with special feature on prescription drugs. Hyattsville (MD): National Center for Health Statistics (US); 2014.
64. Pratt LA, Brody DJ, Gu Q. Antidepressant use in persons aged 12 and over: United States, 2005-2008. NCHS data brief. 2011;76:1–8.
65. Ried LD, Tueth MJ, Jia H. A pilot study to describe antidepressant prescriptions dispensed to veterans after stroke. Research in social & administrative pharmacy : RSAP. 2006;2(1):96–109.
66. Paasche-Orlow MK, Parker RM, Gazmararian JA, Nielsen-Bohlman LT, Rudd RR. The prevalence of limited health literacy. J Gen Intern Med. 2005;20(2): 175–84.
67. Institute of Medicine Committee on Health L. In: Nielsen-Bohlman L, Panzer AM, Kindig DA, editors. Health literacy: a prescription to end confusion. Washington (DC): National Academies Press (US) Copyright 2004 by the National Academy of Sciences. All rights reserved; 2004.
68. Dewalt DA, Berkman ND, Sheridan S, Lohr KN, Pignone MP. Literacy and health outcomes: a systematic review of the literature. J Gen Intern Med. 2004;19(12):1228–39.
69. Santiago CD, Kaltman S, Miranda J. Poverty and mental health: how do low-income adults and children fare in psychotherapy? J Clin Psychol. 2013; 69(2):115–26.
70. Olfson M, Marcus SC, Tedeschi M, Wan GJ. Continuity of antidepressant treatment for adults with depression in the United States. Am J Psychiatry. 2006;163(1):101–8.
71. Mikami K, Jorge RE, Adams HP Jr, Davis PH, Leira EC, Jang M, Robinson RG. Effect of antidepressants on the course of disability following stroke. Am J Geriatr Psychiatry. 2011;19(12):1007–15.
72. Rost K, Nutting P, Smith J, Coyne JC, Cooper-Patrick L, Rubenstein L. The role of competing demands in the treatment provided primary care patients with major depression. Arch Fam Med. 2000;9(2):150–4.
73. Richardson K, Bennett K, Kenny RA. Polypharmacy including falls risk-increasing medications and subsequent falls in community-dwelling middle-aged and older adults. Age Ageing. 2015;44(1):90–6.
74. Spina E, Santoro V, D'Arrigo C. Clinically relevant pharmacokinetic drug interactions with second-generation antidepressants: an update. Clin Ther. 2008;30(7):1206–27.
75. Greenblatt DJ, von Moltke LL, Harmatz JS, Shader RI. Drug interactions with newer antidepressants: role of human cytochromes P450. The Journal of clinical psychiatry. 1998;59(Suppl 15):19–27.
76. Luppino FS, de Wit LM, Bouvy PF, Stijnen T, Cuijpers P, Penninx BW, Zitman FG. Overweight, obesity, and depression: a systematic review and meta-analysis of longitudinal studies. Arch Gen Psychiatry. 2010;67(3):220–9.
77. Raeder MB, Bjelland I, Emil Vollset S, Steen VM. Obesity, dyslipidemia, and diabetes with selective serotonin reuptake inhibitors: the Hordaland health study. The Journal of clinical psychiatry. 2006;67(12):1974–82.
78. Pratt LA, Brody DJ. Depression and smoking in the U.S. household population aged 20 and over. NCHS data brief. 2005-2008;2010(34):1–8.
79. Hughes JR, Stead LF, Hartmann-Boyce J, Cahill K, Lancaster T. Antidepressants for smoking cessation. The Cochrane database of systematic reviews. 2014;1:CD000031.
80. Rost K, Fortney J, Fischer E, Smith J. Use, quality, and outcomes of care for mental health: the rural perspective. Medical care research and review : MCRR. 2002;59(3):231–65. discussion 266-271
81. Ziller EC, Anderson NJ, Coburn AF. Access to rural mental health services: service use and out-of-pocket costs. The Journal of rural health : official journal of the American Rural Health Association and the National Rural Health Care Association. 2010;26(3):214–24.
82. The Darthmouth Atlas of Medicare Prescription Drug Use. A report of the Darthmouth Atlas Project. http://www.dartmouthatlas.org/downloads/reports/Prescription_Drug_Atlas_101513.pdf. Accessed 14 July 2017.

6

Social differences in diagnosed depression among adolescents in a Swedish population based cohort

Therese Wirback[1*], Jette Möller[1], Jan-Olov Larsson[2] and Karin Engström[1]

Abstract

Background: Population based research regarding social differences in diagnosed depression in adolescence is sparse. In this study unique material containing in-and outpatient data was used to determine if low social position in childhood increases the risk of diagnosed depression in adolescence. To further examine this association, gender differences and interactions were explored.

Methods: The study population was extracted from the Stockholm Youth Cohort (SYC), a register based cohort containing psychiatric care for all young people in Stockholm County and information about social position. For the purpose of this study, all in the SYC who turned 13 years old during 2001–2007, in total 169,262 adolescents, were followed up in 2005–2011 for diagnoses of depression until age 18. Associations were estimated with Cox regression models and presented as Hazard Ratios (HR).

Results: The risk of diagnosed depression was higher for adolescents with parents with low education (HR = 1.1, CI = 1.0–1.2) and medium education (HR = 1.1, CI = 1.1–1.2) compared to high as well as for those with lower household income (for example, medium low, HR = 1.2, CI = 1.1–1.3) and for those with parents who received an unemployment benefit (HR = 1.3, CI = 1.2–1.4). No differences were found for those with the lowest household income compared to those with the highest level. Adolescents with parents born outside the Nordic countries had a lower risk of diagnosed depression (HR = 0.7, CI = 0.6–0.7). An interaction effect was found between gender and parental education.

Conclusions: Social differences were found but the magnitude was modest and gender differences small.

Keywords: Socioeconomic status, Cohort study, Depression, Adolescence, Gender

Background

Depression is a leading cause of years lived with disabilities (YLDs) [1, 2] and often originates early in life [3, 4]. The prevalence of adolescents treated for depression in Sweden has increased during the past two decades, and is more common among females [5]. Much research points at higher risks of poor mental health among adolescents with low social position [e.g. 6–18], though some studies found no association [19, 20]. There are likely several mechanisms behind social differences, including differential exposure to determinants of depression [21, 22] as well as negative psychosocial factors which can cluster in persons with low social position. How people describe depressive symptoms and where people seek care can further vary depending on for example academic background [23, 24]. Moreover, children of parents with depression can be at a higher risk for depression [25] both because of social and genetic influence. Overall, the results of studies investigating social differences in depression are hard to summarize due to methodological differences such as the measures used to assess depression as well as social position [7, 9, 11, 14, 15, 17–20, 26, 27]. So far most studies on social position and poor mental health in adolescence have been based on psychiatric disorders overall [14, 16, 28, 29], poor mental health overall [6, 8, 10, 12, 13, 16, 30, 31], or self-reported depressive symptoms [7, 9, 11, 15–17, 19, 26,

* Correspondence: therese.wirback@ki.se
[1]Department of Public Health Sciences, Karolinska Institutet, Solnavägen 1E, 113 65 Stockholm, Sweden

32]. Only a few studies focus on diagnosed depression or mood disorders specifically [18, 20, 27, 33]. McLaughlin et al. [18] show in their study from the United States that financial hardship in childhood increases the risk of diagnosed mood disorders in adolescence, but low parental education and lower status occupation do not. A Finish study with a focus on late adolescence reports that both low parental income and education increase the risk of depression, but education to a lesser extent [27]. Two less recent studies, one from New Zealand and one from the United States, found no increased risk of depression [20] or mood disorders [33] among groups with low socioeconomic status. Gender-specific risks in relation to social position and mental health problems show inconclusive results [16]. Some studies indicate that girls are more vulnerable [17, 30, 34] whereas others point to boys' vulnerabilities [10, 31, 32], and some report no gender differences [6, 11, 15]. Only one study looked at gender differences in relation to social position and diagnosed depression [27], and they found merely small differences.

To add to the limited knowledge of social differences in diagnosed depression among adolescents - in a setting where free mental health services are available - this Swedish population based cohort study was performed. It will also increase knowledge on whether boys and girls are equally affected. Registers with several measures of social position and with diagnoses set by professionals within clinical settings was used. The aim was to determine if low social position in childhood increases the risk of diagnosed depression in adolescence (13–17 year olds), and if there are gender-specific differences.

Methods

Setting and material

The material derives from Sweden, a country with a relatively strong redistributive system with mental health services for adolescents primarily financed by tax. The public Child and Adolescent Mental Health Service (CAMHS; In Swedish, BUP) is free of charge for the patient. Children and adolescents can be referred to CAMHS from primary care, seek care directly themselves or via their parents. Primary care with public general practitioners, counsellors and therapists, internet-based psychiatric help and psychiatric emergency units (free for children and adolescents) is also available, as well as private therapists (high fee but mainly targeting adults).

This study is based on The Stockholm Youth Cohort (SYC), a register-based cohort containing information of psychiatric care of children and adolescents in Stockholm County Council (SLL) as well as several measures of social position. SYC includes all individuals aged 0–17 residing in Stockholm County at any point in time during 2001 and 2011, ascertained from the Swedish register of the total population [35]. The SYC is built up with linkage to several different health care and administrative registers by the personal identification number for each individual (recoded for research use). The SYC database is held by the Department of Public Health Sciences at Karolinska Institute. The registers used for the current study were: CAMHS, which includes public psychiatric in-and out-patient care in Stockholm County; The Cause of Death Register [36] with dates and causes of death, according to ICD (International Classification of Disease), for Swedish residents; The National Patient Register which initially included all patients treated in psychiatric care and some somatic care at public hospitals, but now includes information about all public in-patient care (from 1984) and out-patient visits to specialized clinics at hospital (from 2001) in Sweden [37], but not primary care; health care registers in SLL (VAL, Swedish acronym) that include in- and outpatient care for residents in Stockholm County, including public and private outpatient care clinics and primary care facilities as well as hospitals for public and private inpatient care, financed by SLL but not private specialists [38]; The Longitudinal Integration Database for Health Insurance and Labour Market Studies (LISA, Swedish acronym) [35], with information about employment, education, income and social benefits for those over 16 years old residing in Sweden; The Multi-generation Register which is part of the Total Population Register and includes connections between index persons and their parents [39].

Study population and design

The study population was extracted from SYC and is defined as adolescents who were residing in Stockholm County the year they turned 13, between 2001 and 2007, i.e. 7 consecutive birth cohorts (born 1988–1994). A total of 169,262 adolescents were followed for 5 years, until they turned 18, in 2005–2011. A closed cohort design was employed. Individuals were censored at whatever occurred first: time of first depression diagnosis, death, moving out of Stockholm County or end of follow up at age of 18. Age was restricted to 18 as individuals in the Swedish health care system are then considered adults and shall seek care at mental health services for adults.

Exposure and outcome

Social position

Parental education and household disposable income was used to assess childhood social position. To capture additional aspects of social position, parental receipt of an unemployment benefit and parental country of origin were assessed. Parents were defined as social parents, i.e. persons that the child lives with, including biological parents, adoptive parents and other adults responsible for the child. *Parental education* was assessed according to the Swedish standard for classification of individual educational programs [40] and was categorized in three groups; low (pre-secondary), medium (upper secondary), and high (post-secondary) based on the parent with the highest education. *Household disposable income* [35] is an individualized weighted average income, i.e. the sum of the family members' disposable income multiplied by the individual consumption weights and divided by their aggregate consumption weight. It was categorized according to the distribution within the study population in quintiles; low, medium-low, medium, medium-high and high. *Receipt of an unemployment benefit* was defined and categorised as, two, or the single parent receiving it once or several times, or not. *Parental country of birth* was categorised into born in Sweden, born in the Nordic countries (but not in Sweden), or born outside the Nordic countries. Adolescents were classified as having non-Swedish parents if the lone or both parents were born outside of Sweden, where the parental country of birth geographically closest to Sweden was used in the categorization. Born in Sweden was the reference category. All measures of social position were assessed at age 12, the year before the start of follow up, and collected from LISA.

Depression

Depression was defined as a first time depression diagnoses registered at CAMHS or in VAL. Diagnoses are clinical and were not established specifically for the aim of this study. Depression was defined as to include major depressive disorder, unspecified depressive disorder and dysthymic disorder (DSM-IV: 296.20–24, 300.4, 296.30–36, 311 including the DSM-IV based diagnostic code 19 used at CAMHS; ICD-10: F32.0–9, F38.0–8, F39, F33.0–9, F34.8–9).

Confounding and mediation

Parental depression was considered a potential confounder since previous research have shown that children of parents with depression have a higher risk for depression [25], and a history of depression has been found to confound the relationship between SES (Socioeconomic Status) and major depression among adults [41]. Information regarding parental depression was collected from the National Patient Register and was taken into consideration if it occurred before the child turned 13. Parental depression was defined as occurring if a parent received a diagnosis in in-or outpatient care according to the following diagnoses from ICD 8, 9 and 10; F32.0–9, F33.0–9, F34.1,8,9, F38.0,1,8, F39, 300E, 296B, 311, 300, 296, 301.10, 302.99, 314.99. In the current study 4% had a mother or father with depression. Measures of social position and psychosocial factors, e.g. childhood adversities such as divorce, which are considered to occur within the causal pathway, were not adjusted for.

Statistical analysis

The Incidence Rate Ratio (IRR) and corresponding 95% confidence intervals (CI) of social position and first time onset of diagnosed depression were calculated using Cox regression models and are presented as Hazard Ratios (HR). Boys and girls were analysed jointly as well as separately to explore possible gender differences. Estimates were calculated for all measures of social position separately. Additionally, adjustments were included for parental depression, country of birth, and education. A test for fulfilment of the proportional hazards assumption was performed with a time dependent variable [42]. There was no indication of a violation of the assumption. Additive interactions were calculated by using the Synergy Index (SI) [43, 44]. SI calculations require dichotomized independent variables. For this purpose the following variables were dichotomized: parental education (low/medium vs. high), household income (low/medium low/medium vs. medium high/high) and parental country of birth (born in Sweden or not). To make use of as much information as possible in the respective analyses, individuals with missing information on respective exposure variable were excluded only for that particular analysis. A sensitivity analysis including complete cases showed no significant differences. All analyses were done using SAS version 9.3 and 9.4 (SAS Institute Inc. Cary, N.C., US.

Results

Most adolescents had parents with high education level and 9% had parents with a low level, which corresponds quite well with the national average [45]. Six percent had received an unemployment benefit and 19% had parents born outside the Nordic countries while 3% had parents born in Nordic countries. Characteristics of the adolescents are presented in Table 1.

During follow-up, 6439 adolescents, 1978 boys (2.3%) and 4461 girls (5.4%), were diagnosed with first time depression. The majority of the cases of depression were identified in the outpatient clinics. Of the adolescents with depression, 242 (3.7%) had been treated in in-patient care (0.14% of the total study population); 84 boys (4.2% of the depressed boys) and 158 girls (3.5% of the depressed girls). The mean age for diagnosis of first time depression was 15.36 for girls and 15.38 for boys. Depression was more common in later adolescence, especially for girls. The largest proportion received a diagnosis at the age of 17 (27%) and the smallest at age 13 (12%). Most adolescents with depression were

Table 1 Characteristics among the adolescents, with and without diagnosed depression, and by gender

	All (*n* = 169,262)		Boys (*n* = 86,888) 51.3%		Girls (*n* = 82,374) 48.7%	
	Depression (*n* = 6439)	No depression (*n* = 162,823)	Depression (*n* = 1978)	No depression (*n* = 84,910)	Depression (*n* = 4461)	No depression (*n* = 77,913)
	%		%		%	
Parental country of origin						
Sweden	67.2	63.4	66.6	63.2	67.4	63.6
Nordic	3.3	2.9	2.8	3.0	3.5	2.8
Outside Nordic	13.2	19.7	14.7	19.7	12.6	19.7
Missing	16.3	14.1	15.9	14.2	16.5	14.0
Parental education						
High	44.9	47.7	46.3	47.8	44.3	47.6
Medium	44.2	41.0	43.4	41.0	44.5	41.0
Low	9.2	9.4	8.3	9.3	9.6	9.4
Missing	1.7	2.0	2.0	2.0	1.6	2.0
Disposable household income						
High	16.2	18.2	15.1	18.2	16.7	18.3
Medium high	20.2	19.7	21.2	19.7	19.7	19.7
Medium	22.5	20.0	23.8	20.0	21.9	20.0
Medium low	22.4	20.4	21.8	20.5	22.7	20.4
Low	17.5	20.4	16.7	20.4	17.8	20.5
Missing	1.3	1.3	1.3	1.3	1.2	1.3
Parental receipt of an unemployment benefit						
Not received	86.3	86.1	85.1	86.1	86.8	86.0
Received	6.7	5.3	7.5	5.4	6.4	5.3
Missing	7.0	8.6	7.4	8.6	6.8	8.7

diagnosed with the CHAMS code 19 (69.4%), followed by major depressive disorder (23.4%), unspecified depressive disorder (6%) and dysthymic disorder (1.2%).

Childhood social position and risk of diagnosed depression in adolescence

Crude and adjusted HRs are shown in Tables 2 and 3. The risk of depression diagnosis was slightly higher for adolescents with parents of a low and medium education compared to high (HR = 1.1). Increased risks were found for adolescents with medium-low (HR = 1.2), medium (HR = 1.3), and medium-high household income (HR = 1.2) when compared to those with the highest. No increased risk was found for those with the lowest income compared to high. Having parents who received an unemployment benefit was associated with a higher risk of diagnosed depression (HR = 1.3). Adolescents with parents born outside the Nordic countries had a lower risk of diagnosed depression (HR = 0.7), whereas those with parents born in the Nordic countries had a marginally increased risk (HR = 1.1) compared to those with Swedish-born parents. The effect estimates remained or decreased marginally when adjusted for parental depression. Results with adjustments for parental depression are therefore only shown in the first model. Overall, the effect estimates increased slightly when adjusting for parental country of origin and education.

Gender differences

Girls had a more than twofold increased risk of diagnosed depression compared to boys (HR = 2.4, CI = 2.3–2.6). Gender stratified associations between social position and diagnosed depression showed minor differences. Risk estimates were slightly higher for boys with a lower household income and parental receipt of an unemployment benefit, and for girls with higher parental education; however with overlapping CIs. See Table 3.

Additive interaction effects of gender and different measures of social position are shown in Table 4. Being a girl and having low educated parents had a synergistic effect of 1.2 (CI = 1.0–1.4).

Discussion

The findings from this population based cohort study from Sweden expand upon and handle some methodological shortcomings of previous research. In the current

Table 2 Crude and adjusted Hazard Ratios (HR) of diagnosed depression in adolescence, by social position, $n = 169{,}262$

Social factors	Crude HR (95% CI)	Adjusted for biological parents depression HR (95% CI)	Adjusted for parental country of origin HR (95% CI)	Adjusted for parental country of origin and education HR (95% CI)
Sex				
Boy	1.0			
Girl	2.4 (2.3–2.6)			
Parental country of origin				
Sweden (ref.)	1.0			
Nordic	1.1 (1.0–1.3)			
Outside Nordic	0.7 (0.6–0.7)			
Parental education				
High (ref.)	1.0	1.0	1.0	
Medium	1.1 (1.1–1.2)	1.1 (1.1–1.2)	1.2 (1.1–1.3)	
Low	1.1 (1.0–1.2)	1.0 (0.9–1.1)	1.2 (1.1–1.4)	
Disposable Household income				
High (ref.)	1.0	1.0	1.0	1.0
Medium high	1.2 (1.1–1.2)	1.1 (1.1–1.2)	1.2 (1.1–1.3)	1.2 (1.1–1.3)
Medium	1.3 (1.2–1.4)	1.3 (1.2–1.4)	1.3 (1.2–1.5)	1.3 (1.2–1.4)
Medium low	1.2 (1.1–1.3)	1.2 (1.1–1.3)	1.4 (1.2–1.5)	1.3 (1.2–1.4)
Low	1.0 (0.9–1.1)	1.0 (0.9–1.1)	1.2 (1.0–1.3)	1.1 (1.0–1.2)
Parental receipt of an unemployment benefit				
Not received (ref)	1.0	1.0	1.0	1.0
Received	1.3 (1.2–1.4)	1.2 (1.1–1.4)	1.4 (1.3–1.6)	1.4 (1.2–1.5)

study it was shown that 3.8% of 13–17 year old adolescents received a diagnosis of depression during a follow-up period of 5 years. The risk of diagnosed depression was higher for adolescents with parents who hold a medium education level, have a lower household income, received an unemployment benefit or were born in the Nordic countries. The social differences were however modest and not found for adolescents with the lowest household income. In addition, adolescents with parents born outside the Nordic countries had a lower risk of diagnosis. No prominent gender differences were found.

The increased risk of diagnosed depression for adolescents with a lower household income or with parents with a lower level of education, found in the current study, is in line with results from recent research from Finland and the US. In comparison however, the current study found smaller differences over all, and no increased risk for those with the very lowest income. The latter contrasts the Finnish study, and an increased risk for those in the group with the lowest income was also found in another Finnish study, where self-reported depressive symptoms were studied [46]. This indicates possible national differences, despite the fact that Finland has a welfare state similar to Sweden. Larger social differences, related to education, have also been noted in another study from Sweden, where self-reports of depressive symptoms were studied [17], which could indicate that groups with low social position seek care to a lower extent. The increased risk of depression for adolescents with parents who received an unemployment benefit are also in line with previous studies [17, 47, 48]. McLaughlin et al. [18] suggests that material deprivation such as financial hardship has a stronger association than relative status, as indicated by education for example, which is supported by the results from the current study as social differences related to low income and receipt of unemployment benefit were more prominent than social differences related to education.

One issue that can explain modest social differences in adolescence, as seen in this study, is the theory of social equalization in adolescence. The theory implies that adolescence is the life period when social differences are expected to be the smallest [13, 49]. Adolescence is a period when youths interact a lot with friends and thereby start to develop their own social position, whereas the social position of younger children depends more on their parents' social position. Differences in the magnitude of social inequalities between different studies cannot be fully explained by this. The Swedish context, with relatively low social differences overall, in combination with a possible social equalization in

Table 3 Gender stratified Hazard Ratios (HR) of diagnosed depression in adolescence, by social position, $n = 169{,}262$

Social factors	Crude HR (95% CI)		Adjusted for parents country of origin HR (95% CI)		Adjusted for parents country of origin and education HR (95% CI)	
	Boys	Girls	Boys	Girls	Boys	Girls
Parental country of origin						
Sweden (ref.)	1.0	1.0				
Nordic	0.9 (0.7–1.2)	1.2 (1.0–1.4)				
Outside Nordic	0.7 (0.6–0.8)	0.6 (0.6–0.7)				
Parental education						
High (ref.)	1.0	1.0	1.0	1.0		
Medium	1.1 (1.0–1.2)	1.2 (1.1–1.2)	1.2 (1.0–1.3)	1.2 (1.1–1.3)		
Low	0.9 (0.8–1.1)	1.1 (1.0–1.2)	1.1 (0.9–1.3)	1.3 (1.2–1.5)		
Disposable household income						
High (ref.)	1.0	1.0	1.0	1.0	1.0	1.0
Medium high	1.3 (1.1–1.5)	1.1 (1.0–1.2)	1.4 (1.2–1.6)	1.1 (1.0–1.3)	1.4 (1.2–1.6)	1.1 (1.0–1.2)
Medium	1.4 (1.2–1.7)	1.2 (1.1–1.3)	1.5 (1.3–1.8)	1.3 (1.1–1.4)	1.5 (1.3–1.8)	1.2 (1.1–1.3)
Medium low	1.3 (1.1–1.5)	1.2 (1.1–1.3)	1.5 (1.2–1.7)	1.3 (1.2–1.5)	1.4 (1.2–1.6)	1.3 (1.1–1.4)
Low	1.0 (0.9–1.2)	1.0 (0.9–1.1)	1.2 (1.0–1.4)	1.2 (1.0–1.3)	1.1 (0.9–1.3)	1.1 (1.0–1.2)
Parental receipt of an unemployment benefit						
Not received (ref)	1.0	1.0	1.0	1.0	1.0	1.0
Received	1.4 (1.2–1.7)	1.2 (1.1–1.4)	1.5 (1.3–1.8)	1.4 (1.2–1.6)	1.5 (1.2–1.8)	1.3 (1.2–1.5)

adolescence, can however add to the explanation as to why a smaller magnitude of social differences were found in the current study. The widespread, and free access to mental health services can further add to the explanation. In addition, it has been shown that the influence of equalization in adolescence can depend on the specific health outcome as well as the measure used for social position [50, 51].

The protective effect of having parents born outside the Nordic countries contrasts earlier findings from a similar population in Sweden, focusing on self-reported depressive symptoms, where no differences between foreign-born and Swedish-born were detected [17, 52]. This indicates that adolescents with parents born outside the Nordic countries may seek care to a lower extent. A previous Swedish study reports that adolescents with parents born in in middle or low-income countries use psychiatric care to a lesser extent than native-born Swedes [53]. Possible explanations can include problems in accessing mental health services or lower health literacy; both in comparison with those whose parents are born in Sweden and in the Nordic countries since Nordic nations have more similar health systems and traditions. Differences can also be related to how depression is expressed and articulated in different cultures [54]. More work is needed to elucidate social differences in care-seeking for depressive symptoms, especially for foreign-born.

As expected, and in line with previous research, both on self-reported depressive symptoms [12, 17, 55] and diagnosed depression [27, 33], girls had an increased risk compared to boys. That girls suffer more from depression can partly depend on the diagnostic criteria or that expressions of depressive symptoms differ between boys

Table 4 Hazard Ratios (HR) and Synergy Index (SI) between gender and social position in diagnosed depression, $n = 169{,}262$

Social factors	Male (95% CI)		Female (95% CI)		Synergy Index (SI) (95% CI)
	Unexposed to social factor	Exposed to social factor	Unexposed to social factor	Exposed to social factor	
Parental education[a] High vs. low/medium	1.0	1.1 (1.0–1.2)	2.3 (2.0–2.6)	2.7 (2.5–3.0)	1.2 (1.0–1.4)
Disposable household income[b] High vs. low	1.0	1.0 (0.9–1.1)	2.3 (2.2–2.5)	2.5 (2.3–2.7)	1.1 (0.9–1.3)
Parental receipt of an unemployment benefit[b] Received vs. not received	1.0	1.4 (1.2–1.7)	2.3 (2.2–2.5)	3.1 (2.7–3.5)	1.2 (0.9–1.5)

[a]Adjusted for parental country of origin
[b]Adjusted for parental country of origin and education

and girls [56]. Boys can for example have succumbed to traditional norms of masculinity and not express their symptoms [57]. Regarding the gender-specific risks in relation to social position, the current study support to some extent the findings from studies that did not detect gender differences [6, 11, 15]. Muntaner [58] mention that different SES indicators can perform inconsistently for men and women, and even though only small gender differences were found in the current study there was some indication of inconsistency depending on the SES indicator. In the current study girls living with low educated parents were found to be somewhat more vulnerable for depression, which parallels the findings from one of the research group's previous studies [17] on depressive symptoms. There are contradictory theoretical models to explain an elevated risk of depression depending on social position, for boys and girls respectively. It has been suggested that low parental education is a more powerful risk factor for depression among boys than girls [59]. Girls may not be affected as much as boys by the added vulnerability of low parental education because they are already so vulnerable to depression. However our results support the theoretical model proposed by Cyranowski et al. [60], which proposes that girls are more vulnerable to depression due to the combination of a more affiliative style in social relations and transition difficulties, which are triggered by negative life events. Further, social position can have different meanings and effects on mental health depending on for example the context and ethnicity [61, 62], which highlights the importance of studies from different countries.

A complex picture of the association between social position and depression is revealed, and it reminds us that the indicators used to define social differences describe different dimensions of social position [63]. Income translates into material and immaterial resources and fluctuates to some extent, whereas education is more stable and relates to, for example, health literacy. These different dimensions are considered to be interconnected, and the cause and effect chain depends on what is being studied [63]. Miech et al. [20] has furthermore concluded that different mental disorders are differently related to social position, which points to the importance of research with measures of specific mental disorders and not overall measures of poor mental health.

There are likely several mechanisms behind the social differences, which are not explored in the current study. There are many different determinants for depression, such as negative social circumstances including low social support and poverty [21, 22], and serious conflict during upbringing [64]. Differential exposure to these determinants can cause inequalities. One additional explanation is that of susceptibility, meaning that some social groups are more vulnerable. Long lasting stress is one factor that can contribute to depression [65] but the same amount of stress can affect people differently. Higher SES groups may have better opportunities for social support and know where to turn for help in handling stress. Furthermore, negative psychosocial factors can cluster in persons with low social position and etiological mechanisms can differ depending on at what age depression is present. For example, juvenile onset depression is more affected by adverse childhood factors than adult onset depression [66].

Strengths and limitations

The possibility to use register-based material, encompassing a large population-based sample of adolescents with both in- and outpatient data, is a great strength of the current study. Including both in- and outpatient data has been found to be important to calculate reliable rates of mental diseases [67]. Population characteristics and the distribution of care utilities are similar to other big cities of Sweden and thus it is possible to generalize to those, as well as to other populations within a similar context. The cohort design allowed an etiological focus and the clinical assessment of diagnoses within CAMHS offered a naturalistic design. Furthermore the diagnostic procedures at CAMHS are based on professional assessment and not on structured instruments to measure depressive symptoms. The use of register-based material decreased problems with self-reported data such as recall bias. Swedish official registers have overall a high standard and are useful for research purposes [68]. Concerning depression, a validation study in Sweden among adults showed 88% agreement when depression diagnosis from out-patient care was compared to a clinical diagnosis from court-ordered inpatient evaluations [69].

One important limitation of this study is possible misclassification of the outcome, where some adolescents who fulfil the criteria of depression are classified as not having a depression. This can be due to that adolescents with depression often do not seek care [70], reluctance by care givers to diagnose children [71], as well as the possibility of misdiagnosis. The incidence presented may therefore underestimate the true levels of depression in the population. Potential social differences in care-seeking introduce further bias [9] though the direction of the bias is not clear. Finnish studies [14, 72] suggest that children of parents with higher socioeconomic position may have better access to care. Differences in care seeking can also apply to gender and ethnic background, where boys in later adolescence and those with parents from ethnic minorities are less likely to seek care [73]. This would result in an underestimation of the risk for those groups in the current study. On the other hand

some care in the private sector was not included in the current analyses, and if those with higher social position to a higher extent seek private care this would lead to an overestimation of the results.

Another possible, but less severe, limitation is misclassification of exposure due to the procedures for registering housing. Children can only be registered at one address, thus only one social context is considered for those with alternate living arrangements. Furthermore, in the current study the second parent was excluded if he or she was not a biological/adoptive parent, since information for those was differential due to housing conditions, which in turn can be related to social position. This misclassification is not likely to be large but can classify adolescents to a lower social position than they should be, and thus may lead to an underestimation of the associations.

A history of own major depression has been found to confound the relationship between SES and major depression among adults [41] but parental depression only marginally affected the results in the current study, which is in line with findings from Modin et al. [74]. Other measures of poor parental mental health could have been used as also other mental disorders can have an impact on SES and offspring depression. One additional measure of parents' mental disease, defined as any mental disorder severe enough for in-patient care, was tested in the current study. Including this as a confounder changed the estimates marginally compared to adjusting for depression. Childhood adversities and psychosocial factors were considered mediators in the current study as they are within the causal pathway between social position and depression. Patterson et al. [75] imply for example that adversities in youth increase the risk of depression more than family history of parental mental disease do, and that the adversity is more related to SES.

Implications

The social differences detected in the current study were modest, and still more work needs to be done to reduce social differences. This is especially important considering that a great number of people are affected by depression, and to a higher extent in groups with lower social position. Disentangling the role of social position in care-seeking can further guide the direction of future research, access to care and mental health promotion.

Conclusion

Social differences in diagnosed depression were found for adolescents in Sweden. The differences were modest and gender differences negligible.

Acknowledgements

Special thanks to Fredrik Mattsson at FM Statistikkonsult for his assistance with data management.

Funding

This study was supported by grants from the Swedish Research Council for Health, Working Life and Welfare (FORTE).

Authors' contributions

TW participated in the design of the study, performed the statistical analyses, interpreted the results and drafted the manuscript. JM participated in the design of the study, interpretation of the results and reviewed the manuscript. J-O L contributed with expertise in psychiatrics and reviewed the manuscript. KE participated in the design of the study, interpretation of the results, supported in drafting the manuscript and reviewed the manuscript. All authors read and approved the final manuscript.

Competing interests

The authors declare that they have no competing interests.

Author details

[1]Department of Public Health Sciences, Karolinska Institutet, Solnavägen 1E, 113 65 Stockholm, Sweden. [2]Department of Women's and Children's Health, Karolinska Institutet, Tomtebodavägen 18A, 171 77 Stockholm, Sweden.

References

1. Vos T, Flaxman AD, Naghavi M, Lozano R, Michaud C, Ezzati M, Shibuya K, Salomon JA, Abdalla S, Aboyans V, et al. Years lived with disability (YLDs) for 1160 sequelae of 289 diseases and injuries 1990-2010: a systematic analysis for the global burden of disease study 2010. Lancet. 2012;380(9859):2163–96.
2. Gore FM, Bloem PJN, Patton GC. Global burden of disease in young people aged 10-24 years: a systematic analysis. Lancet. 2011;378(9790):486.
3. Fryers T, Brugha T. Childhood determinants of adult psychiatric disorder. Clin Pract Epidemiol : CP & EMH. 2013;9:1–50.
4. Gilman SE, Kawachi I, Fitzmaurice GM, Buka SL. Socioeconomic status in childhood and the lifetime risk of major depression. Int J Epidemiol. 2002; 31(2):359–67.
5. National Board of Health and Welfare. Public Health Report 2009. Stockholm: National Board of Health and Welfare; 2009.
6. Amone-P'Olak K, Burger H, Ormel J, Huisman M, Verhulst FC, Oldehinkel AJ. Socioeconomic position and mental health problems in pre- and early-adolescents: the TRAILS study. Soc Psychiatry Psychiatr Epidemiol. 2009; 44(3):231–8.
7. Lemstra M, Neudorf C, D'Arcy C, Kunst A, Warren LM, Bennett NR. A systematic review of depressed mood and anxiety by SES in youth aged 10-15 years. Can J Public Health Revue canadienne de sante publique. 2008;99(2):125–9.
8. Rajmil L, Herdman M, Ravens-Sieberer U, Erhart M, Alonso J. Socioeconomic inequalities in mental health and health-related quality of life (HRQOL) in children and adolescents from 11 European countries. Int J Public Health. 2013;59(1):95-105
9. Goodman E, Huang B. Socioeconomic status, depression, and health service utilization among adolescent women. Women's Health Issues. 2001;11(5): 416–26.
10. Huisman M, Araya R, Lawlor DA, Ormel J, Verhulst FC, Oldehinkel AJ. Cognitive ability, parental socioeconomic position and internalising and externalising problems in adolescence: findings from two European cohort studies. Eur J Epidemiol. 2010;25(8):569–80.
11. Jackson B, Goodman E. Low social status markers: do they predict depressive symptoms in adolescence? Race Soc Probl. 2011;3(2):119–28.

12. Piko B, Fitzpatrick KM. Does class matter? SES and psychosocial health among Hungarian adolescents. Soc Sci Med. 2001;53(6):817–30.
13. Sonego M, Llacer A, Galan I, Simon F. The influence of parental education on child mental health in Spain. Qual Life Res. 2013;22(1):203–11.
14. Paananen R, Ristikari T, Merikukka M, Gissler M. Social determinants of mental health: a Finnish nationwide follow-up study on mental disorders. J Epidemiol Community Health. 2013;67(12):1025–31.
15. Aslund C, Leppert J, Starrin B, Nilsson KW. Subjective social status and shaming experiences in relation to adolescent depression. Arch Pediatr Adolesc Med. 2009;163(1):55–60.
16. Reiss F. Socioeconomic inequalities and mental health problems in children and adolescents: a systematic review. Soc Sci Med. 2013;90(0): 24–31.
17. Wirback T, Moller J, Larsson JO, Galanti MR, Engstrom K. Social factors in childhood and risk of depressive symptoms among adolescents - a longitudinal study in Stockholm, Sweden. Int J Equity Health. 2014;13 https://doi.org/10.1186/s12939-014-0096-0.
18. McLaughlin KA, Breslau J, Green JG, Lakoma MD, Sampson NA, Zaslavsky AM, Kessler RC. Childhood socio-economic status and the onset, persistence, and severity of DSM-IV mental disorders in a US national sample. Soc Sci Med. 2011;73(7):1088–96.
19. Twenge JM, Nolen-Hoeksema S. Age, gender, race, socioeconomic status, and birth cohort differences on the children's depression inventory: a meta-analysis. J Abnorm Psychol. 2002;111(4):578–88.
20. Miech RA, Caspi A, Moffitt TE, Wright BRE, Silva PA. Low socioeconomic status and mental disorders: a longitudinal study of selection and causation during young adulthood. Am J Sociol. 1999;104(4):1096–131.
21. Molarius A, Berglund K, Eriksson C, Eriksson HG, Linden-Bostrom M, Nordstrom E, Persson C, Sahlqvist L, Starrin B, Ydreborg B. Mental health symptoms in relation to socio-economic conditions and lifestyle factors–a population-based study in Sweden. BMC Public Health. 2009;9:302.
22. Ostberg V, Lennartsson C. Getting by with a little help: the importance of various types of social support for health problems. Scand J Public Health. 2007;35(2):197–204.
23. Danielsson U. Träffad av blixten eller långsam kvävning: genuskodade uttryck för depression i en primärvårdskontext. Umeå: Umeå university; 2010.
24. Wallerblad A, Moller J, Forsell Y. Care-seeking pattern among persons with depression and anxiety: a population-based study in Sweden. Int J Fam Med. 2012;2012:895425.
25. Beardslee WR, Keller MB, Lavori PW, Staley J, Sacks N. The impact of parental affective disorder on depression in offspring: a longitudinal follow-up in a nonreferred sample. J Am Acad Child Adolesc Psychiatry. 1993;32(4):723–30.
26. Joinson C, Kounali D, Lewis G. Family socioeconomic position in early life and onset of depressive symptoms and depression: a prospective cohort study. Soc Psychiatry Psychiatr Epidemiol. 2017;52(1):95–103.
27. Korhonen K, Remes H, Martikainen P. Education as a social pathway from parental socioeconomic position to depression in late adolescence and early adulthood: a Finnish population-based register study. Soc Psychiatry Psychiatr Epidemiol. 2017;52(1):105–16.
28. Spady DW, Schopflocher DP, Svenson LW, Thompson AH. Prevalence of mental disorders in children living in Alberta, Canada, as determined from physician billing data. Arch Pediatr & Adolesc Med. 2001;155(10):1153–9.
29. Tonge BJ, Hughes GC, Pullen JM, Beaufoy J, Gold S. Comprehensive description of adolescents admitted to a public psychiatric inpatient unit and their families. Aust N Z J Psychiatry. 2008;42(7):627–35.
30. Leve LD, Kim HK, Pears KC. Childhood temperament and family environment as predictors of internalizing and externalizing trajectories from ages 5 to 17. J Abnorm Child Psychol. 2005;33(5):505–20.
31. Due P, Lynch J, Holstein B, Modvig J. Socioeconomic health inequalities among a nationally representative sample of Danish adolescents: the role of different types of social relations. J Epidemiol Community Health. 2003;57(9): 692–8.
32. Frojd S, Marttunen M, Pelkonen M, von der Pahlen B, Kaltiala-Heino R. Perceived financial difficulties and maladjustment outcomes in adolescence. Eur J Pub Health. 2006;16(5):542–8.
33. Roberts RE, Roberts CR, Xing Y. Rates of DSM-IV psychiatric disorders among adolescents in a large metropolitan area. J Psychiatr Res. 2007;41(11):959–67.
34. Mendelson T, Kubzansky LD, Datta GD, Buka SL. Relation of female gender and low socioeconomic status to internalizing symptoms among adolescents: a case of double jeopardy? Soc Sci Med. 2008;66(6):1284–96.
35. Statistics Sweden. Background facts, labour and education statistics 2011: 4. Stockholm: Integrated database for labour market research; 2011.
36. The National Board of Health and Welfare. 2016. Available from: http://www.socialstyrelsen.se/register/dodsorsaksregistret [cited 2016 March 8].
37. The National Board of Health and Welfare. 2016. Available from: http://www.socialstyrelsen.se/register/halsodataregister/patientregistret/inenglish [cited 2016 March 8].
38. Stockholm County Council. VAL databaserna - datalager för uppföljning av vårdhändelser i SLL. Stockholm läns landsting: Stockholm; 2014.
39. Statistics Sweden: Background Facts, Population and Welfare Statistics 2011:2, Multi-generation register 2010. A description of contents and quality 2011.
40. Statistics Sweden: SUN. Swedish standard for classification of individual educational programs 2000.
41. Wang JL, Schmitz N, Dewa CS. Socioeconomic status and the risk of major depression: the Canadian National Population Health Survey. J Epidemiol Community Health. 2010;64(5):447–52.
42. Paul A. Survival analysis using SAS: a practical guide; second edition [electronic resource]: North Carolina: SAS Institute; 2010.
43. Lundberg M, Fredlund P, Hallqvist J, Diderichsen F. A SAS program calculating three measures of interaction with confidence intervals. Epidemiol. 1996;7(6):655–6.
44. Rothman KJ. In: GS RKJ, Lash TL, editors. Modern epidemiology. 3rd ed. Philadelphia: Lippincott Williams & Wilkins; 2008.
45. Finding statistics. Population statistics http://www.statistikdatabasen.scb.se/pxweb/sv/ssd/START__UF__UF0506/Utbildning/?rxid=1f210474-5ffe-452d-b3f9-cd9d0499962f [cited 2017 November 7].
46. Elovainio M, Pulkki-Raback L, Jokela M, Kivimaki M, Hintsanen M, Hintsa T, Viikari J, Raitakari OT, Keltikangas-Jarvinen L. Socioeconomic status and the development of depressive symptoms from childhood to adulthood: a longitudinal analysis across 27 years of follow-up in the young Finns study. Soc Sci Med. 2012;74(6):923–9.
47. Kaltiala-Heino R, Rimpela M, Rantanen P, Laippala P. Adolescent depression: the role of discontinuities in life course and social support. J Affect Disord. 2001;64(2–3):155–66.
48. Aslund C, Nilsson KW, Starrin B, Sjoberg RL. Shaming experiences and the association between adolescent depression and psychosocial risk factors. Eur Child Adolesc Psychiatry. 2007;16(5):298–304.
49. West P. Health inequalities in the early years: is there equalisation in youth? Soc Sci Med. 1997;44(6):833–58.
50. Chen E, Martin AD, Matthews KA. Socioeconomic status and health: do gradients differ within childhood and adolescence? Soc Sci Med. 2006;62(9): 2161–70.
51. Spencer NJ. Social equalization in youth: evidence from a cross-sectional British survey. Eur J Pub Health. 2006;16(4):368–75.
52. Swedish National Institute of Public Health: Survey of mental health among children and adolescents. Results of the national total population study in grades 6 and 9, autumn 2009. Mölnlycke: Swedish National Institute of Public Health; 2011.
53. Ivert AK, Merlo J, Svensson R, Levander MT. How are immigrant background and gender associated with the utilisation of psychiatric care among adolescents? Soc Psychiatry Psychiatr Epidemiol. 2013;48(5):693–9.
54. Niemi ME, Falkenberg T, Nguyen MTT, Nguyen MTN, Patel V, Faxelid E. The social contexts of depression during motherhood: a study of explanatory models in Vietnam. J Affect Disord. 2010;124(1–2):29–37.
55. SBU. Treatment of Depression. A Systematic Review. Stockholm: The Swedish Council on Technology Assessment in Health Care (SBU); 2004.
56. Mackenbach JP. Health inequalities : Europe in profile. London: Produced by COI for the Dept. of Health; 2006.
57. Wirback T, Forsell Y, Larsson J-O, Engstrom K, Edhborg M. Experiences of depression and help-seeking described by young Swedish men. Psychol Men Masc. Advance online publication 2017.

58. Muntaner C, Eaton WW, Miech R, O'Campo P. Socioeconomic position and major mental disorders. Epidemiol Rev. 2004;26:53–62.
59. Ritsher JE, Warner V, Johnson JG, Dohrenwend BP. Inter-generational longitudinal study of social class and depression: a test of social causation and social selection models. British J Psychiatry Suppl. 2001;40:s84–90.
60. Cyranowski JM, Frank E, Young E, Shear MK. Adolescent onset of the gender difference in lifetime rates of major depression: a theoretical model. Arch Gen Psychiatry. 2000;57(1):21–7.
61. Courtenay WH. Constructions of masculinity and their influence on men's well-being: a theory of gender and health. Soc Sci Med. 2000;50(10):1385–401.
62. Ochi M, Fujiwara T, Mizuki R, Kawakami N, Grp WMHJS. Association of socioeconomic status in childhood with major depression and generalized anxiety disorder: results from the world mental health Japan survey 2002-2006. BMC Public Health. 2014;14 https://doi.org/10.1186/1471-2458-14-359.
63. Geyer S, Hemstrom O, Peter R, Vagero D. Education, income, and occupational class cannot be used interchangeably in social epidemiology. Empirical evidence against a common practice. J Epidemiol Community Health. 2006;60(9):804–10.
64. Fors S, Lennartsson C, Lundberg O. Childhood living conditions, socioeconomic position in adulthood, and cognition in later life: exploring the associations. J Gerontol Ser B Psychol Sci Soc Sci. 2009; 64(6):750–7.
65. Socialstyrelsen. Folkhälsorapport 2009. Stockholm: Socialstyrelsen; 2009.
66. Jaffee SR, Moffitt TE, Caspi A, Fombonne E, Poulton R, Martin J. Differences in early childhood risk factors for juvenile-onset and adult-onset depression. Arch Gen Psychiatry. 2002;59(3):215–22.
67. Jorgensen L, Ahlbom A, Allebeck P, Dalman C. The Stockholm non-affective psychoses study (snaps): the importance of including out-patient data in incidence studies. Acta Psychiatr Scand. 2010;121(5):389–92.
68. Allebeck P. The use of population based registers in psychiatric research. Acta Psychiatr Scand. 2009;120(5):386–91.
69. Fazel S, Wolf A, Chang Z, Larsson H, Goodwin GM, Lichtenstein P. Depression and violence: a Swedish population study. Lancet Psychiat. 2015; 2(3):224–32.
70. Essau CA. Frequency and patterns of mental health services utilization among adolescents with anxiety and depressive disorders. Depressn Anxiety. 2005;22(3):130–7.
71. Wasserman D: Depression-en vanlig sjukdom. Stockholm: Natur och Kultur; 2010.
72. Paananen R, Santalahti P, Merikukka M, Ramo A, Wahlbeck K, Gissler M. Socioeconomic and regional aspects in the use of specialized psychiatric care–a Finnish nationwide follow-up study. Eur J Pub Health. 2013;23(3): 372–7.
73. Zwaanswijk M, Verhaak PF, Bensing JM, van der Ende J, Verhulst FC. Help seeking for emotional and behavioural problems in children and adolescents: a review of recent literature. Eur Child Adolesc Psychiatry. 2003; 12(4):153–61.
74. Modin B, Ostberg V, Almquist Y. Childhood peer status and adult susceptibility to anxiety and depression. A 30-year hospital follow-up. J Abnorm Child Psychol. 2011;39(2):187–99.
75. Patterson V, Mackenzie L, Zwicker A, Drobinin V, Cumby J, Abidi S, Bagnell A, Propper L, Alda M, Uher R. Adversity, parental mental illness, and risk of depression in youth. Eur Psychiat. 2017;41:S220.

7

Outcomes of an integrated care pathway for concurrent major depressive and alcohol use disorders

Andriy V. Samokhvalov[1,2,3,4*], Charlotte Probst[3,8,9], Saima Awan[1], Tony P. George[1,2,4], Bernard Le Foll[1,2,3,4,5], Peter Voore[1,4] and Jürgen Rehm[1,2,3,4,5,6,7,8,9]

Abstract

Background: In 2013, an Integrated Care Pathway (ICP) for concurrent Major Depressive (MDD) and Alcohol Use (AUD) Disorders was developed at the Centre for Addiction and Mental Health (CAMH), Toronto, Ontario, Canada. The ICP was further implemented at 8 other clinical sites across Ontario (the DA VINCI Project) in 2015–2017. The goal of this study was to systematically describe and analyze the main clinical outcomes of the project.

Methods: Data on a non-randomized cohort of patients receiving ICP-based treatment were collected prospectively at nine clinical sites in a variety of clinical settings. Statistical methods: descriptive statistics, t-test, chi-square, ANOVA, generalized linear models.

Results: Two hundred forty-six patients were enrolled, 58.8% males, mean age was 45.6 years, 170 patients received treatment at academic health centres (AHC), 49 – at community hospitals (CH) and 27 – in family health teams (FHT). There were no major differences in anamnestic parameters and depression severity between the three settings, but there were differences in baseline drinking patterns between subgroups ($F = 4.271$, $df = 2$, $p = 0.015$). Overall completion rate was 70.7% with no significant variation between settings ($\chi^2 = 3.35$, $df = 2$, $p = 0.19$). Treatment duration in AHC was the longest, and completion rates were the highest. There was a statistically significant and clinically meaningful reduction in the number of drinking days per week (1.81, $t = 8.78$, $p < 0.001$). The cohort overall demonstrated significant and meaningful reduction in severity of cravings (Penn Alcohol Craving Scale: 4.42, $t = 8.63$, $p < 0.001$) and depressive symptoms (Quick Inventory of Depressive Symptomatology: 4.25, $t = 11.26$, $p < 0.001$). While some of the baseline patient characteristics and treatment parameters varied between the settings, the variation in clinical outcomes was mostly insignificant, though clinical improvement was more pronounced in academic setting and with individual therapy.

Conclusions: The study demonstrated that ICP is a feasible and effective treatment for concurrent AUD and MDD that delivers meaningful clinical improvement in a variety of settings. A randomized controlled study is needed to properly compare the treatment outcomes between ICP model and treatment as usual and to further explore the role of various factors on treatment outcomes.

Keywords: Concurrent disorders, Alcohol use disorder, Major depressive disorder, Care pathway, Pharmacotherapy, Psychotherapy, Integrated treatment

* Correspondence: andriy.samokhvalov@camh.ca
[1]Addictions Division, Centre for Addiction and Mental Health (CAMH), 33 Russell Street, Office T519, Toronto, ON M5S 2S1, Canada
[2]Institute for Medical Science, University of Toronto, Toronto, ON, Canada
Full list of author information is available at the end of the article

Background

In 2013, an Integrated Care Pathway (ICP) for concurrent Major Depressive (MDD) and Alcohol Use (AUD) Disorders was developed at the Centre for Addiction and Mental Health (CAMH), Toronto, Ontario, Canada [1]. These two conditions were chosen as both of them are highly prevalent in Canada and worldwide [2, 3] and often are comorbid with each other, which significantly complicates their effective treatment [4]. Both conditions are also associated with high socioeconomic burden [5, 6] and there is a lack of well-established evidence-based treatments for the treatment of concurrent MDD and AUD [7]. The ICP was created in order to address this systemic shortcoming and after a short pilot stage showed promising clinical results [8, 9]. In 2015 the ICP received support through a joint funding program Adopting Research To Improve Care (ARTIC) in order to implement this ICP at multiple clinical sites across the province of Ontario. The 22-month project was named DA VINCI (Depression and Alcoholism: Validation of an Integrated Care Initiative) and was completed in January 2017 with the ICP fully implemented at nine clinical sites including CAMH.

The goal of this study was to summarize the main clinical outcomes of the implementation of ICP in a variety of clinical settings and to explore the determinants of clinical improvement in patients receiving treatment within the ICP paradigm.

Objectives of the study were to evaluate the treatment completion rate as well as the changes in severity of depressive symptoms, cravings for alcohol and patterns of drinking over the course of treatment.

The primary hypothesis was that patients receiving treatment through the ICP would have a retention rate significantly higher than the retention rate in patients who received treatment as usual (TAU) as previously reported for the central site (CAMH, 42.0 and 30.9% 12- and 16-week retention rates, respectively) [9].

Secondary hypotheses 1–3: There would be a significant reduction in 1) severity of depressive symptoms, 2) severity of cravings, and 3) weekly alcohol consumption levels over the course of ICP treatment.

Methods

Design: The study is observational in nature and had one prospective cohort of patients receiving ICP treatment at multiple sites. There was no control group. Patients were not randomized into treatment (convenience sample). Data were collected through a review of the clinical charts of all patients enrolled into the ICP since its inception in December 2013 and until September 30th, 2016. The latter time limit was set in order to ensure that all patients had at least 16 weeks to complete the ICP by the time the data collection was completed (January 20th, 2017). No post-treatment follow-up data were collected.

Eligibility criteria: Patients were considered eligible for the ICP when they had concurrent AUD and MDD and were never diagnosed with bipolar disorder. Cases of alcohol-induced depressive disorder were excluded. Patients were diagnosed with alcohol-induced depressive disorder if there was a clear temporal association between the onset of depressive symptoms and alcohol intoxication or withdrawal. Alcohol-induced depressive disorder was ruled out if the onset of depressive symptoms preceded the onset of excessive alcohol use, the symptoms persisted for a substantial period of time after the cessation of alcohol use or there was a clear history of non-alcohol-related depressive episodes as per DSM-5 diagnostic criteria and guidelines for differential diagnosis [10]. There were no age restrictions and patients with a wide variety of sociodemographic and clinical characteristics were included to ensure delivery of treatment to a broader population of eligible patients. Patients who required medical alcohol withdrawal management received it first and then were reassessed and enrolled into the project.

Setting: The project was carried out at 8 sites in Ontario in addition to CAMH, or 9 in total. These sites included 2 academic health centres (AHC): Royal Ottawa Mental Health Centre, Toronto Western Hospital / University Health Network; 3 community hospitals (CH): Trillium Health Partners, North Bay Regional Health Centre, and William Osler Health System and 3 large family health teams (FHT): Hamilton FHT, Village FHT and Inner City FHT.

Intervention: The ICP model includes several crucial components: Pharmacotherapy for both MDD and AUD - treatment was provided by trained physicians who followed the manualized treatment algorithm, which included several antidepressants of different pharmacological classes (sertraline, fluoxetine, venlafaxine and mirtazapine) [11–13] and several medications for the treatment of AUD (naltrexone, acamprosate and topiramate) [7, 12, 14] (See Additional file 1 for details). The algorithm was based on several clinical measures to monitor patients' therapeutic responses and justify the changes of medications and/or their dosages [15, 16]. These measures included quick inventory of depressive symptomatology (QIDS) [17], Penn alcohol craving scale (PACS) [18] and patterns of drinking operationalized via the following four indicators: number of standard drinks consumed on weekly basis (SD/w), number of drinking days per week (DD/w), number of heavy drinking days per week (HDD/w), and the number of standard drinks consumed per drinking day (SD/DD). Standard drink was defined as any alcoholic beverage containing 13.6 g of ethanol as per the Canada's Low-Risk

Drinking Guidelines [19]. Another important component of the ICP was a 16-week manualized psychotherapy protocol which combined empirically supported treatments for both MDD and AUD such as cognitive behavior therapy (CBT) and motivational interviewing [20]. Initial sessions (1–2) focused on building therapeutic alliance, introduction of the treatment model and motivational enhancement, sessions 3–5 focused on behavioral components and gradually transitioned to cognitive techniques in sessions 6–10. Starting with session 11 protocol focused on relapse prevention, strengthening and rehearsal of the skills acquired during treatment, preparation for transition into community [1, 8]. Psychotherapy was provided weekly by trained clinicians in group or individual format depending on the setting. Also, where possible the ICP was supported by pharmacists and nurses who monitored patients' medication compliance and provided psychoeducation when necessary. Finally, all clinicians involved in the ICP were meeting on weekly basis to increase the cohesion and integrative collaboration of the clinical team.

Outcome measures:

1. ICP completion rates: the treatment was considered completed if patients had received at least 12 core ICP psychotherapy sessions while being enrolled into the pathway or, in few cases, when they have completed the psychotherapy manual in accelerated pace and demonstrated significant clinical improvement (achieved remission from both MDD and AUD).
2. Severity of depressive symptoms: Measured by 16-item Quick Inventory of Depressive Symptomatology (QIDS-SR_{16} [17]) at baseline and biweekly throughout the treatment.
3. Severity of cravings was measured by Penn Alcohol Cravings Scale (PACS [18]) biweekly.
4. Drinking patterns: Self-reported at each biweekly clinical visit and included number of drinking days per week (DD/w), number of standard drinks per week (SD/w), number of standard drinks per drinking day (SD/d) and number of heavy drinking days (HDD) per week (HDD/w).
5. Severity of depressive symptoms and cravings and drinking patterns were measured at baseline and at the end of treatment (or last clinical visit for patients who dropped out).

Data collection: Data were extracted from clinical charts by three independent raters. Clinical characteristics included medical history, drug use history, alcohol use and AUD history, history of depressive symptoms and MDD, history of treatments for conditions, current drinking patterns and comorbidities. The data from 10 charts were extracted by two raters simultaneously in order to ensure reliable data extraction and inter-rater agreement was evaluated for key variables. Furthermore, data extracted by one rater were randomly checked by other raters for potential extraction errors. In cases of disagreement, the principal investigator reviewed the issue and a consensus on extraction was reached.

Statistical methods: All analyses were performed in R v.3.3.1 [21]. Means and proportions were used to describe the baseline and end-of-treatment characteristics of the sample, which were then compared using paired t-test. ANOVA was used to compare the difference between subgroups of subjects based on the type of clinical settings (AHC, HC, FHT), and type of therapy they received (group or individual). Chi-square test for homogeneity was used for between-group comparisons of categorical variables. A series of linear models were calculated to evaluate the impact of setting and therapy format on clinical outcomes. All tests were bidirectional and based on alpha error of 5%. For non-completers intent-to-treat approach was used [22]. Missing data were imputed using last observation carried forward [23].

Research ethics board: The study received approval from CAMH REB (protocol #053–2016).

Results

Patient characteristics

A total of 396 patients with concurrent MDD and AUD were enrolled into ICP across the 9 sites including 44 patients who started their treatment before the DA VINCI project was funded (pilot group) and the 81 patients included into previous report [24]. Out of these, we have selected 246 patients who received treatment within the specified timeframe – 170 patients received treatment in academic health centres (AHC), 49 – in community hospitals (CH) and 27 – in family health teams (FHT). Overall, 58.8% of the samples were men, with the CH subgroup having almost equal distribution of men and women, insignificantly higher proportion of men in AHC and lower – in FHT. Mean age was 45.6 years, there were no significant differences between subgroups ($F = 0.364$, $df = 2$, $p = 0.695$). More than half of patients were tobacco smokers (52.4%); majority of them (70.7%) used cannabis in the past month.

On average patients had 14.85 years of AUD history and 12.39 years of MDD history, with no significant difference between settings ($F = 0.47$, $df = 2$, $p = 0.625$, and $F = 1.22$, $df = 2$, $p = 0.299$, respectively). While severity of depressive symptoms as per QIDS did not vary much between subgroups with the average score of 15.02 (SD = 5.12), the severity of cravings varied insignificantly (17.94, SD = 8.35, $F = 2.363$, $df = 2$, $p = 0.096$), and there were significant differences in patterns of drinking (see Table 1). The average number of SD consumed weekly was 34.37 (SD = 35.13), the average number of drinking

Table 1 Baseline characteristics of study participants

Characteristic	AHC[a] ($n = 169$)	CH[b] ($n = 49$)	FHT[c] ($n = 27$)	Test statistic	All subjects ($n = 246$)
Sex, %					
Men	63.3%	51.0%	44.4%	$\chi^2 = 4.94$, df = 2, $p = 0.08$	58.8%
Women	36.7%	49.0%	55.6%		41.2%
Age, mean (SD)	45.42 (11.37)	46.80 (13.83)	44.63 (11.75)	F = 0.364, df = 2, $p = 0.695$	45.61 (11.75)
Smokers, %	51.8%	61.2%	40.7%	$\chi^2 = 3.02$, df = 2, $p = 0.22$	52.4%
Cannabis users[d], %	70.6%	77.6%	59.3%	$\chi^2 = 2.81$, df = 2, $p = 0.25$	70.7%
AUD history, years, mean (SD)	14.29 (11.65)	15.56 (12.60)	16.52 (12.88)	F = 0.47, df = 2, $p = 0.625$	14.85 (11.99)
Drinking patterns:					
SD/w, mean (SD)	37.28 (37.27)	20.96 (26.34)	41.78 (26.86)	F = 4.271, df = 2, $p = 0.015$	34.37 (35.13)
SD/d, mean (SD)	6.59 (5.38)	4.31 (4.46)	7.89 (3.43)	F = 4.509, df = 2, $p = 0.012$	6.24 (5.16)
HDD/w, mean (SD)	3.68 (3.13)	2.60 (2.95)	4.06 (2.57)	F = 2.481, df = 2, $p = 0.086$	3.50 (3.07)
DD/w, mean (SD)	4.11 (2.99)	3.14 (2.92)	5.11 (2.25)	F = 3.325, df = 2, $p = 0.038$	4.00 (2.96)
PACS, mean (SD)	17.73 (8.95)	16.90 (7.10)	21.07 (5.86)	F = 2.363, df = 2, $p = 0.096$	17.94 (8.35)
MDD history, years, mean (SD)	13.47 (11.37)	9.71 (8.51)	11.53 (9.66)	F = 1.22, df = 2, $p = 0.299$	12.39 (10.61)
QIDS, mean (SD)	15.03 (5.23)	14.39 (5.07)	16.41 (4.22)	F = 1.185, df = 2, $p = 0.307$	15.02 (5.12)

[a]*AHC* Academic health centre
[b]*CH* Community hospital
[c]*FHT* Family Health Team
[d]Cannabis users were defined as those who used cannabis at least once in the past year

days per week was 4.00 (SD = 2.96), and the average number of standard drinks per drinking day was 6.24 (SD = 5.16). Overall, the lowest alcohol consumption was reported in patients receiving treatment in community hospitals and the highest in family health teams. The only drinking-related parameter that did not differ significantly between settings was the number of heavy drinking days per week (3.50, SD = 3.07, on average in the whole sample).

Treatment parameters

Average treatment duration varied between 99.31–103.11 days in community settings and 134.09 in AHC, which was significantly longer (F = 3.527, df = 2, $p = 0.031$) than treatment at FHT. There were significant differences between settings in terms of number of physician visits with an average of 7.26 visits across the whole cohort (F = 4.183, df = 2, $p = 0.016$). The largest number was observed in community hospitals, followed by FHT and the lowest in academic settings. There were no significant differences in the number of psychotherapy sessions (F = 1.209, df = 2, $p = 0.300$).

Clinical outcomes

The data on clinical outcomes are presented in Table 2. One hundred seventy-four (70.7%) of patients completed their treatment, with some insignificant variation between sites ($\chi^2 = 3.35$, df = 2, $p = 0.19$). On average, there were statistically significant and clinically meaningful reductions in the number of drinking days per week (1.81, $t = 8.78$, $p < 0.001$), number of heavy drinking days per week (2.32, $t = 10.95$, $p < 0.001$), average number of SD per drinking day (3.23, $t = 8.65$, $p < 0.001$) and weekly alcohol consumption (22.19, $t = 9.53$, $p < 0.001$). The drinking patterns changed the most in academic settings with the only parameter significantly varying between settings being DD/w (2.12, F = 3.511, df = 2, $p = 0.032$). The cohort overall demonstrated significant and meaningful reduction in severity of cravings (Reduction in PACS score of 4.42, $t = 8.63$, $p < 0.001$) and depressive symptoms (reduction of QIDS score of 4.25, $t = 11.26$, $p < 0.001$).

Determinants of clinical improvement

Only the reductions in number of SD/w and DD/w were significantly associated with the format of therapy – individual therapy was associated with better outcomes ($\beta = 9.785$, 95%CI: 0.371–19.199, $p = 0.042$ and $\beta = 1.051$, 95%CI: 0.220–1.882, $p = 0.013$). Correlations between the type of setting and clinical outcomes were in line with the descriptive analyses – treatment in a community hospital and being a patient of FHT was associated with less pronounced reduction in drinking ($\beta = -11.957$, 95%CI: -0.446- -23.468, $p = 0.042$ and $\beta = -1.678$, 95%CI: -0.199- -1.908, $p = 0.026$, respectively).

Discussion

The study demonstrated that the ICP paradigm is capable of ensuring high treatment retention rates in complex clinical populations and in a variety of settings.

Table 2 Summary of the clinical outcomes in the ICP patients

Outcome	AHC[a] ($n = 169$)	HC[b] ($n = 49$)	FHT[c] ($n = 27$)	Test statistic	All subjects ($n = 246$)	Base vs. EoT (paired t-test)[d]
Completion rate, %	74.1%	65.3%	59.3%	$\chi^2 = 3.35$, df = 2, $p = 0.19$	70.7%	–
Treatment duration, mean (SD)	134.09 (106.51)	99.31 (43.26)	103.11 (30.23)	F = 3.527, df = 2, $p = 0.031$	123.76 (92.36)	
Number of physician visits, mean (SD)	7.65 (4.19)	5.88 (2.64)	6.89 (3.30)	F = 4.183, df = 2, $p = 0.016$	7.26 (3.89)	
Number of therapy sessions, mean (SD)	10.95 (6.03)	12.45 (4.47)	11.41 (6.54)	F = 1.209 df = 2, $p = 0.300$	11.30 (5.82)	
Changes in clinical parameters						
Reduction in SD/w, mean (SD)	25.35 (37.06)	13.39 (26.01)	16.08 (24.03)	F = 2.407, df = 2, $p = 0.093$	22.19 (34.46)	t = 9.53, $p < 0.001$
Reduction in SD/d, mean (SD)	3.57 (6.09)	2.08 (4.05)	3.03 (2.93)	F = 1.251, df = 2, $p = 0.288$	3.23 (5.56)	t = 8.65, $p < 0.001$
Reduction in HDD/w, mean (SD)	2.63 (3.34)	2.06 (2.98)	1.11 (2.64)	F = 2.107, df = 2, $p = 0.124$	2.39 (3.24)	t = 10.95, $p < 0.001$
Reduction in DD/w, mean (SD)	2.12 (3.16)	1.23 (2.85)	0.44 (1.86)	F = 3.511, df = 2, $p = 0.032$	1.81 (3.05)	t = 8.78, $p < 0.001$
Reduction in PACS, mean (SD)	4.57 (8.29)	4.27 (7.38)	3.78 (6.35)	F = 0.128, df = 2, $p = 0.880$	4.42 (7.88)	t = 8.63, $p < 0.001$
Reduction in QIDS, mean (SD)	4.17 (6.22)	4.74 (4.94)	3.77 (3.84)	F = 0.262, df = 2, $p = 0.77$	4.25 (5.76)	t = 11.26, $p < 0.001$

[a] *AHC* Academic health centre
[b] *HC* Community hospital
[c] *FHT* Family Health Team
[d] the difference between the baseline and the end-of-treatment parameters for the whole sample

Also, it yielded significant and meaningful clinical improvement in patterns of drinking, severity of cravings and severity of depressive symptoms. Despite the differences in baseline characteristics of patients receiving treatment in the three major types of settings the observed reductions in patterns of drinking, severity of cravings and depressive symptoms were quite similar with slightly better improvements observed in academic settings, likely due to higher availability of clinical resources and higher level of training and specialization of personnel. Also, individual format of therapy and academic settings were associated with significantly better improvement in specific aspects of drinking patterns.

These findings corroborate our preliminary reports on ICP – at the pilot stage, with a small sample or patients ($n = 28$) we reported 80% retention rate at 12 weeks, which is in line with our current definition of ICP completion, and a tendency of reduction in depressive symptoms and alcohol consumption [8]. Later on, in a larger sample of $n = 81$ patients restricted to CAMH only we have demonstrated that ICP patients have significantly higher retention rates in comparison to a convenience sample of matched historical controls (81.5% vs.30.9%) as well as significant and clinically meaningful reduction in depressive symptoms, cravings and alcohol consumption [9]. Thus, with the expansion of the pathway to a variety of settings and despite rather rapid implementation model the ICP still yielded good clinical outcomes comparable to those presented in literature [25].

As the ICP was created and tailored to specific settings and clinical population there are no data on pathways of the same design. At the same time our data are in line with the findings from several randomized clinical trials (RCT) testing effectiveness of several antidepressants and anti-craving medications in depressed alcoholics [11–13, 26]. Out of these the most relevant would be the study of Pettinati and colleagues testing the effectiveness of a combination of naltrexone and sertraline in similar population [12]. Despite less rigorous design and no financial incentives our study yielded retention rates higher than in that RCT (70.7% vs. 57.1%). At the same time the effect sizes for all clinical outcomes in our cohort were significantly smaller than the ones observed in that trial.

In addition to clinical trials of pharmaceuticals there are at least two clinical trials investigating the effects of structured CBT-based clinical pathways [27, 28]. The studies were smaller ($n = 73$ and $n = 37$, respectively), utilized only psychotherapy, but at the same time yielded clinical data comparable to our findings.

In addition, the comparisons to existing literature are complicated due to several methodological limitations of our study, specifically, absence of control group, non-randomized observational design as well as heterogeneity of clinical settings. While the latter aspect of our study allowed to illustrate the impact of the clinical setting on treatment outcomes, the limitations warrant further research aimed to compare the ICP-based treatment to TAU or other treatment models. In addition, the data collection is based on chart review, which though being thorough still leads to a substantial amount of missed data.

Nevertheless, the overall outcomes of the study were positive and corroborate both our previous findings and the results of several studies with similar treatment protocols. Also, as the study is based on a project whose main goal was to broadly implement the ICP protocol in a variety of clinical settings with minimalistic eligibility criteria, we can assume that similar results may be expected in future adaptation and implementation of the ICP protocol in other provinces of Canada as well as internationally.

Conclusion

The study demonstrated that ICP is a feasible and effective treatment for concurrent AUD and MDD that delivers meaningful clinical improvement in a variety of settings. There was a significant variation in baseline patient characteristics and to some degree – in specific clinical outcomes depending on the setting and format of therapy. Controlled study is needed to properly compare the treatment outcomes between ICP model and treatment as usual as well as to further explore the role of various factors on treatment outcomes.

Abbreviations

AHC: Academic Health Centre; ANOVA: Analysis of Variance; ARTIC: Adopting Research to Improve Care; AUD: Alcohol Use Disorder; CAMH: Centre for Addiction and Mental Health; CBT: Cognitive Behavior Therapy; CH: Community Hospital; DA VINCI: Depression and Alcoholism – Validating an Integrated Care Initiative; DD/w: Number of drinking days per week; FHT: Family Health Team; PACS: Penn Alcohol Craving Scale; QIDS: Quick Inventory of Depressive Symptomatology; QIDS-SR16: Quick Inventory of Depressive Symptomatology – Self-Rated, 16-item; RCT: Randomized Clinical Trial; REB: Research ethics board; SD: Standard deviation; SD/DD: Number of standard drinks per drinking day; SD/w: Number of standard drinks consumed on weekly basis; HDD/w: Number of heavy drinking days per week; ICP: Integrated Care Pathway; MDD: Major Depressive Disorder TAU Treatment as usual

Acknowledgements

The authors would like to acknowledge the work of Steve Perrotta, Amanda Carpenter, Leena Rahman, and Muna Osman who performed the chart review. Also, we would like to acknowledge the work of a number of clinicians, scientists and administrators involved in creation and implementation of the ICP and directly involved it patient care including the ICP MDAD working group, CAMH ICP program personnel and CAMH AMS clinicians and administrators. Also, we would like to thank our colleagues from all clinical sites for their contribution to implementation of the pathway and their dedication to provision of excellent clinical care to the ICP patients.

Funding

Two authors, Dr. Samokhvalov and Ms.Awan, are co-leads of the DA VINCI project which was supported by the Adopting Research to Improve Care (ARTIC) Program, a proven model that accelerates the spread and implementation of evidence-based health care interventions across Ontario. ARTIC is co-led by the Council of Academic Hospitals of Ontario (CAHO) and Health Quality Ontario (HQO), and is funded by the Ministry of Health and Long-term Care. The grant was exclusively covering implementation aspects and no research activities were funded, including this study and this paper. Neither CAHO, nor HQO had any influence on the manuscript preparation or the way the data are being presented and interpreted by the authors.

Authors' contributions

AVS was the Co-Lead for the DA VINCI project and the Principal Investigator for this study, he designed the study, organized data collection and analyzes, drafted and finalized the manuscript. CP and JR have contributed substantially to study conceptualization, data analyses and manuscript preparation. SA was the Co-lead of the DA VINCI Project and substantially contributed to data collection, interpretation and manuscript preparation. BLF, PV and TG have substantially contributed to the interpretation of clinical data and manuscript preparation. All authors have reviewed and approved the final manuscript for submission.

Competing interests

Dr. George has served on Data Safety and Monitoring Boards for Novartis, and has had a grant and contract funding from Pfizer in the past 2 years. Dr. Le Foll has received grant and salary support from Pfizer and Bioprojet. He received speaker fees or has been consultant for Richter Pharmaceuticals, Lundbeck, Ethypharm, Mettrum and Allergan. Drs. George, Le Foll and Rehm held multiple grants from CIHR, NIH and other organizations. None of these activities are related to this study, thus the authors report no conflicts of interest. The authors alone are responsible for the content and writing of this paper.

Author details

[1]Addictions Division, Centre for Addiction and Mental Health (CAMH), 33 Russell Street, Office T519, Toronto, ON M5S 2S1, Canada. [2]Institute for Medical Science, University of Toronto, Toronto, ON, Canada. [3]Institute for Mental Health Policy Research, CAMH, Toronto, ON, Canada. [4]Division of Brain and Therapeutics, Department of Psychiatry, University of Toronto, Toronto, ON, Canada. [5]Campbell Family Mental Health Research Institute, Toronto, ON, Canada. [6]Division of Adult Psychiatry and Health Systems, Department of Psychiatry, University of Toronto, Toronto, ON, Canada. [7]Dalla Lana School of Public Health, University of Toronto, Toronto, ON, Canada. [8]Institute for Clinical Psychology and Psychotherapy, Technische Universität Dresden, Dresden, Sachsen, Germany. [9]WHO Collaborating Centre on Mental Health and Addiction, Toronto, ON, Canada.

References

1. Awan S, Samokhvalov AV, Aleem N, Hendershot CS, Irving JA, Kalvik A, Lefebvre L, Le Foll B, Quilty L, Voore P: Development and implementation of an ambulatory integrated care pathway for major depressive disorder and alcohol dependence. Psychiatr Serv (Washington, DC) 2015: https://doi.org/10.1176/appi.ps.
2. Pearson C, Janz T, Ali J. Mental and substance use disorders in Canada. In: Health at a Glance. Ottawa: Statistics Canada; 2013.
3. Patten SB, Wang JL, Williams JV, Currie S, Beck CA, Maxwell CJ, El-Guebaly N. Descriptive epidemiology of major depression in Canada. Can J Psychiatr. 2006;51(2):84–90.
4. Currie SR, Patten SB, Williams JV, Wang J, Beck CA, El-Guebaly N, Maxwell C. Comorbidity of major depression with substance use disorders. Can J Psychiatr. 2005;50(10):660–6.
5. Whiteford HA, Degenhardt L, Rehm J, Baxter AJ, Ferrari AJ, Erskine HE, Charlson FJ, Norman RE, Flaxman AD, Johns N, Burstein R, Murray CJ, Vos T. Global burden of disease attributable to mental and substance use disorders: findings from the global burden of disease study 2010. Lancet. 2013;382(9904):1575-86.
6. Samokhvalov AV, Popova S, Room R, Ramonas M, Rehm J. Disability associated with alcohol abuse and dependence. Alcohol Clin Exp Res. 2010;34(11):1871–8.
7. Beaulieu S, Saury S, Sareen J, Tremblay J, Schutz CG, McIntyre RS, Schaffer A. The Canadian network for mood and anxiety treatments (CANMAT) task force recommendations for the management of patients with mood disorders and comorbid substance use disorders. Ann Clin Psychiatry : Official J Am Acad Clin Psychiatrists. 2012;24(1):38–55.
8. Samokhvalov AV, Awan S, Voore P. Early outcomes of the integrated care pathway for concurrent major depressive disorder and alcohol dependence. Eur Psychiatry. 2015;30(**Supplement 1**):1088.
9. Samokhvalov A, Awan S, George T, Irving J, Le Foll B, Perrotta S, Probst C, Voore P, Rehm J. Integrated care pathway for co-occurring major depressive and alcohol use disorders: outcomes of the first two years. Am J Addict. 2017;
10. Diagnostic and Statistical Manual of Mental Disorders. DSM-5. 5th ed. Arlington, VA: American Psychiatric Association; 2013.
11. Kranzler HR, Mueller T, Cornelius J, Pettinati HM, Moak D, Martin PR, Anthenelli R, Brower KJ, O'Malley S, Mason BJ, et al. Sertraline treatment of co-occurring alcohol dependence and major depression. J Clin Psychopharmacol. 2006;26(1):13–20.

12. Pettinati HM, Oslin DW, Kampman KM, Dundon WD, Xie H, Gallis TL, Dackis CA, O'Brien CP. A double-blind, placebo-controlled trial combining sertraline and naltrexone for treating co-occurring depression and alcohol dependence. Am J Psychiatry. 2010;167(6):668–75.
13. Cornelius JR, Salloum IM, Ehler JG, Jarrett PJ, Cornelius MD, Perel JM, Thase ME, Black A. Fluoxetine in depressed alcoholics. A double-blind, placebo-controlled trial. Arch Gen Psychiatry. 1997;54(8):700–5.
14. Anton RF, O'Malley SS, Ciraulo DA, Cisler RA, Couper D, Donovan DM, Gastfriend DR, Hosking JD, Johnson BA, LoCastro JS, et al. Combined pharmacotherapies and behavioral interventions for alcohol dependence: the COMBINE study: a randomized controlled trial. Jama. 2006;295(17):2003–17.
15. Trivedi MH, Rush AJ, Crismon ML, Kashner TM, Toprac MG, Carmody TJ, Key T, Biggs MM, Shores-Wilson K, Witte B, et al. Clinical results for patients with major depressive disorder in the Texas medication algorithm project. Arch Gen Psychiatry. 2004;61(7):669–80.
16. Guo T, Xiang YT, Xiao L, Hu CQ, Chiu HF, Ungvari GS, Correll CU, Lai KY, Feng L, Geng Y, et al. Measurement-based care versus standard Care for Major Depression: a randomized controlled trial with blind raters. Am J Psychiatry. 2015;172(10):1004–13.
17. Rush AJ, Trivedi MH, Ibrahim HM, Carmody TJ, Arnow B, Klein DN, Markowitz JC, Ninan PT, Kornstein S, Manber R, et al. The 16-item quick inventory of depressive symptomatology (QIDS), clinician rating (QIDS-C), and self-report (QIDS-SR): a psychometric evaluation in patients with chronic major depression. Biol Psychiatry. 2003;54(5):573–83.
18. Kavanagh DJ, Statham DJ, Feeney GF, Young RM, May J, Andrade J, Connor JP. Measurement of alcohol craving. Addict Behav. 2013;38(2):1572–84.
19. Butt P, Beirness D, Cesa F, Gliksman L, Paradis C, Stockwell T. Alcohol and health in Canada: a summary of evidenceand guidelines for low-risk drinking. Ottawa, ON: Canadian Centre on Substance Abuse; 2012.
20. Riper H, Andersson G, Hunter SB, de Wit J, Berking M, Cuijpers P. Treatment of comorbid alcohol use disorders and depression with cognitive-behavioural therapy and motivational interviewing: a meta-analysis. Addiction. 2014;109(3):394–406.
21. R Development Core Team. R: A language and environment for statistical computing. Vienna: R Foundation for Statistical Computing; 2008.
22. Gupta SK. Intention-to-treat concept: a review. Pers Clin Res. 2011;2(3):109–12.
23. Little RJ, D'Agostino R, Cohen ML, Dickersin K, Emerson SS, Farrar JT, Frangakis C, Hogan JW, Molenberghs G, Murphy SA, et al. The prevention and treatment of missing data in clinical trials. N Engl J Med. 2012;367(14):1355–60.
24. Samokhvalov AV, Awan S, George TP, Irving J, Le Foll B, Perrotta S, Probst C, Voore P, Rehm J. Integrated care pathway for co-occurring major depressive and alcohol use disorders: outcomes of the first two years. Am J Addict. 2017;26(6):602–9.
25. Rotter T, Kinsman L, James E, Machotta A, Gothe H, Willis J, Snow P, Kugler J. Clinical pathways: effects on professional practice, patient outcomes, length of stay and hospital costs. Cochrane Database Syst Rev. 2010;3:Cd006632.
26. Adamson SJ, Sellman JD, Foulds JA, Frampton CM, Deering D, Dunn A, Berks J, Nixon L, Cape G. A randomized trial of combined citalopram and naltrexone for nonabstinent outpatients with co-occurring alcohol dependence and major depression. J Clin Psychopharmacol. 2015;35(2):143–9.
27. Hunter SB, Watkins KE, Hepner KA, Paddock SM, Munjas B, Osilla KC, Perry S. Treating depression and substance use: a randomized controlled trial. J Subst Abus Treat. 2012;43(2):137–51.
28. Morley KC, Baillie A, Leung S, Sannibale C, Teesson M, Haber PS, Specialized Integrated I. Treatment for comorbid anxiety, depression and alcohol dependence better than treatment as usual in a public hospital setting? Alcohol Alcohol (Oxford, Oxfordshire). 2016;51(4):402–9.

Facilitators and barriers to modifying dietary and hygiene behaviours as adjuvant treatment in patients with depression in primary care

B. Olivan-Blázquez[1,2,3*], J. Montero-Marin[2,3], M. García-Toro[2,4], E. Vicens-Pons[2,5], M. J. Serrano-Ripoll[4], A. Castro-Gracia[4], M. C. Sarasa-Bosque[6], J. M. Mendive-Arbeloa[7], Y. López-del-Hoyo[1,2,3] and J. Garcia-Campayo[2,3,6,8]

Abstract

Background: Major depression is a highly prevalent condition. Its pathogenesis is related to a wide variety of biological and psychosocial factors and among these is factors related to lifestyle. Lifestyle-based interventions seem to be appropriate strategies as coadjutant treatment. The objective of this study is to explore and identify expectations and experiences of both patients and healthcare professionals that can point to the main barriers and facilitators with regard to the promotion of healthy dietary and hygiene behaviours in patients suffering from major depression.

Methods: A qualitative design was used to collect information from a wide range of purposefully and theoretically guided samples of depressed patients and health professionals from Primary Care (PC). Both in-depth interviews and discussion groups were used. A standardized protocol was designed to guide the interviews and groups, including the preparation of a topic list to be addressed, with previously tested, open suggestions that could be of interest. A thematic analysis was performed from grounded theory in order to explore, develop and define until saturation the emergent categories of analysis derived from the individual interview and group data.

Results: Both patients as well as PC professionals noted a series of central aspects with respect to the implementation of a programme for the acquisition of healthy dietary and hygiene habits for depressive patients, which may be organized around 'personal', 'programmatic', and 'transversal' aspects. As for the personal aspects, categories regarding 'patient history', and 'disposition' were found; the programmatic aspects included categories such as 'presentation and monitoring', and modification of 'cognitive' and 'behavioural' habits; whereas the transversal aspects comprised the possibilities of 'social support' and defining categories of 'objectives'.

Conclusion: The implementation of intervention programmes that combine dietary and hygiene-related factors in patients with depression is complex, given the nature of the disorder itself, and its symptoms such as apathy and feelings of guilt or incompetence. Key issues exist for the success of the intervention, such as the simplicity of guidelines, tailoring through motivational interviewing, prolonged and intense monitoring throughout the different stages of the disorder, and the provision of adequate feedback and social support. PC could be an appropriate level in which to implement these interventions.

Keywords: Depression, Lifestyle, Intervention programmes, Facilitators, Barriers

* Correspondence: bolivan@unizar.es
[1]Department of Psychology and Sociology, University of Zaragoza, Violante de Hungria 23, 50009 Zaragoza, Spain
[2]Research Network on Preventive Activities and Health Promotion (Red de Investigación en Actividades Preventivas y Promoción de la Salud - RedIAPP), Barcelona, Spain
Full list of author information is available at the end of the article

Background

Major depression Disorder (MDD) is a highly prevalent condition and has become the second most common cause of disease-induced disability in our society [1–3]. Its pathogenesis is related to a wide variety of biological and psychosocial factors. Among these are factors related to lifestyle, as diverse studies claim [4–9].

The relationship between depression, diet and obesity is well established [10], as is that between eating style, weight gain and depression [11]. The comorbidity of obesity and depression is highly significant, with depression being up to 20–45% more prevalent in obese individuals [12]. A systematic review of prospective studies describes a reciprocal cause-effect relationship between depression and obesity [12]. Furthermore, weight loss in the obese has been found to reduce symptoms of depression [13], and similarly an improvement in short-term depression has been associated with weight loss, not only in females [14], but also in the general population [15]. A poor diet, obesity and/or metabolic syndrome predispose individuals to metabolic changes that interact with cerebral function through very complex mechanisms, probably having an individualized effect on each patient [10, 16–18]. The alteration of certain metabolic mechanisms has been associated with a poor outcome for depression, but this phenomenon also occurs in the opposite direction, creating a vicious circle of illness [10, 19]. Lee et al. [20] highlight the complex relationship between antidepressant drugs, MDD and weight gain. Hypothalamic-pituitary-adrenal (HPA) axis activation occurs during states of stress; concurrently, the HPA axis is also dysregulated in obesity and metabolic syndrome, making it the best understood shared common pathophysiological pathway with MDD.

Given this close relationship, lifestyle – more specifically dietary and hygiene behaviours – could play a major role in the initiation, maintenance and treatment of depression, at least as an adjuvant [4, 7, 19, 21]. The combination of different lifestyle-based interventions (diet, exercise, sun exposure, and sleep hygiene) appears to be an appropriate strategy to increase their effectiveness [19, 22], although it has been poorly investigated and has had varied results [4, 19, 23]. Furthermore, no studies exist regarding the difficulties and opportunities for change and how the healthcare system could help patients suffering from depression to modify their dietary and hygiene behaviours, as compared to other medical conditions such as diabetes [24, 25], Crohn's disease [26] or cardiovascular disease [27].

Primary Care (PC) is the most accessible healthcare service, offering comprehensive and continuous patient-centred care, and it is the most frequently used by citizens. Therefore, it is an ideal scenario for conducting individual, group and community interventions to change behaviours [28]; in this case, those related to the treatment of depression [19] or even its prevention [29].

Thus, the objective of this study is to explore and identify facilitators and barriers to the promotion of healthy dietary and hygiene habits in patients suffering from major depression from the expectations and experiences of both patients and healthcare professionals. This study was developed in PC centres and those attending to the most important aspects when implementing behaviour modification programmes in this population.

Methods

A qualitative design was used to collect information from a wide range of purposefully and theoretically guided samples of depressed patients and health professionals from PC. With the intention of increasing the consistence of the study, both in-depth interviews (with depressed patients) and discussion groups (with depressed patients and health professionals, separately) were used to access the subjectivity and the processes involved in generating ideas and concepts [30]. This triangulation of techniques and informants has been used in other works [31], with the assumption that qualitative research is inherently multi-method [32]. In-depth interviews were conducted by a single interviewer, and discussion groups were moderated by an interviewer and an observer, both of them female psychologists and researchers with previous experience in the field and no previous contact with participants.

Patients were recruited from the Spanish autonomous regions of Aragon and the Balearic Islands during their visits to PC, taking advantage of their participation in a research project (randomized controlled trial, RCT) on lifestyle change recommendations in patients with major depression [10, 23, 33]. This RCT consisted of a series of written dietary and hygiene-related lifestyle recommendations to improve their depressive symptoms and quality of life with low socio-sanitary costs. Through a randomized, double-blinded, multicentre, two arm-parallel clinical trial, with 12 month follow-up, and a sample of 273 PC patients, it was observed that just giving written lifestyle recommendations is not enough for depressive patients to benefit from them. Therefore, there seems to be a need for deeper understanding into the patient and professional expectations and experiences that might point to the barriers and facilitators to the implementation of these kinds of programmes. For this purpose, a subsample of patients was created, selected after stratification based on the variables of age, (18–40; 41–60; > 60), sex, level of education (primary, secondary, tertiary), occupation (paid, unpaid, no occupation) and level of depression at the basal assessement of the RCT using the Beck depression inventory [34] (mild, moderate, severe), treatment group in the study (active vs control), and city (Palma, Zaragoza). Health professionals were contacted by telephone, based on their age (18–40; 41–60; > 60), sex, occupation (general practitioner vs nurse), years of experience (< 15; 15–30; > 30), type of work contract (temporary vs permanent), participation in the study (participation vs not participation) and city (Palma, Zaragoza), in order to gather plentiful and varied information. Both patients and professionals were aware of the research project about lifestyle change recommendations, but none of them had any knowledge on the group to which patients were assigned. Every contacted patient and health professional initially agreed to be interviewed, but a number of them eventually did not keep the appointment owing to incompatible schedules. Table 1 outlines the main characteristics of the final 41 participants (11 patients and 30 professionals). The profile of a participating patient is a woman, between 40 and 60 years of age, with primary studies and mild or moderate depression. The profile of a participating health professional is a woman, between 40 and 60 years of age, general practitioner, with a permanent contract and more than 15 years of professional experience. The interviews were conducted between November 2014 and January 2015.

A standardized protocol was designed to guide the interviews and groups, including the preparation of a topic list to be addressed, with previously tested, open suggestions that could be of interest. The topic list was compiled from the experience of a panel of expert researchers who had developed and conducted a previous study on hygienic-dietary recommendations as adjuvant treatment in depression [19, 35] and taking into account the NICE behaviour change recommendations [36]. This topic list, shown in Table 2, comprised the following: previous knowledge of lifestyle recommendations (diet, physical exercice, sun exposure, sleep hygiene) as an adjuvant treatment for depression; where there was compliance with instructions: difficulties, feelings; in case of non-compliance with recommendations: causes, feelings; perception of efficacy; aspects that facilitate compliance with recommendations; appropriate level or means to change behaviour; ability of health system to help patients to change their behaviour and mood; proposals by health professionals when consulted about a mood problem; type of proposals that health professionals give and their characteristics; type of proposals that can be given; effectiveness of the proposals. After a short introduction about the study, patients and health professionals were asked open, general questions in order to raise a response and begin discussion. More direct questions were asked when specific topics did not spontaneously arise in the discourse. These are given in Table 3.

The objectives of the study were indirectly raised and questions asked about the topics in an open and progressive way. The interviewers and/or moderators were introduced to the participants as research psychologists and assumed a minimally orientative role, limiting their interventions to addressing the topics in the script. The

Table 1 Characterístics of patients and health care professionals

Variables	Patients ($n = 11$)
Age	
20–40 years	1 (9.1%)
41–60 years	6 (54.5%)
> 60 years	4 (36.4%)
Sex	
Male	3 (27.3%)
Female	8 (72.7%)
Education	
Primary	6 (54.5%)
Secondary	4 (36.5%)
Tertiary	1 (9.1%)
Occupation	
Paid	2 (18.2%)
Unpaid	4 (36.4%)
No occupation	5 (45.5%)
Level of depression	
Mild	4 (36.4%)
Moderate	4 (36.4%)
Severe	3 (27.3%)
Group	
Active	6 (54.5%)
Control	5 (45.5%)
Variables	Professionals ($n = 30$)
Age	
20–40 years	8 (26.6%)
41–60 years	17 (56.7%)
> 60 years	5 (16.7%)
Sex	
Male	11 (36.7%)
Female	19 (63.3%)
Occupation	
General practitioner	23 (76.7%)
Nurse	7 (23.3%)
Experience	
< 15 years	9 (30%)
15–30 years	10 (33.3%)
> 30 years	11 (36.7%)
Type of work contract	
Temporary	10 (33.3%)
Permanent	20 (66.7%)
Group	
Participation	16 (53.3%)
No participation	14 (46.7%)
City	
Zaragoza	26 (86.7%)
Palma	4 (13.3%)

Table 2 Topic list

- Previous knowledge of lifestyle recommendations (diet, physical exercise, sun exposure, sleep hygiene) as an adjuvant treatment for depression.
- Compliance with instructions.
  - Difficulties
  - Feelings
  - In case of non-compliance with recommendations: causes, feelings.
  - Perception of efficacy
- Aspects that facilitate compliance with recommendations
- Appropriate level or means to change behaviour.
- Ability of healthcare system to help patients change their behaviour and mood.
- Proposals by health professionals when consulted about a mood problem
- Type of proposals that health professionals offer and their characteristics.
- Type of proposals that can be made.
- Effectiveness of the proposals

settings for data collection were a neutral room in the different health centres at which the patients were registered, without the presence of non-participants. In-depth interviews lasted between 35 and 55 min and the discussion groups lasted 50–75 min. All of them were digitally audio-recorded and a verbatim transcription made in order to obtain the final set of qualitative data for the analysis, which was revised by the participants and added to the field notes made during and after the interviews/groups. An inductive thematic content analysis was performed from grounded theory in order to explore, develop and define the emergent categories of analysis derived from the individual interview and group data until saturation [37–40].

The type of analysis used was therefore of a qualitative, vertical and interpretative nature, with stratified and projected sampling aimed at gathering plentiful and varied information, and with an emerging and non-frequential design for the analysis categories [41, 42]. The aplication of the 'constant comparative method' strategy enabled conceptual categories to be systematically generated, and analysis and explicit coding to be combined with theory building, highlighting significant properties and relationships among all of them [43]. Specifically, we used 'open coding' to develop the first provisional interpretations; 'axial coding' to deepen and discover properties and relationships in each category; and also a 'core category', which was able to integrate and summarize all the emergent categories by means of 'selective coding' that finally provided the esential framework [44, 45]. Theory integration throughout the design, implementation and evaluation of the previously mentioned parallel RCT intervention also provided valuable insight into how these emergent categories contribute to effectiveness in changing behavioral outcomes [46].

All the analyses were performed iteratively using Maxqda-2007 software in agreement between two researchers (BOB, JMM), and the interpretations made from the data were discussed with interviewers (PR, PHM) and participants to obtain their approval [47]. This methodological triangulation was able to increase consistency and rigour by combining multiple techniques and maximizing the breadth and depth of perspectives.

Participants provided written informed consent to participate in the study. No interview/group was repeated. As previously explained, this study forms part of a research project that includes an RCT on the effectiveness of a lifestyle change recommendation programme in depressed patients [10, 23, 33]. Once the clinical trial stage was completed, this qualitative study was carried out to analyse the facilitators and barriers that patients with depression experience with regard to modifying their dietary and hygiene behaviours. The project was independently approved by the Research Ethics Committee of Aragon

Table 3 Questions asked to patients and healthcare professionals

Patients	Professionals
- Do you know anything about lifestyle modification (diet, exercise, etc.) in order to change your mood and depression? - All of you have taken part in a research project about modifying lifestyles. Did these recommendations that were given to you show you something new that you did not know? - Did you follow the recommendations for modifying lifestyles? If NOT, why didn't you follow them? - How did you feel when you followed the recommendations? And when you didn't? - What difficulties did you encounter in implementing the recommendations? - Do you think these recommendations helped you? - What do you think about the doctor's role? - And about the way of carrying out this modification? - Do you think another type of intervention would have helped you? Would an educational group or another kind of intervention have helped you? - Do you think there is something more that can be done to help you to modify your lifestyle when depressed?	- How do you think you should make recommendations for modifying life styles? - And to a patient with depression? - Do you know how this intervention can help him/her? - Do you think these recommendations can be effective? And do you believe the patient thinks that they work? - What difficulties do you think depressed patients have in changing their behaviour? - And what feelings do they have? - And as for modifying lifestyles, do you work in a different way in the case of a depressed patient? - What do you think is necessary in order to be effective when modifying lifestyles? - What do you think about educational groups? - And about follow-up? - Do you think these interventions are feasible from PC? - What difficulties do you encounter when giving this type of advice? - What is the appropriate level (or department or system) to implement this kind of interventions?

(PI12/0022) and the Research Ethics Committee of the Balearic Islands (PI11/1563), Spain, on March 2012.

Results

Both patients and PC professionals noted a series of central aspects with respect to the implementation of a programme for depressive patients to acquire healthy dietary and hygiene habits, which may be organized around 'personal', 'programmatic', and 'transversal' aspects. In relation to personal aspects, from the patients' perspective, topics regarding their 'personal history' and their personal readiness or 'disposition' were found. On the other hand, the programmatic aspects included topics such as programme 'presentation and monitoring', from both the patients and professionals' perspective; the modification of 'cognitive habits', from patients' perspective; and the modification of 'behavioural habits', from professional's point of view. All of them were interconnected in a synergetic manner towards the achievement of the transversal aspects, which were delimited by the possibilities of 'social support', from patients' perspective, and definition of 'objectives', from professional's point of view. Figure 1 provides a graphic representation of the core aspects that configure the central category (e.g., personal, programmatic, and transversal), and the main categories for the implementation programme for patients with major depression to acquire healthy dietary and hygiene habits. Table 4 provides quotes (Q) in which the properties or characteristics that make up each of the emerged categories are explained in the participants' own words.

Conceptualization of the discourse

Personal aspects

Personal aspects emerged from the patients' discourse, revolving around their 'personal history', including subtopics, such as 'history and comorbidity', in relation to patient background and development (Q1), and with reference to comorbidities with other physical illnesses that prevent behaviour modification (Q2). Within the patients' 'personal history', 'life changes' were also noted, whereby lifestyle modifications would have significant effects on the course of the illness (Q3). Personal 'disposition' also appeared, with subtopics that function as general 'facilitators', such as the simplicity of instructions (Q4), as well as general 'barriers', including aspects that hinder participation in and commitment to the programme, such as apathy (Q5), one of the symptoms of the illness.

Programmatic aspects

Programmatic aspects included topics such as programme 'presentation and monitoring' or follow up, which from the patient's perspective meant receiving appropriate 'instructions' on the quantity of information and stimuli (Q6). However, from a professional perspective, it took on the form of a suitable 'assessment', as reflected in its interest as a form of objectifying the level of programme adherence and change in mood (Q7). On the other hand, programme 'presentation and monitoring' for patients also included the idea of 'supervision' throughout the intervention process (Q8). However, for the professionals, the idea of also explaining the pharmacological treatment, and how habit modification could improve it, was found to be more relevant. The appropriate monitoring or follow-up of 'pharmaceutical' consumption would be essential from their point of view (Q9). Programmatic aspects also included the patients' handling of 'cognitive habits', such as the idea of 'agency' in the sense of determination and motivation (Q10) or 'ruminations', which are negative thoughts that hinder the implementation of a new, healthier life style (Q11). Other subtopics were found within the 'cognitive habits' category, such as 'avoidance', considered to be cognitive avoidance of responsibilities (Q12), as well as the cognitive 'restructurings' that take place throughout the new lifestyle implementation process (Q13). Finally, the differences that lead to the implementation of new lifestyle based on dietary and hygiene behaviours generated a certain sense of 'guilt' in patients (Q14). Programmatic aspects for the professionals also included the handling of 'behavioural habits', including the idea of

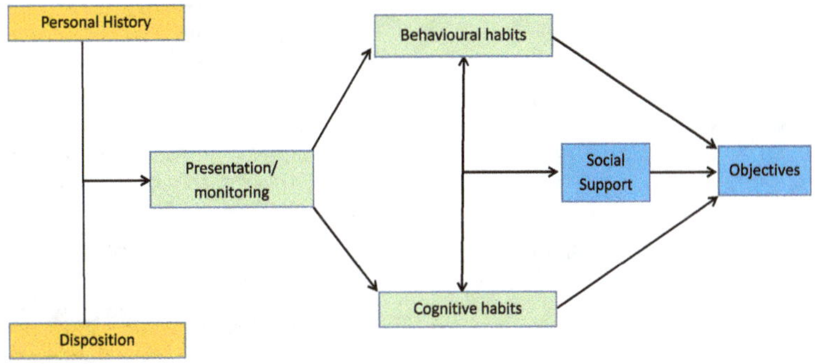

Fig. 1 Categories for the implementation of a programme for the acquisition of healthy dietary and hygiene habits in patients with major depression. Note: 'Personal' aspects are in orange. 'Programmatic' aspects are in green. 'Transversal' aspects are in blue

Table 4 Quotes regarding the results and relationships with emergent categories

Core aspects	Categories	Properties	Quotes
Personal aspects	Personal History (patient's perspective)	-History and comorbidity	*Q1: "While my husband was ill [with cancer], I didn't cry… But when he died, my life changed completely…. I was not the same person…, I withdrew into myself…"* (Patient 7) *Q2: "I have osteoarthritis... and chronic lower back pain… a lot of pain".* (Patient 6)
		-Vital changes	*Q3:"When you have a problem, if you don't change the way you live, you don't solve it". (Patient 9)*
	Disposition (patient's perspective)	-General facilitators (e.g. simplicity)	*Q4: "…very simple and effective things… very easy to do things, and they don't involve anything out of the ordinary".* (Patient 3)
		-General barriers (e.g. apathy)	*Q5:"You read the recommendations several times and yes, you see that they're good… but you aren't going to follow them every day. You are stuck and wound up and you can't pick yourself up... There are always things that make you lose heart".* (Patient 4)
Program aspects	Presentation and monitoring	-Instructions (patient's perspective)	*Q6: "I would have appreciated receiving more information and more encouragement".* (Patient 1)
		-Assessment (professional's perspective)	*Q7: "The degree of compliance has to be objectified and measured in some way in order to obtain clear conclusions about the intervention and the change in mood".* (General practitioner 8)
		-Supervision (patient's perspective)	*Q8: "The fact that the psychologist would phone me and ask me how I was doing and about whether I was following instructions was a big help for me".* (Patient 8)
		-Pharmaceutical consumption (professional's perspective)	*Q9: "You have to explain what the drugs are, the possible side effects, how long it will take to feel an effect and how long the treatment can last".* (General practitioner 25)
	Cognitive habits (patient's perspective)	-Agency	*Q10: "Motivation, will, determination. It costs a lot of work and you go as you can, but you end up improving".* (Patient 11)
		-Ruminations	*Q11: "You feel useless, absolutely useless… why should you do anything if there's no point? I don't think that any more, but at the time I couldn't help but feel that way."* (Patient 9)
		-Avoidance	*Q12: "The only thing that saved me was reading; it blocked everything out and I found some relief."* (Patient 3)
		-Restructurings	*Q13: "I see that when other people don't feel like doing something, they don't, and nothing happens. Why should it be different for me? Well, I also have to get on with things my way."* (Patient 4)
		-Guilt	*Q14: -So you are blaming yourself for failing…* *-Yes, that's right.* *-Guilt is the first problem in this illness…* *-Guilt is very difficult…* *-It's a very important factor…* (Interactions of several patients in a focus group)
	Behavioural habits (professional's perspective)	-Activation	*Q15: "We have to motivate our patients to go out and stay in touch with people, but gradually, with a guide, for instance by avoiding situations of conflict at the beginning, because they have to make a great effort at this stage".* (General practitioner 21)
		-Empowerment	*Q16:"When dealing with a person suffering from depression, we're starting with a very low level of motivation".* (General practitioner 12) *Q17:"A person with depression has their ups and downs; if you want your advice to have an effect, you have to wait until the right moment, when the person is open to it".* (General practitioner 18)

Table 4 Quotes regarding the results and relationships with emergent categories *(Continued)*

Core aspects	Categories	Properties	Quotes
		-Time pressure	Q18:"...*high-speed medicine, which means you have to get eight messages across to them in five minutes*". (General practitioner 18)
		-Habit control	Q19:"*There's no doubt about it that if you're going to change your eating habits, you must have control over your diet. You have to do it yourself, because if you eat out for work or if somebody prepares your meals for you, it's more complicated*". (General practitioner 5)
		-Opportunities	Q20:"*One difficulty that patients may find when changing their habits, especially with regard to food, is cost... eating certain foods is more expensive than eating others*". (General practitioner 8) Q21: "*Patients should be able to go for a walk or do exercise in nice places, in a pleasant urban environment that is well looked after*". (General practitioner 23)
Transversal aspects	Social Support (patient's perspective)	-Group format of intervention	Q22:"*The (intervention) group helped a lot because you realize that there are other people who are in the same situation as you.*" (Patient 5)
		-Contact with others	Q23: "*Having contact with others has been very useful for me. Going out for coffee with someone, people phoning me and showing interest in me, regaining face-to-face contact*". (Patient 8) Q24:"*When you're depressed, you need somebody to help you along, and your family and friends are there for that. But when you're really down, your family can lose patience, friends too; so it's important to have someone from outside to lend you a hand.*" (Patient 2) Q25:"*The group is a good thing, but then you need to have your personal, more private space....*" (Patient 8)
	Objectives (professional's perspective)	-Adjustment	Q26:"...*because you can't ask people to do something they've never done before or something that is very difficult for them*". (General practitioner 11). Q27: "*I believe that this programme would obtain better results by applying it to prevent recurrences in patients who have already improved their depression (...) that is, to acquire this lifestyle and maintain it.*" (General practitioner 21).
		-Intervention level	Q28: "*When it comes to personal level intervention, healthcare professionals should be the ones to do it, but if we're talking about a mass intervention, the media – radio, television, press – should be involved.*" (General practitioner 15) Q29: "...*in schools for young children... I think schools should teach children healthy lifestyle habits from a very young age*". (General practitioner 17)

behaviour 'activation' (Q15) and patient 'empowerment' (Q16, Q17), and also noting the 'time pressure' as a difficulty in carrying out patient care at this level (Q18). Other subtopics were also included such as 'habit control' (Q19) and the influence of the acquisitive power or 'opportunities' (Q20, Q21).

Transversal aspects

Transversal aspects emerged as an area dependent on all the above properties, which included the possibilities of 'social support' and defining the 'objectives' categories. The 'social support' category emerged from the patients' discourse and included the social possibilities of the 'group format' interventions, which are well accepted (Q22), although without losing individual 'contact with others', especially face-to-face contact beyond family members and friends, in order to gain a more private support space (Q23, Q24, Q25). Finally, the category of defining 'objectives' appeared as an assessment that was also dependent on all of the above, when considering the difficulty of implementing a programme of this sort. According to the professionals, the need for 'adjustment' to the specifics of each patient property included – the notion that this type of programme could perhaps better improve the prevention of recurrences in patients who have already improved (Q26, Q27). The 'intervention level' property showed that the programme should be implemented at PC level –in coordination with the general practitioner and nurse – while also noting the advertising campaigns that have a great influence on the patients and their decision to follow specific lifestyle patterns (Q28), and the importance of education – beginning at primary level – on the acquisition of healthy lifestyle habits (Q29).

Table 5 shows the theoretical definitions for the basic properties of the model based on the results, summarizing the main influencing factors that both patients and healthcare professionals highlighted, in order to change behaviours of depressed patients, with especial emphasis on modifications to dietary and hygiene behaviour in order to adopt a healthier lifestyle.

Discussion

According to the results of this study, certain personal, programmatic and transversal properties affect the general objective of modifying dietary and hygiene behaviours. These characteristics, which may act as barriers or facilitators, are all interrelated.

The properties particularly emphasized for modifying dietary and hygiene behaviours in patients suffering from depression include the need to conduct a simple and motivating intervention at the appropriate moment when the patient is receptive and capable of overcoming apathy. For this, the patient must receive the support and supervision of a healthcare professional. Thus, PC may be an appropriate level at which to implement lifestyle modification programmes in individuals suffering from depression, since the conditions for effective change can be provided by patient-centred care that is accessible, comprehensive and ongoing [28]. The intervention might be planned between a general practitioner/nurse and the patient, using a motivational interview, because health professionals are trained in the field of changing habits, and a tailored intervention can be set up [48, 49] based on their knowledge of the patient. Moreover, they are in a position to motivate and enable, assess patient evolution and provide constant feedback [50, 51].

The main barriers faced by patients are of a psychological nature and are directly related to the symptoms of depression: apathy, feelings of guilt or incompetence, intrusive thoughts, cognitive avoidance and the need for cognitive restructuring [3, 6]. These barriers reduce motivation and hinder compliance, which is why interventions must be appropriate and timely, and should take into account the course of the disorder [52]. Time pressures in medical consultations [53], the possible inability to implement recommendations, and more particularly, not having the purchasing power to implement and maintain healthy habits are also perceived barriers to changing habits by professionals, who highlight the importance of driving modifications from a behavioural point of view. As expressed by some participants, by way of example, a healthy diet is more expensive than an unhealthy one. In fact, several studies conducted on the general population highlight a relationship between affordable or lower prices and the consumption of fruits and vegetables, and the resulting impact on body weight [54–57]. This relationship is also evidenced in the opposite direction, i.e. a tax on certain types of food and drinks reduce their consumption [54–57]. Furthermore, it has been demonstrated that specific changes in diet are maintained while there is purchasing power [55], so this is a particularly important factor when implementing an intervention for the modification of dietary and hygiene behaviours.

On the other hand, facilitators are factors that enable programme adherence, such as the simplicity of recommendations, which do not require instrumentation and are largely dependent on only the patients themselves, the tailoring of recommendations to their situation and the importance of motivating patients. These factors are consistent with several studies [24, 36] that highlight the importance of giving simple, progressive and tailored messages depending on the evolution of the disorder, and frequent repetition [58]. Behaviour modification is a process that usually requires successive approaches to learning, and it is important for patients to play a proactive role in change. The new experiences must be beneficial but also rewarding, since this increases the probability of repetition [59]. Supervision and assessment of compliance have been considered facilitators by patients and health professionals, respectively. ICTs (mobile apps, software, etc.) are an option to improve monitoring or its intensity, and they may be able to serve as support and complementary tools for both patients and health professionals in this regard [36]. Another important facilitator category is the perceived social support provided by the social network, or even better, that provided by the programme itself, as affirmed by patients. The social support provided by family, friends, associations, groups, etc. helps to create an appropriate environment in which patients feel capable of changing their habits and behaviours [36]. Social support has been defined as a protective factor against depression [60, 61], but it is modulated by the subjects' perceptions of the support that they receive; and for certain mental illnesses, it is known that depressed patients perceive less social support than they in fact have [62] . Thus, as has been observed by patients, professionals should try to create an intimate, trusting atmosphere in which patients feel entirely supported.

As discussed, general agreement exists regarding the idea that PC is the optimum level at which to implement lifestyle programmes for the modification of dietary and hygiene behaviours with depressive patients. However, other studies reveal that excessive workloads and time constraints to which health professionals are subjected make it difficult to implement these types of interventions in real practice, and continuous implementation is

Table 5 Theoretical definitions for the properties of the model

Core aspects	Categories/Properties	Definitions
Personal aspects	Personal history	
	-History and comorbidity	History, aetiology, course, severity of depressive disorder and comorbidity that determines psychological capacity.
	-Vital changes	Modifications in forms and lifestyles with significant effects for the subject.
	Disposition	
	-G. Facilitators	Personal or environmental aspects that encourage participation and engagement with the programme, like the feeling of improvement, the practice of certain activities, or the ease and simplicity of compliance.
	-G. Barriers	Personal or environmental aspects that complicate participation and commitment to the programme, such as the symptoms of the actual disorder, and apathy.
Program aspects	Presentation and monitoring	
	-Instructions	Clear presentation and explanation of the recommendations that make up the programme, using different channels and giving them the importance that they deserve, but with some flexibility, progressiveness and tailoring so that they are possible to implement.
	-Assessment	Assessment of compliance with the specific programme recommendations, with appropriate monitoring and support suited to the characteristics of patients and their disorder.
	-Supervision	Regular reminders and visits to a professional specialist in a personal and intimate context, which allows patients to converse in confidence.
	-Pharmaceutical	Managing of the antidepressant drugs, of possible improvement and their side effects.
	Cognitive habits	
	-Agency	Determination, personal effort when carrying out the program instructions, search for security and self-confidence.
	-Ruminations	Negative thoughts that hinder the implementation of the habits proposed in the programme.
	-Avoidance	Evasion of responsibilities via distracting activities on a cognitive level.
	-Restructurings	Modification of the values and ways of thinking in the sense of facilitating potential inclusion of the programme recommendations within the activities of daily life.
	-Guilt	Feelings of guilt derived from the failure to comply with the recommendations.
	Behavioural habits	
	-Activation	Mobilization of resources towards the carrying out of activities, breaking with inactivity and attempting to achieve behavioural objectives, little by little, generalized to all spheres.
	-Empowerment	To enable patients to lead their recovery.
	-Time pressure	Difficulties for giving instructions regarding change of habits in a short consultation.
	-Habit control	Personal ability to implement habit requirements and recommendations.
	-Opportunities	Socio-economic capacity to acquire certain foods, to follow certain instructions, and to carry out physical and pleasant activities.
Transversal aspects	Social support	
	-Group format of intervention	Social support coming from the group format of intervention, which helps to realize one is not alone when facing difficulties, in order to cope with depression and change habits.
	-Contact with others	People in the patient's close social context – apart from family members and friends – that provide face-to-face contact and the opportunity for the acquisition of recommendations.
	Objectives	
	-Adjustment	Fit of the programme to the situation of each patient, with special interest in the prevention of recurrences once the patient has improved depression.
	-Intervention level	Special affinity of the programme with a level of individual intervention integrated in healthcare systems, although with possible connections with the media and educational systems.

still sub-optimal [63, 64]. Educational, legislative and fiscal measures regarding food prices, environmental planning, and communication and marketing campaigns are important factors that have been highlighted by healthcare professionals to help assure the success of the intervention. This idea is consistent with results from other studies: fiscal measures regarding food prices help to regulate consumption [54–57] and marketing campaigns and audio-visual messages broadcast on television, in particular, have demonstrated their effectiveness in changing habits at a community level [65] through the use of emotional drivers to encourage behaviour change [66], such as affiliation, the presentation of aversive stimuli, etc. Nevertheless, at this time the role of the education system is still in question given the inconsistent results from several studies [67].

This study has certain limitations, mainly arising from the complexity of establishing a theoretical framework and taxonomy for changing lifestyles [68]. On the contrary, the main strength of this study is the triangulation of information related to the techniques of individual and group interviews, including the complementarity of patients and healthcare professionals, and therefore providing result with greater perspective. As for the generalizability of the results, the selection criteria for participants were defined with pragmatic intention; thus they are wide and relatively unrestrictive. This increases the heterogeneity of the sample and brings it closer to the real population of depressed patients served by PC professionals, while also allowing for the collection of a wide range of opinions.

Conclusions

The implementation of intervention programmes that combine dietary and hygiene factors in patients with depression is complex, given the nature of the disorder itself and that of some of its main symptoms, such as apathy, the feeling of guilt, or ruminations on incompetence. However, key points exist for the success of the intervention, such as the simplicity of the guidelines, the tailoring of the intervention through motivational interviewing, and the prolonged and intense monitoring throughout the different stages of the disorder and the provision of adequate feedback. Taking into account its own limitations (e.g. time pressure), PC could be an appropriate level at which to implement these interventions, although educational, legislative and fiscal measures, environmental planning, and communication and marketing campaigns may be important factors that should also be considered.

Abbreviations

ICT: Information and communications technology; PC: Primary Care

Acknowledgements

We wish to thank the Instituto de Salud Carlos III of the Spanish Ministry of Health for funding the study (FIS n° PI11/01392). We thank the Research Network on Preventive Activities and Health promotioP ("Red de Investigación en Actividades Preventivas y de Promoción de la Salud - RedIAPP") for its support in the development of the study.

Funding

We received a specific grant from Instituto de Salud Carlos III of the Spanish Ministry of Health (FIS No. PI11/01392) for developing a randomized controlled trial on the effectiveness of recommendations for healthy dietary and hygiene behaviours as an adjuvant treatment in patients with depression in Primary Care.

Authors' contributions

BOB, MGT and MCSB were responsible for the study design. BOB, MSB, MGT, MJSR and AC collected the data from the interviews and groups. BOB and JMM were responsible of the qualitative analysis. All the authors interpreted the data. BOB and JMM wrote the first version of the manuscript and all authors participated in the review of the manuscript. All authors read and approved the final manuscript.

Consent for publication

Not applicable because the data are anonymous and there are no individual images.

Competing interests

The authors declare that they have no competing interests.

Author details

[1]Department of Psychology and Sociology, University of Zaragoza, Violante de Hungria 23, 50009 Zaragoza, Spain. [2]Research Network on Preventive Activities and Health Promotion (Red de Investigación en Actividades Preventivas y Promoción de la Salud - RedIAPP), Barcelona, Spain. [3]Promosam Network, Red de Excelencia PSI2014-56303-REDT PROMOSAM: (Investigación en procesos, mecanismos y tratamientos psicológicos para la promoción de la salud mental), Economy and Competitiveness Ministry, Madrid, Spain. [4]Institut Universitari d'Investigació en Ciències de la Salut (IUNICS), Universitat de les Illes Balears (UIB), Palma de Mallorca, Spain. [5]Departamento de Psiquiatría, Parc Sanitari San Joan de Déu, Sant Boi de Llobregat, Spain. [6]Aragones Health Service, Zaragoza, Spain. [7]Institut Català de la Salut, Barcelona, Spain. [8]Department of Medicine and Psychiatry, University of Zaragoza, Zaragoza, Spain.

References

1. Ferrari AJ, Charlson FJ, Norman RE, Patten SB, Freedman G, Murray CJ, Vos T, Whiteford HA. Burden of depressive disorders by country, sex, age, and year: findings from the global burden of disease study 2010. PLoS Med. 2013;10: e1001547. https://doi.org/10.1371/journal.pmed.1001547.
2. Gabilondo A, Rojas-Farreras S, Vilagut G, Haro JM, Fernández A, Pinto-Meza A, Alonso J. Epidemiology of major depressive episode in a southern

European country: results from the ESEMeD-Spain project. J Affect Disord. 2010;120(1–3):76–85. https://doi.org/10.1016/j.jad.2009.04.016.

3. Stegmann ME, Ormel J, de Graaf R, Haro JM, de Girolamo G, Demyttenaere K, Kovess V, Matschinger H, Vilagut G, Alonso J, Burger H, ESEMED/MHEDEA Investigators. Functional disability as an explanation of the associations between chronic physical conditions and 12-month major depressive episode. J Affect Disord. 2010;124(1–2):38–44. https://doi.org/10.1016/j.jad.2009.10.026.
4. Sarris J, O'Neil A, Coulson CE, Schweitzer I, Berk M. Lifestyle medicine for depression. BMC Psychiatry. 2014;10(14):107. https://doi.org/10.1186/1471-244X-14-107.
5. Hidaka BH. Depression as a disease of modernity: explanations for increasing prevalence. J Affect Disord. 2012;140(3):205–14. https://doi.org/10.1016/j.jad.2011.12.036.
6. Kupfer DJ, Frank E, Phillips ML. Major depressive disorder: new clinical, neurobiological, and treatment perspectives. Lancet. 2012;379(9820):1045–55. https://doi.org/10.1016/S0140-6736(11)60602-8.
7. Lopresti AL, Hood SD, Drummond PD. A review of lifestyle factors that contribute to important pathways associated with major depression: diet, sleep and exercise. J Affect Disord. 2013;148:12–27. https://doi.org/10.1016/j.jad.2013.01.014.
8. Oliver-Quetglas A, Torres E, March S, Socias IM, Esteva M. Risk factors of depressive syndrome in young adults. Actas Esp Psiquiatr. 2013;41(2):84–96.
9. Patten SB, Kennedy SH, Lam RW, O'Donovan C, Filteau MJ, Parikh SV, Ravindran AV. Clinical guidelines for the management of major depressive disorder in adults. I. Classification, burden and principles of management. J Affect Disord. 2009;117(Suppl 1):5–14. https://doi.org/10.1016/j.jad.2009.06.044.
10. García-Toro M, Vicens-Pons E, Gili M, Roca M, Serrano-Ripoll MJ, Vives M, Leiva A, Yáñez AM, Bennasar-Veny M, Oliván-Blázquez B. Obesity, metabolic syndrome and Mediterranean diet: impact on depression outcome. J Affect Disord. 2016;19(194):105–8. https://doi.org/10.1016/j.jad.2015.12.064.
11. Van Strien T, Konttinen H, Homberg JR, Engels RC, Winkens LH. Emotional eating as a mediator between depression and weight gain. Appetite. 2016; 18 https://doi.org/10.1016/j.appet.2016.02.034.
12. Luppino FS, De Wit LM, Bouvy PF, Stijnen T, Cuijpers P, Penninx B, et al. Overweight, obesity, and depression: a systematic review and meta-analysis of longitudinal studies. Arch Gen Psychiatry. 2010;67(3):220–9. https://doi.org/10.1001/archgenpsychiatry.2010.2.
13. Fabricatore AN, Wadden TA, Higginbotham AJ, Faulconbridge LF, Nguyen AM, Heymsfield SB, Faith MS. Intentional weight loss and changes in symptoms of depression: a systematic review and meta-analysis. Int J Obes. 2011;35(11):1363–76. https://doi.org/10.1038/ijo.2011.2.
14. Simon GE, Rohde P, Ludman EJ, Jeffery RW, Linde JA, Operskalski BH, et al. Association between change in depression and change in weight among women enrolled in weight loss treatment. Gen Hosp Psychiatry. 2010;32(6):583–9. https://doi.org/10.1016/j.genhosppsych.2010.09.010.
15. Pagoto S, Bodenlos JS, Schneider KL, Olendzki B, Spates CR, Ma Y. Initial investigation of behavioral activation therapy for co-morbid major depressive disorder and obesity. Psychotherapy. 2008;45(3):410–5. https://doi.org/10.1037/a0013313.
16. Pan A, Sun Q, Czernichow S, Kivimaki M, Okereke OI, Lucas M, Manson JE, Ascherio A, Hu FB. Bidirectional association between depression and obesity in middle-aged and older women. Int J Obes. 2012;36(4):595–602. https://doi.org/10.1038/ijo.2011.111.
17. Preiss K, Brennan L, Clarke D. A systematic review of variables associated with the relationship between obesity and depression. Obes Rev. 2013; 14(11):906–18. https://doi.org/10.1111/obr.12052.
18. Quirk SE, Williams LJ, O'Neil A, Pasco JA, Jacka FN, Housden S, Berk M, Brennan SL. The association between diet quality, dietary patterns and depression in adults: a systematic review. BMC Psychiatry. 2013;27(13):175. https://doi.org/10.1186/1471-244X-13-175. 13, 175.
19. García-Toro M, Ibarra O, Gili M, Serrano MJ, Oliván B, Vicens E, Roca M. Four hygienic-dietary recommendations as add-on treatment in depression: a randomized-controlled trial. J Affect Disord. 2012;140:200–3. https://doi.org/10.1016/j.jad.2012.
20. Lee SH, Paz-Filho G, Mastronardi C, Licinio J, Wong ML. Is increased antidepressant exposure a contributory factor to the obesity pandemic? Transl Psychiatry. 2016;6:e759. https://doi.org/10.1038/tp.2016.25.
21. Walsh R. Lifestyle and mental health. Am Psychol. 2011;66(7):579–2. https://doi.org/10.1037/a0021769.
22. Daubenmier JJ, Weidner G, Sumner MD, Mendell N, Merritt-Worden T, Studley J, Ornish D. The contribution of changes in diet, exercise, and stress management to changes in coronary risk in women and men in the multisite cardiac lifestyle intervention program. Ann Behav Med. 2007; 33(1):57–68.
23. Serrano Ripoll MJ, Oliván-Blázquez B, Vicens-Pons E, Roca M, Gili M, Leiva A, García-Campayo J, Demarzo MP, García-Toro M. Lifestyle change recommendations in major depression: do they work? J Affect Disord. 2015; 1(183):221–8. https://doi.org/10.1016/j.jad.2015.04.059.
24. Price P. How can we improve adherence? Diabetes Metab Res Rev. 2016; 32(S1):201–5. https://doi.org/10.1002/dmrr.2744.
25. Laranjo L, Neves AL, Costa A, Ribeiro RT, Couto L, Sá AB. Facilitators, barriers and expectations in the self-management of type 2 diabetes–a qualitative study from Portugal. Eur J Gen Pract. 2015;21(2):103–10. https://doi.org/10.3109/13814788.2014.1000855.
26. García-Sanjuán S, Lillo-Crespo M, Sanjuán-Quiles Á, Richart-Martínez M. Dietary habits and feeding beliefs of people with Crohn's disease. Nutr Hosp. 2015;32(6):2948–55. https://doi.org/10.3305/nh.2015.32.6.9894.
27. Cole JA, Smith SM, Hart N, Cupples ME. Do practitioners and friends support patients with coronary heart disease in lifestyle change? a qualitative study. BMC Fam Pract. 2013;28(14):126. https://doi.org/10.1186/1471-2296-14-126.
28. Green L, Fryer GJ, Yawn B, Lanier D, Dovey S. The ecology of medical care revisited. N Engl J Med. 2001;344(26):2021–5.
29. van't Veer-Tazelaar PJ, van Marwijk HW, van OP, van der Horst HE, Smit F, Cuijpers P, et al. Prevention of late-life anxiety and depression has sustained effects over 24 months: a pragmatic randomized trial. Am J Geriatr Psychiatry. 2011;19(3):230–9.
30. Pope C, Mays N, editors. Qualitative Research in Health Care. London: BMJ books; 2000. p. 168.
31. Montero-Marín J, Prado-Abril J, Botella C, Mayoral-Cleries F, Baños R, Herrera-Mercadal P, Romero-Sanchiz P, Gili M, Castro A, Nogueira R, García-Campayo J. Expectations among patients and health professionals regarding web-based interventions for depression in primary care: a qualitative study. J Med Internet Res. 2015;17(3):e67. https://doi.org/10.2196/jmir.3985.
32. Denzin N, Lincoln Y. Introduction: Entering the field of qualitative research. In: Denzin N, Lincoln Y, editors. Handbook of Qualitative Research. California: Sage; 1994. p. 1–18.
33. García-Toro M, Roca M, Monzón S, Vives M, Oliván B, Vicens E, Salva J, Gili M. Hygienic-dietary recommendations for major depression treatment: study protocol of a randomized controlled trial. BMC Psychiatry. 2012;12:201. https://doi.org/10.1186/1471-244X-12-201.
34. Beck AT, Steer RA, Brown GK. BDI-II –Beck depression inventory manual, volume second. San Antonio: The Psychological Corporation; 1996.
35. García-Toro M, Ibarra O, Gili M, Serrano MJ, Vives M, Monzón S, Bauzá N, Oliván B, Vicens E, Roca M. Adherence to lifestyle recommendations by patients with depression. Rev Psiquiatr Salud Ment. 2012;5(4):236–40. https://doi.org/10.1016/j.rpsm.2012.04.003.
36. NICE public health guidance [PH49]. Behaviour change: individual approaches. 2014. https://www.nice.org.uk/guidance/ph49. Accessed 12 Oct 2016.
37. Strauss A, Corbin J. Basics of qualitative research. 2nd ed. London: Sage; 1998.
38. Strauss A. Qualitative analysis for social scientists. Cambridge: Cambridge University Press; 1987.
39. Glaser BG, Strauss AL. The discovery of grounded theory. Chicago: Aldine; 1967.
40. Alonso LE. A qualitative approach to sociology. An interpretative approach. Madrid: Editorial Fundamentos; 1998.
41. Gaitán JA, Piñuel JL. Técnicas de Investigación en comunicación social (Research techniques in social communication). Madrid: Síntesis; 1998. p. 281–311.
42. Vallés MS. Técnicas Cualitativas de Investigación Social (Qualitative Social Research Techniques). Madrid: Síntesis Sociología; 2003.
43. Rapley T. Doing conversation, discourse and document analysis. London: Sage; 2007.
44. Gibbs G. The analysis of qualitative data in qualitative research. Madrid: Morata; 2012.
45. Callejo Gallego J, Val Cid C, Gutiérrez BritoJ, Viedma Rojas A. Introduction to social research techniques. Madrid: Ed. Ramón Areces; 2017.
46. Bluethmann SM, Bartholomew LK, Murphy CC, Vernon SW. Use of theory in behavior change interventions. Health Educ Behav. 2017;44(2):245–53. https://doi.org/10.1177/1090198116647712.
47. Phillips N, Hardy C. Discourse analysis. Investigating processes of social construction. Thousand Oaks: Sage; 2002. p. 104.
48. Jameson JL, Longo DL. Precision medicine–personalized, problematic, and promising. N Engl J Med. 2015;372(23):2229–34. https://doi.org/10.1056/NEJMsb1503104.
49. Patel V. Rethinking personalised medicine. Lancet. 2015;385(9980):1826–7. https://doi.org/10.1016/S0140-6736(15)60917-5.

50. Johnson MJ, May CR. Promoting professional behaviour change in healthcare: what interventions work, and why? A theory-led overview of systematic reviews. BMJ Open. 2015;5(9):e008592. https://doi.org/10.1136/bmjopen-2015-008592.
51. Tuccero D, Railey K, Briggs M, Hull SK. Behavioral health in prevention and chronic illness management: Motivational Interviewing. Prim Care. 2016; 43(2):191–202. https://doi.org/10.1016/j.pop.2016.01.006.
52. Post RM. Heading off depressive illness evolution and progression to treatment resistance. Dialogues Clin Neurosci. 2015;17(2):105–9.
53. Molina Siguero A, García Pérez MA, Alonso González M, Cecilia Cermeño P. Prevalence of worker burnout and psychiatric illness in primary care physicians in a health care area in Madrid. Aten Primaria. 2003;31(9):564–71.
54. Powell LM, Chriqui JF, Khan T, Wada R, Chaloupka FJ. Assessing the potential effectiveness of food and beverage taxes and subsidies for improving public health: a systematic review of prices, demand and body weight outcomes. Obes Rev. 2013;14(29):110–28. https://doi.org/10.1111/obr.12002.
55. Powell LM, Kumanyika SK, Isgor Z, Rimkus L, Zenk SN, Chaloupka FJ. Price promotions for food and beverage products in a nationwide sample of food stores. Prev Med. 2016;86:106–13. https://doi.org/10.1016/j.ypmed.2016.01.011.
56. Epstein LH, Finkelstein E, Raynor H, Nederkoorn C, Fletcher KD, Jankowiak N, Paluch RA. Experimental analysis of the effect of taxes and subsides on calories purchased in an on-line supermarket. Appetite. 2015;95:245–51. https://doi.org/10.1016/j.appet.2015.06.020.
57. Le HN, Gold L, Abbott G, Crawford D, McNaughton SA, Mhurchu CN, Pollard C, Ball K. Economic evaluation of price discounts and skill-building strategies on purchase and consumption of healthy food and beverages: the SHELf randomized controlled trial. Soc Sci Med. 2016;159:83–91. https://doi.org/10.1016/j.socscimed.2016.04.015.
58. Bombardier CH, Ehde DM, Gibbons LE, Wadhwani R, Sullivan MD, Rosenberg DE, Kraft GH. Telephone-based physical activity counseling for major depression in people with multiple sclerosis. J Consult Clin Psychol. 2013;81(1):89–99. https://doi.org/10.1037/a0031242.
59. Marqués Molias F, Cabezas C, Camarelle F, Córdoba R, Gómez- Puente J, Muñoz E. Recommendations about lifestyles. Preventive activities program and health promotion PAPPS. Update. Health education group. Barcelona: Spanish Society of Family Medicine Society. 2009. http://www.papps.es/upload/file/08%20PAPPS%20ACTUALIZACION%202009.pdf. Accessed 11 June 2017.
60. Goldberg D, Kendler K, Sirovatka P, Regier D. Diagnostic Issues in Depression and Generalized Anxiety Disorder Refining the Research Agenda for DSM-V. Arlington: American Psychiatric Association; 2010.
61. Santini ZI, Koyanagi A, Tyrovolas S, Mason C, Haro JM. The association between social relationships and depression: a systematic review. J Affect Disord. 2015;175:53–64. https://doi.org/10.1016/j.jad.2014.12.049.
62. Leskelä US, Melartin TK, Lestelä-Mielonen PS, Rytsälä HJ, Sokero TP, Heikkinen ME, Isometsä ET. Life events, social support, and onset of major depressive episode in finnish patients. J Nerv Ment Dis. 2004;192(5):373–81.
63. Brotons C, Björkelund C, Bulc M, Ciurana R, Godycki-Cwirko M, Jurgova E, et al. Prevention and health promotion in clinical practice: the views of general practitioners in Europe. Prev Med. 2005;40(5):595–601.
64. Rubio-Valera M, Pons-Vigués M, Martínez-Andrés M, Moreno-Peral P, Berenguera A, Fernández A. Barriers and facilitators for the implementation of primary prevention and health promotion activities in primary care: a synthesis through meta-ethnography. PLoS One. 2014;9(2):e89554. https://doi.org/10.1371/journal.pone.0089554.
65. White S, Schmidt W, Sahanggamu D, Fatmaningrum D, van Liere M, Curtis V. Can gossip change nutrition behaviour? Results of a mass media and community-based intervention trial in east java, Indonesia. Tropical Med Int Health. 2016;21(3):348–64. https://doi.org/10.1111/tmi.12660.
66. Aunger R, Curtis V. Behavior Centred Desig. London: London School of Hygiene and Tropical Medicine; 2015.
67. Moore GF, Littlecott HJ, Turley R, Waters E, Murphy S. Socioeconomic gradients in the effects of universal school-based health behaviour interventions: a systematic review of intervention studies. BMC Public Health. 2015;17(15):907. https://doi.org/10.1186/s12889-015-2244-x.
68. Michie S, Wood CE, Johnston M, Abraham C, Francis JJ, Hardeman W. Behaviour change techniques: the development and evaluation of a taxonomic method for reporting and describing behaviour change interventions (a suite of five studies involving consensus methods, randomised controlled trials and analysis of qualitative data). Health Technol Assess. 2015;19(99):1–188. https://doi.org/10.3310/hta19990.

9

Factors associated with hospitalization after self-poisoning in France: special focus on the impact of alcohol use disorder

Juliette Salles[1,2,3*], Julie Calonge[1], Nicolas Franchitto[1,3], Emmanuelle Bougon[1,2] and Laurent Schmitt[1,2]

Abstract

Background: Previous studies have identified factors associated with admission to hospital after suicide spectrum behaviors. In this study, we aim to identify specific factors associated with psychiatric hospitalization after self-poisoning. Given earlier findings suggesting that alcohol use disorder is not associated with hospital admission, we also aim to consider its impact, as well as blood alcohol concentrations, on hospitalization decisions after a suicide attempt.

Methods: We studied the association between demographic features, suicide intent, psychiatric characteristics and admission to hospital in self-poisoning patients in an emergency department in France.

Results: Suicide intent, a past history of suicide attempts, bipolar disorder and depression were associated with psychiatric hospital admissions. Despite alcohol use disorder being known to be associated with a suicide risk, it was not linked with psychiatric hospitalization. A positive blood alcohol concentration in the emergency department likewise had no association with admission to a psychiatric ward for inpatient care.

Conclusions: Our findings were similar to those reported for other suicide spectrum behaviors. Alcohol use disorder was not associated with admission for inpatient psychiatric care, whereas depression clearly was. The cause of this discrepancy must be determined in future research.

Keywords: Suicide, Epidemiology, Hospitalization, Alcohol use disorder

Background

Suicide is a major global public health concern and in Europe represents 1.5% of all deaths [1]. The causes of suicide are multiple and complex and can be linked to psychological, environmental and cultural factors. Among the psychological factors, mental illnesses such as mood disorders, schizophrenia, anxiety disorders, post-traumatic stress and substance abuse [2–6] play an important role and must be regarded as specific suicide risk factors.

In terms of suicide care, 80% of patients receiving medical help after a suicide attempt are admitted to the emergency ward. In France, every patient hospitalized for an attempted suicide benefits from a psychiatric assessment [7]. This assessment is an opportunity to evaluate the suicide risk, initiate treatment if required and prevent future self-harm. The assessment of suicide spectrum behaviors in the emergency department is a key factor in preventing suicide [8]. The suicidal patient may be discharged or hospitalized based on the assessment. There are many guidelines on how suicide assessments should be conducted, but none are universally accepted [9–11]. The referral of patients for hospitalization or discharge is a crucial clinical decision, and most guidelines recommend that direct discharge from the emergency department should be considered if an after-care plan can be arranged before the patient leaves hospital. In France, attempted suicide by self-poisoning represents 81.7% of all suicide attempts. Overall, 66% of self-poisoned patients are women versus 63% for the entire population of suicide attempters versus 45% for other methods. The frequency of self-poisoning versus other suicide methods decreases with age [12]. Compared with other methods, previous

* Correspondence: juliette.salles@hotmail.fr
[1]Université de Toulouse III, F-31000 Toulouse, France
[2]CHU Toulouse, Service de Psychiatrie eSt Psychologie, Psychiatrie, F-31000 Toulouse, France

studies have found that patients who self-poison are less often psychotic and more often have an anxiety or affective disorder than those admitted following the use of violent methods such as hanging, cutting, jumping, and the use of firearms. However, no differences in demographic characteristics (age, marital status, living conditions, educational status and employment status) and a past history of suicide attempts have been identified [13].

Hospitalization is recommended if there is an imminent risk of suicide. Admission policies for suicide treatment have been associated with clinical and psychological factors such as older age, male gender, poor physical health, psychosis, high suicidal intent, a plan to use a lethal method, previous psychiatric hospitalization, a past history of suicide attempts and a low expectation of being found after an attempt [8, 14]. Hospitalization is generally indicated if the attempt was violent or premeditated, precautions were taken to avoid rescue, distress is increased, the patient regrets surviving, the patient has limited social support, there is current impulsive behavior or a refusal of help is evident, and the patient has a change in mental status with a metabolic, toxic, infectious or other etiology requiring further workup in a structured setting. However, when considering hospitalization, the risk of suicide is not the only factor to take into account, as admission to hospital could reinforce dependency and regressive behaviors. Psychiatric inpatients and their relatives may also have unrealistic expectations and hospitalization can be associated with disillusionment and may contribute to feelings of hopelessness. Moreover, in cases of personality disorder, it may lead to a vicious circle of intensifying suicidal thoughts that require more restrictive care [15].

Within psychiatric disorders, alcohol use disorder (AUD) is particularly associated with an increased suicide mortality rate, which is six times higher than in the general population [16]. A literature review put the suicide risk over a lifetime at 3.4% in AUD populations in the USA [17], while a meta-analysis found a strong association between suicide attempts and alcohol consumption (OR = 3.1) [18].

Despite the impact that acute alcohol consumption has on decision making, AUD appears to not be related to clinicians' decisions to hospitalize, even though the association between AUD and suicide is largely documented. Indeed, one study [19] specifically addressed the issue of clinical decision-making with respect to hospitalization in a population of patients demonstrating suicide spectrum behaviors, including suicidal ideation, non-suicidal injuries and suicide attempts. This research found that AUD was not associated with admission for inpatient psychiatric care, whereas schizophrenia and depression were. The authors hypothesized that clinicians' decisions about hospitalization could be more related to drug or alcohol consumption associated with suicide attempts than to AUD [20].

Previous data on factors associated with hospital admissions are available for suicide spectrum behaviors, especially in Spain [8, 19]. However, there is a difference between countries concerning care management, which is why we sought to replicate those results in France. In particular, we aimed to identify factors associated with psychiatric hospitalization, especially in a population of self-poisoning suicide attempters. Regarding previous results, we also aimed to pay specific attention to the impact of AUD and blood alcohol concentrations (BAC) on clinicians' decisions concerning hospitalization.

Methods

Participants

The study took place in Toulouse University Hospital, which is located in the south of France. This hospital benefits from an emergency room that is specifically set up to deal with self-poisoning patients. This ward is a medical department directed by an emergency team in which a psychiatric liaison team ensures that appropriate psychiatric assessments are carried out. This team consists of a nurse and a psychiatrist working 7 days a week, 24 h a day. All patients who attempt suicide by self-poisoning are referred to this unit.

The WHO definition of a suicide attempt was used, namely: any "act with a non-fatal outcome, in which an individual deliberately initiates a non-habitual behavior that without intervention from others will cause self-harm or deliberately ingests a substance in excess of the prescribed or generally recognized therapeutic dosage" [21].

This article is based on data initially collected between November 2016 and April 2017 for an Intent of Suicide and Alcohol (ISA) study. Patients were excluded if they were under 18 years old, because of the legal liability for research participation. Patients with a diagnosis of mild or severe mental disability and mild or severe neurocognitive impairment were also excluded to ensure the quality of responses. We used administrative data to compare included attempters versus non-included attempters. During the relevant period, 98 patients did not meet the inclusion criteria. In total, 519 patients were recruited, but three were excluded because of incomplete data (Fig. 1).

Measurements

The data collected included patients' sociodemographic and clinical features, personal and familial history of suicide attempts and type of follow-up (inpatient or outpatient care).

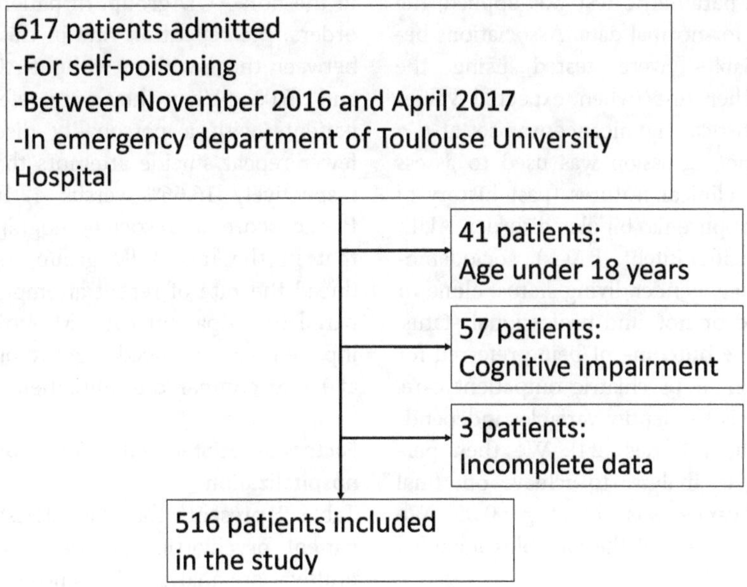

Fig. 1 Flow chart

Sociodemographic characteristics consisted of age, gender, living status (alone or not) and employment status.

Clinical features comprised psychiatric diagnoses according to the DSM IV criteria, which were assessed by referring to the Mini International Neuropsychiatry Interview (MINI) subset (A-I) [22].

Data on prior mental health-care included previous psychiatric follow-up by a psychiatrist, a history of suicide attempts and a personality disorder diagnosis. This data was collected from the information in patient assessments or the emergency database concerning previous medical involvement.

Data concerning suicide attempts included information obtained from the Intent of Suicide Assessment, which is based on the Pierce Scale [23]. The Pierce Scale is a 12-item questionnaire designed to assess the severity of suicide intent associated with an episode of self-harm. Each item scores 0–3, giving a total score of 0–25. The questionnaire is divided into three sections: the first six items constitute the "circumstances" section and are concerned with the objective circumstances of the act of self-harm; the following four items constitute the "self--report" section and are based on patients' own reconstructions of their feelings and thoughts at the time of the act; finally the remaining two items constitute the "risk" section and are concerned with the medical risk of self-harm relative to the lethality of the suicide method.

Blood samples were taken systematically at the time of admission to the emergency unit in order to determine blood alcohol concentrations (BACs).

Referrals were separated into two pathways:

-Outpatient psychiatric care: this consisted of an at-home psychiatric appointment with a primary psychiatrist, information to make an appointment with a psychiatrist in public medical psychological centers (CMPs) or an appointment with a psychiatrist in a brief therapy center (CTB).

-Inpatient psychiatric care: this consisted of either voluntary or forced hospitalization in a psychiatric department.

The psychiatric assessments were performed in an emergency ward that enabled all patients to be evaluated, including those who were severely intoxicated. Evaluations were performed after cognitive assessments and negative BACs were obtained to ensure that patients were capable of being assessed.

Referrals were systematically determined by a psychiatrist during a psychiatric assessment.

We also collected data relating to repeat suicide attempts at 1 year from the administrative database of Toulouse University's emergency department.

Data analysis

We compared sociodemographic characteristics and clinical features according to the referral after the psychiatric assessment. Quantitative variables are described using the mean (+/− standard deviation) and/or median (+/− interquartile range) according to their distributions.

The Shapiro-Wilk test was performed to evaluate the normality distribution of the data. In cases of non-normal data, the Wilcoxon non-parametric test was applied; the Student T test was used for normal data. Associations between qualitative variables were tested using the chi-squared or the Fischer test (when expected values were less than five). Statistical significance was set at $p <$ 0.05. Multinomial logistic regression was used to assess the association between clinical features (past history of suicide, depression, schizophrenia, bipolar disorder, AUD, personality disorder, suicide intent, BACs), sociodemographic characteristics (age, gender, living status: alone or not, living status: housed or not, and professional status: employed or not), and the outcome of being referred for psychiatric hospitalization or psychiatric outpatient care. We used a logistic analysis to identify variables independently associated with the referrals [24]. We then performed backward stepwise analyses to achieve our final model. Statistical significance was set at $p < 0.05$. We tested the interactions between all the variables included in the final model.

The statistical analyses were performed using the R-Studio software, version 14R (StataCorp LP, College Station, TX, USA).

Results

Sample description

A total of 165 men (31.9%) and 351 women (68.1%) were included in the sample. The mean age was 40.5 (SD = 14.8) and the median age 42 (IQ = 27–51). Overall, during self-poisoning, 38.58% of patients ingested two medications, 10.85% ingested three and 1.16% ingested more than three. The most common medications used were benzodiazepines, with 85% of patients ingesting at least one of these. Paracetamol accounted for 8.91% of the ingested drugs and opioids 3.68%. The characteristics of the overall sample are described in Table 1.

Most of the patients did not live alone (65.1%), 38.0% were employed and 92.0% had a home. More than half of the patients had a history of suicide attempts (59.7%) and 17.8% had a family history of suicide. In our sample, according to the DSM IV criteria, the AUD prevalence was 30.0%, the mood disorder prevalence 44.0%, including 33.0% with depression and 11.0% with bipolar disorder, and the schizophrenia prevalence was 3%. Thirty-four percent of patients had a previous diagnosis of a personality disorder, mostly borderline personality (58.2%).

After psychiatric assessment, 32.9% of patients were referred for inpatient psychiatric care and 67.1% to outpatient care. Compulsory inpatient admissions comprised 9% of the total admissions.

The repeat suicide attempt rate within the one-year follow-up period was 25.51%: 24.69% for inpatient care and 28.10% for outpatient care. Patients suffering from AUD had a higher rate of repetition of 38%, versus 24% in the non-AUD group. In patients with personality disorders, the repetition rate in this sub-group was similar between those with or without AUD: respectively 34.53% and 36.0%. When they were referred for inpatient care, patients with a personality disorder and AUD made fewer repeat suicide attempts than those without AUD: respectively 16.66% versus 42.10%. Adjusting for the Pierce score and sociodemographic factors, we found that in the non-AUD group inpatient orientation reduced the rate of repeat attempts by 2% at 1 year compared to outpatient care. Moreover, in the AUD group, inpatient care reduced the rate of repeat attempts by 5% at 1 year compared to outpatient care.

Factors associated with referral for psychiatric hospitalization

Table 2 presents the characteristics associated with inpatient psychiatric care determined by univariate and multivariate analyses. We chose to include variables previously associated with a suicide risk in the model.

In the univariate analysis, age ($p \leq 0.001$) and depression ($p \leq 0.001$) were significantly associated with psychiatric hospitalization, whereas personality disorder ($p \leq 0.001$) was associated with outpatient care.

In the multivariate analysis, compared to those who had no depression, those who were depressed were more often hospitalized in the psychiatric department (OR = 3.6, 95% CI = 2.18–6.05). Bipolar disorder (OR = 3.16; 1.57–6.33), a history of suicide attempts (OR = 1.53; 0.95–2.47) and suicide intent (OR = 1.18; 0.13–1.24) were also associated with a higher rate of hospitalization.

The association of a personality disorder or schizophrenia with hospitalization was not significant.

Although AUD was significantly related to a suicide risk, patients suffering from the condition did not have a higher likelihood of being referred to inpatient care (OR = 0.87; 0.49–1.54) ($p = 0.65$). BACs were also not associated with a clinician's decision to hospitalize a patient (OR = 0.87; 0.64–1.18), ($p = 0.39$) (Fig. 1).

As the presence of a personality disorder often affected the referral decision, we performed a regression analysis on patients that excluded this as a variable. The results were similar to those observed in the overall sample. Indeed, we noted that depressive episodes (OR = 3.58, 95% CI = 1.93–6.80) ($p < 0.001$), bipolar disorder (OR = 2.36, 95% CI = 1.02–5.44) ($p = 0.04$), the Pierce score (OR = 1.17, 95% CI = 1.11–1.23) ($p < 0.001$) and housing status (OR = 3.21, 95% CI = 1.87–16.97) ($p < 0.001$) were associated with inpatient referrals Fig. 2.

Discussion

The main finding of our study was that AUD was not associated with psychiatric admissions. This also underlined a discrepancy in the consideration of AUD and

Table 1 Descriptive characteristics of the study population

	N	%
Age		
18-39 years	233	45.16
40-59 years	242	46.90
more than 60 years	41	7.95
Gender		
Men	165	31.98
Women	351	68.02
Number of medication used		
One	516	100
Two	199	38.56
Three	56	10.85
More than three	6	1.16
Type of drug used		
Benzodiazepine	439	85
Paracetamol	46	8.91
Non-steroidal anti-inflammatory Drugs	25	4.84
Neuroleptic	46	8.91
Antidepressant	26	5.03
Opioids	19	3.68
Others	35	6.78
Not known	10	1.93
Past history of suicide	308	59.69
Family past history of suicide	92	17.83
Psychiatric disorder	351	68.02
Depression	170	32.95
Schizophrenia	18	3.49
Bipolar disorder	59	11.43
Alcohol use disorder (AUD)	155	30.04
AUD and depression	54	34.83
AUD and bipolar disorder	13	8.38
AUD and schizophrenia	4	2.58
AUD and personality disorder	65	41.93
Borderline	23	14.83
Dependent	31	20.00
Avoiding	2	1.29
Histrionic	1	0.64
Narcissistic	1	0.64
Obsessive	1	0.64
Antisocial	6	3.87
Personality disorder	178	34.50
Borderline	104	20.16
Dependent	45	8.72
Avoiding	1	0.19
Histrionic	6	1.16

Table 1 Descriptive characteristics of the study population *(Continued)*

	N	%
Narcissistic	3	0.58
Obsessive	2	0.39
Antisocial	17	3.29
Single	179	34.69
Employed	198	38.37
Housing	474	91.86

other psychiatric diagnoses such as depression and bipolar disorders, which were associated with more inpatient referrals.

Admission rate

The total admission rate of 32.9% in our sample is higher than that previously described in Spain (26.8%) [19] or Finland (24%) [25], but is lower than the rate in Switzerland, England or the WHO/Euro Multicentre Study on Parasuicide, in which almost half of patients were admitted for inpatient care after a suicide attempt [9, 26, 27].Those differences in hospitalization rates could be explained by differences in patient characteristics, care organizations and clinical practices.

Factors associated with psychiatric hospitalization

Depression was the main predictive factor of psychiatric inpatient care. Depression is also the most common psychiatric disorder in suicide attempters [28, 29]. This was also the case in our study, with it accounting for 48% of all psychiatric diagnoses. Bipolar disorder was independently associated with increased hospitalization. This is unsurprising, as it is known to be associated with suicide attempts or death by suicide [30]. Contrary to a previous study [19], schizophrenia and personality disorder were not associated with psychiatric inpatient care in our sample. In relation to the former, this could be due to the small representation (only 3% of patients) of this diagnosis in our study.

In our sample, 20.16% of patients suffered from a borderline personality disorder. This is relevant because, personality disorders, especially borderline personality, are commonly observed among individuals who attempt suicide. We found no association between personality disorder and inpatient referral. This could be explained by the fact that the role of hospitalization after suicide attempts has generated controversy. One group advocates that hospitals keep patients safe and are appropriate for the treatment of co-morbidities, diagnosis clarifications and simplifying prescription medications [31, 32]. Others point out that minimal evidence exists concerning the efficacy of hospitalization for chronic suicidality. Moreover, hospitalization can result in

Table 2 Characteristics associated with psychiatric hospitalization

	Hospitalization				
	Univariate comparison			Multivariate logistic regression	
	Yes(*n*=162)	No(*n*=354)	p	OR [95%IC]	p
Sociodemographics					
Age (years)	43.9	38.8	**<0.001**	1.01 [0.99-1.02]	0.12
Gender Men (*n*=165)	48 (29.6)	117 (33)	0.65	0.91 [0.55-1.53]	0.74
Living status (*n*=474) Housing or not	155 (95.6)	319 (90.1)	0.69	1.16[0.45-3.38]	0.76
Living status (*n*=179) Alone or not	58 (35.8)	121 (34.1)	0.85	1.23 [0.77-1.98]	0.37
Professional status (*n*=198) Employee or not	68 (41.9)	130 (36.7)	0.49	1.25 [0.78-2.01]	0.34
Psychopathology and care characteristics					
Depression (*n*=170)	89 (54.9)	81 (22.8)	**<0.001**	3.6 [2.18-6.05]	**<0.001**
Schizophrenia (*n*=18)	5 (3.1)	13 (3.7)	0.95	1.63 [0.43-5.4]	0.43
Bipolar disorder (*n*=59)	23 (14.2)	36 (10.1)	0.29	3.16 [1.57-6.33]	**<0.001**
Alcohol use disorder(*n*=155)	43 (26.5)	112 (31.6)	0.45	0.87 [0.49-1.54]	0.65
Personality disorder(*n*=178)	29 (17.9)	150 (42.3)	**<0.001**	1.03 [0.62-1.71]	0.89
Suicidal intentionnality (Pierce Score)	9.8 (5.7)	4.5 (4.4)	**<0.001**	1.18 [1.13-1.24]	**<0.001**
Past history of suicide (*n*=308)	107 (66.1)	201 (59.3)	0.34	1.53 [0.95-2.47]	**0.07**
Blood alcohol concentration (BAC) mean (SD)	0.63 (0.93)	0.62 (0.92)	0.11	0.87 [0.64-1.18]	0.39

negative consequences for patients with a borderline personality, including behavioral regression [33].

In terms of the data regarding suicide characteristics, and in parallel with the results of [8], we found that a previous suicide attempt was associated with impatient care, as was suicidal intent.

Surprisingly, we found no association with sociodemographic characteristics, despite previous studies finding a link between male gender and psychiatric inpatient care. One explanation could be a recruitment bias among suicide attempters, as we only recruited the self-poisoning population, which comprised a large majority of women (68%). However, the careful evaluation of other important clinical variables (suicide intent, psychiatric disorder and sociodemographic) has tempered the gender effect.

BACs were not associated with inpatient orientation, which is probably explained by the fact that the patient assessment is only performed when the estimated BAC is below 0.05 g/L.

AUD is also a well-recognized suicide risk factor, but was not associated with psychiatric inpatient care decisions in our sample. We also found no association between BACs and the decision to hospitalize.

This finding underlines the fact that, in our center, AUD is considered differently to depression in clinician decisions, whereas previous studies found a similar suicidal risk increase with a depression or AUD diagnosis (respectively OR = 2.2 and OR = 2.4) [34]. Since the decision to treat a suicide attempter as an outpatient is often due to these diagnoses, we performed an analysis on the sample excluding personality disorders and achieved a similar result to that for the entire population. This tends to confirm that AUD is considered differently to depression, even if patients do not suffer from a personality disorder.

Comparing patients with depression and co-morbid AUD, we found that they were less often referred for inpatient care than non-AUD patients (46.4% versus 53.5%).

Moreover, care referrals depended on the level of the risk of repetition, and AUD is related to multiple suicide attempts [35, 36] and rapid reattempts, as 50% of patients plan their suicide attempt less than 1 week before it takes place [37–39], although unplanned suicide attempts can still be deadly [40]. In addition, alcohol intoxication could promote a suicide attempt because of its disinhibitory effect [38, 39], and patients with AUD are at risk of alcohol consumption, including after a suicide attempt.

A longer period of follow-up is the most protective factor when it comes to preventing another suicide attempt [41], which is why, in practice, a psychiatric evaluation needs to assess the effectiveness of outpatient care. Inpatient care after a suicide attempt does not lead to any reduction in the long-term suicide rate compared to outpatient care; in fact, the main protective factors

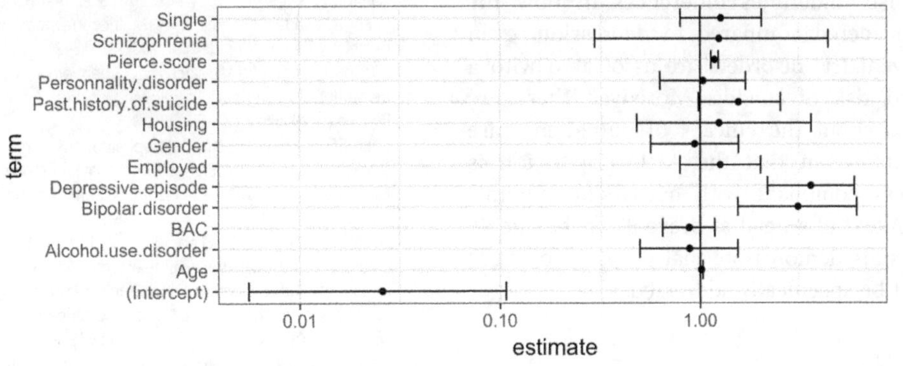

Fig. 2 Factors associated with hospitalization. The figure represents the OR as an estimate. On the x-axis part of the figure, the left of the y-axis represents outpatient care and the right part inpatient care

consist of a care program independent of inpatient or outpatient modalities [28, 42, 43]. However, it has been shown that patients suffering from substance abuse, including AUD, have difficulty engaging in outpatient care [44, 45]. This could therefore mean that inpatient care should be specifically considered during a suicide crisis in order to place the patient at a distance from alcohol, thereby reducing impulsivity, improving mood and promoting follow-up observance [46, 47].

In our database, we found that patients with AUD had a higher risk of repetition than those without AUD. We also found that outpatient care reduced the repetition rate at 1 year in the AUD versus the non-AUD population. This result also led to consideration of inpatient referrals in this group. However, the study was not designed to evaluate repetition rates and we therefore only report retrospective descriptive data concerning the evolution at 1 year. This finding must therefore be confirmed by future studies that specifically focus on this issue.

The discrepancy between the impact of AUD and depression on clinician decisions also needs to be addressed. It could partly be explained by the stigmatization of patients with AUD. Indeed, AUD is the most judged behavior compared with other health conditions such as obesity, depression or schizophrenia [48]. Previous studies reported in the literature demonstrated that AUD was less commonly regarded as a mental illness than depression or schizophrenia [49]. Nevertheless, a previous study showed that holding a conception of AUD as a mental illness increased treatment access [50]. In addition, a study including internal medicine residents found a lower regard for AUD patients than those with other common conditions [51]. Further, previous data suggest that patients hospitalized for suicide risk who are judged to have a risk related to alcohol intoxication are discharged sooner than those who are not perceived to have a substance-related risk [52]. This knowledge led to consideration of whether AUD is stigmatized and its implications for a clinician's decision-making, including by psychiatrists, when it comes to treating suicide attempters. In our study, it is possible to hypothesize that different views of AUD and other psychiatric disorders could partly lead to care discrimination through a clinician's decision not to associate AUD with admission to hospital.

A limitation of this study is that we did not take the types of care for other addictions into account. Other addictions are reported on less, suggesting that practitioners do not consider them when deciding the type of care that a patient requires. Another limitation is that this was a single center study and, despite this center evaluating patients using international guidelines, our observations could not be generalized to all patients seen in France after a self-poisoning suicide attempt. Despite self-poisoning accounting for 82% of suicide attempts in France, this population is very specific. For example, other groups, such as those who attempt suicide by hanging or the use of firearms, are mostly represented by men and are suicide methods associated with greater lethality. Moreover, previous studies have referred to heterogeneity in a population with AUD that is explained by different settings and different populations, leading us to emphasize that our findings are limited to patients with AUD who attempted suicide by self-poisoning [33]. Another limitation is the study's cross-sectional design, which does not enable us to argue that there is a causal relationship. Despite these limitations, the strength of the study is the exhaustiveness of the data, as all eligible patients (expect for three) admitted during the study period were systematically screened. Well-designed intervention studies are now needed to better characterize the possible implications of AUD stigmatization after a suicide attempt and to provide effective strategies to improve AUD consideration in self-poisoning patients.

Conclusion

Our study confirms previous data, which underline the lack of consideration of AUD co-morbidity in suicide attempters. It also underlines differences in how the condition is considered compared to depression, even though both psychiatric disorders are associated with a similar increased risk of suicide. Moreover, there are specific concerns about the efficacy of outpatient care for AUD patients, given that the AUD population is known to be less compliant with outpatient appointments. In the context of a need to prevent repeat suicide attempts, our results demonstrate that the issue of AUD and suicide must be specifically addressed.

Funding

This research did not receive any specific funding from agencies in the public, commercial, or not-for-profit sectors.

Authors' contributions

JS and LS initiated the study. JS, JC and EB recruited the participants. JS and JC contributed to the analysis. JS, JC, EB and NF were involved in writing the publication.

Consent for publication

Not applicable

Competing interests

The authors declare that they have no competing interests.

Author details

[1]Université de Toulouse III, F-31000 Toulouse, France. [2]CHU Toulouse, Service de Psychiatrie eSt Psychologie, Psychiatrie, F-31000 Toulouse, France. [3]CHU Toulouse, Service d'addictologie clinique, urgences réanimation médecine, F-31000 Toulouse, France.

References

1. Murray CJL, Lopez AD. Measuring the global burden of disease. N Engl J Med. 2013;369:448–57.
2. Kessler RC, Borges G, Walters EE. Prevalence of and risk factors for lifetime suicide attempts in the National Comorbidity Survey. Arch Gen Psychiatry. 1999;56:617–26.
3. Kuo WH, Gallo JJ, Tien AY. Incidence of suicide ideation and attempts in adults: the 13-year follow-up of a community sample in Baltimore. Maryland Psychol Med. 2001;31:1181–91.
4. Kelly TM, Cornelius JR, Clark DB. Psychiatric disorders and attempted suicide among adolescents with substance use disorders. Drug Alcohol Depend. 2004;73:87–97.
5. Bernal M, Haro JM, Bernert S, Brugha T, de Graaf R, Bruffaerts R, et al. Risk factors for suicidality in Europe: results from the ESEMED study. J Affect Disord. 2007;101:27–34.
6. Sareen J, Houlahan T, Cox BJ, Asmundson GJG. Anxiety disorders associated with suicidal ideation and suicide attempts in the National Comorbidity Survey. J Nerv Ment Dis. 2005;193:450–4.
7. Haute Autorité de Santé - La crise suicidaire: reconnaître et prendre en charge. [cité 11 avr 2018]. Disponible sur: https://www.has-sante.fr/portail/jcms/c_271964/fr/la-crise-suicidaire-reconnaitre-et-prendre-en-charge
8. Baca-García E, Diaz-Sastre C, Resa EG, Blasco H, Conesa DB, Saiz-Ruiz J, et al. Variables associated with hospitalization decisions by emergency psychiatrists after a patient's suicide attempt. Psychiatr Serv Wash DC. 2004;55:792–7.
9. Bennewith O, Gunnell D, Peters T, Hawton K, House A. Variations in the hospital management of self harm in adults in England: observational study. BMJ. 2004;328:1108–9.
10. Hawton K, Bergen H, Casey D, Simkin S, Palmer B, Cooper J, et al. Self-harm in England: a tale of three cities. Multicentre study of self-harm. Soc Psychiatry Psychiatr Epidemiol. 2007;42:513–21.
11. Olfson M, Gameroff MJ, Marcus SC, Greenberg T, Shaffer D. Emergency treatment of young people following deliberate self-harm. Arch Gen Psychiatry. 2005;62:1122–8.
12. Chan CC, & Jezewski-Serra D. Hospitalisations et recours aux urgences pour tentative de suicide en France métropolitaine à partir du PMSI-MCO 2004–2011 et d'Oscour® 2007–2011. Saint-Maurice: Institut de veille sanitaire. 2014; 25-34.
13. Persett PS, Grimholt TK, Ekeberg O, Jacobsen D, & Myhren H. Patients admitted to hospital after suicide attempt with violent methods compared to patients with deliberate self-poisoning -a study of background variables, somatic and psychiatric health and suicidal behavior. BMC Psychiatry, 2018; 18(1):21. https://doi.org/10.1186/s12888-018-1602-5.
14. Goldberg JF, Ernst CL, Bird S. Predicting hospitalization versus discharge of suicidal patients presenting to a psychiatric emergency service. Psychiatr Serv. 2007;58:561–5.
15. American Psychiatric Association (APA). Practice guideline for the assessment and treatment of patients with suicidal behaviors. 2010.
16. Inskip HM, Harris EC, Barraclough B. Lifetime risk of suicide for affective disorder, alcoholism and schizophrenia. Br J Psychiatry J Ment Sci. 1998;172:35–7.
17. Murphy GE, Wetzel RD. The lifetime risk of suicide in alcoholism. Arch Gen Psychiatry. 1990;47:383–92.
18. Darvishi N, Farhadi M, Haghtalab T, Poorolajal J. Alcohol-Related Risk of Suicidal Ideation, Suicide Attempt, and Completed Suicide: A Meta-Analysis. PLoS ONE. 2015:10. [cité 30 juill 2017] Disponible sur: http://www.ncbi.nlm.nih.gov/pmc/articles/PMC4439031/
19. Jiménez-Treviño L, Saiz PA, Corcoran P, Burón P, García-Portilla MP, Chinea ER, et al. Factors associated with hospitalization after suicide spectrum behaviors: results from a multicenter study in Spain. Arch Suicide Res Off J Int Acad Suicide Res. 2015;19:17–34.
20. Baca-García E, Perez-Rodriguez MM, Basurte-Villamor I, Saiz-Ruiz J, Leiva-Murillo JM, de Prado-Cumplido M, et al. Using data mining to explore complex clinical decisions: a study of hospitalization after a suicide attempt. J Clin Psychiatry. 2006;67:1124–32.
21. Platt S, Bille-Brahe U, Kerkhof A, Schmidtke A, Bjerke T, Crepet P, et al. Parasuicide in Europe: the WHO/EURO multicentre study on parasuicide. I. Introduction and preliminary analysis for 1989. Acta Psychiatr Scand. 1992; 85:97–104.
22. Sheehan DV, Lecrubier Y, Sheehan KH, Amorim P, Janavs J, Weiller E, et al. The Mini-International Neuropsychiatric Interview (M.I.N.I.): the development and validation of a structured diagnostic psychiatric interview for DSM-IV and ICD-10. J Clin Psychiatry. 1998;59(Suppl 20): 22–33. quiz 34–57
23. Pierce DW. Suicidal intent in self-injury. Br J Psychiatry J Ment Sci. 1977;130: 377–85.
24. Barros AJD, & Hirakata VN. Alternatives for logistic regression in cross-sectional studies: an empirical comparison of models that directly estimate the prevalence ratio. BMC Medical Research Methodology. 2003;3:21. https://doi.org/10.1186/1471-2288-3-21.
25. Suominen K, Lönnqvist J. Determinants of psychiatric hospitalization after attempted suicide. Gen Hosp Psychiatry. 2006;28:424–30.
26. Hepp U, Moergeli H, Trier SN, Milos G, Schnyder U. Attempted suicide: factors leading to hospitalization. Can J Psychiatry Rev Can Psychiatr. 2004; 49:736–42.
27. Schmidtke A, Bille-Brahe U, DeLeo D, Kerkhof A, Bjerke T, Crepet P, et al. Attempted suicide in Europe: rates, trends and sociodemographic characteristics of suicide attempters during the period 1989-1992. Results of the WHO/EURO multicentre study on Parasuicide. Acta Psychiatr Scand. 1996;93:327–38.
28. Waterhouse J, Platt S. General hospital admission in the management of parasuicide. A randomised controlled trial. Br J Psychiatry J Ment Sci. 1990; 156:236–42.
29. Marquet RL, Bartelds AIM, Kerkhof AJFM, Schellevis FG, van der Zee J. The epidemiology of suicide and attempted suicide in Dutch general practice 1983-2003. BMC Fam Pract. 2005;6:45.
30. Malhi GS, Outhred T, Das P, Morris G, Hamilton A, Mannie Z. Modeling suicide in bipolar disorders. Bipolar Disord. 2018;20(4):334-348.
31. Goodman M, Roiff T, Oakes AH, Paris J. Suicidal risk and management in borderline personality disorder. Curr Psychiatry Rep. 2012;14:79–85.

32. Vijay NR, Links PS. New frontiers in the role of hospitalization for patients with personality disorders. Curr Psychiatry Rep. 2007;9:63–7.
33. Paris J. Is hospitalization useful for suicidal patients with borderline personality disorder? J Personal Disord. 2004;18:240–7.
34. Darvishi N, Farhadi M, Haghtalab T, Poorolajal J. Alcohol-related risk of suicidal ideation, suicide attempt, and completed suicide: a meta-analysis. PLoS One. 2015;10:e0126870.
35. Monnin J, Thiemard E, Vandel P, Nicolier M, Tio G, Courtet P, et al. Sociodemographic and psychopathological risk factors in repeated suicide attempts: gender differences in a prospective study. J Affect Disord. 2012;136:35–43.
36. Perquier F, Duroy D, Oudinet C, Maamar A, Choquet C, Casalino E, et al. Suicide attempters examined in a Parisian emergency department: contrasting characteristics associated with multiple suicide attempts or with the motive to die. Psychiatry Res. 2017;253:142–9.
37. Conner KR, Hesselbrock VM, Schuckit MA, Hirsch JK, Knox KL, Meldrum S, et al. Precontemplated and impulsive suicide attempts among individuals with alcohol dependence. J Stud Alcohol. 2006;67:95–101.
38. Suokas J, Lönnqvist J. Suicide attempts in which alcohol is involved: a special group in general hospital emergency rooms. Acta Psychiatr Scand. 1995;91:36–40.
39. Hufford MR. Alcohol and suicidal behavior. Clin Psychol Rev. 2001;21:797–811.
40. Simon OR, Swann AC, Powell KE, Potter LB, Kresnow MJ, O'Carroll PW. Characteristics of impulsive suicide attempts and attempters. Suicide Life Threat Behav. 2001;32:49–59.
41. Guthrie E, Patton GC, Kapur N, Mackway-Jones K, Chew-Graham C, Moorey J, et al. Randomised controlled trial of brief psychological intervention after deliberate self poisoningCommentary: another kind of talk that works? BMJ. 2001;323:135.
42. Bostwick JM, Pankratz VS. Affective disorders and suicide risk: a reexamination. Am J Psychiatry. 2000;157:1925–32.
43. Paris J. Chronic suicidality among patients with borderline personality disorder. Psychiatr Serv. 2002;53:738–42.
44. Simpson DD, Joe GW, Rowan-Szal GA, Greener JM. Drug abuse treatment process components that improve retention. J Subst Abus Treat. 1997;14:565–72.
45. Joe GW, Simpson DD, Broome KM. Retention and patient engagement models for different treatment modalities in DATOS. Drug Alcohol Depend. 1999;57:113–25.
46. Davidson M, Galderisi S, Weiser M, Werbeloff N, Fleischhacker WW, Keefe RS, et al. Cognitive effects of antipsychotic drugs in first-episode schizophrenia and schizophreniform disorder: a randomized, open-label clinical trial (EUFEST). Am J Psychiatry. 2009;166:675–82.
47. Ruusa J, Bergman B, Sundell M-L. Alcohol withdrawal, psychological symptoms, and treatment success. Subst Abuse. 2000;21:129–35.
48. Ronzani TM, Higgins-Biddle J, Furtado EF. Stigmatization of alcohol and other drug users by primary care providers in Southeast Brazil. Soc Sci Med. 2009;69:1080–4.
49. Link BG, Phelan JC, Bresnahan M, Stueve A, Pescosolido BA. Public conceptions of mental illness: labels, causes, dangerousness, and social distance. Am J Public Health. 1999;89:1328–33.
50. Pescosolido BA, Martin JK, Long JS, Medina TR, Phelan JC, Link BG. « a disease like any other »? A decade of change in public reactions to schizophrenia, depression, and alcohol dependence. Am J Psychiatry. 2010;167:1321–30.
51. Meltzer EC, Suppes A, Burns S, Shuman A, Orfanos A, Sturiano CV, et al. Stigmatization of substance use disorders among internal medicine residents. Subst Abuse. 2013;34:356–62.
52. Ries RK, Yuodelis-Flores C, Comtois KA, Roy-Byrne PP, Russo JE. Substance-induced suicidal admissions to an acute psychiatric service: characteristics and outcomes. J Subst Abus Treat. 2008;34:72–9.

10

Depressive disorders among patients with gastric cancer in Taiwan

Li-Yu Hu[2,3,4], Chia-Jen Liu[4,5], Chiu-Mei Yeh[6], Ti Lu[1], Yu-Wen Hu[4,7], Tzeng-Ji Chen[4,6], Pan-Ming Chen[8], Shyh-Chyang Lee[9,10] and Cheng-Ho Chang[1*]

Abstract

Background: In cancer patients, depressive disorder comorbidity is associated with greater suicide risk and poorer treatment outcomes, quality of life, and adherence to treatment. The aim of the study was to evaluate the incidence of newly-diagnosed depressive disorders after a gastric cancer diagnosis compared with a matched cohort using the National Health Insurance Research Database in Taiwan.

Methods: We conducted a retrospective cohort study of 57,506 patients (28,753 patients with gastric cancer and 28,753 matched patients) selected from the National Health Insurance Research Database. Patients were observed for a maximum of 12 years to determine the incidence of newly-diagnosed depressive disorders. Also, a Cox regression analysis which included death as an independent censor was performed to identify the potentially predictive variables for developing subsequent depressive disorders following a cancer diagnosis among the patients suffering from gastric cancer.

Results: The cumulative incidence of depressive disorders in the gastric cancer patients was significantly higher compared to those in the matched cohort ($p < .001$). The adjusted hazard ratio was 1.54 (95% confidence interval, CI = 1.39–1.70, $P < .001$) in the gastric cancer cohort compared with the matched cohort. Independent predictive variables for developing subsequent depressive disorders among the patients with gastric cancer included female sex and hypertension.

Conclusions: In the study, higher incidence of new-onset depression, being defined by the records of the diagnostic codes combining antidepressants use in a nationwide database, was noted in the gastric cancer patients compared with the matched cohort. In addition, female sex and comorbid hypertension may be predictive variables for the subsequent depression among the patients with gastric cancer. Further clinical prospective studies were necessary to confirm these findings.

Keywords: Depression, Epidemiology, Gastric neoplasms, Risk factor

Background

Although the incidence of gastric cancer has declined over the last few decades in many countries [1–4], it is still one of the most common cancers in the world. In 2012, an estimated 951,600 newly diagnosed gastric cancer patients and 723,100 deaths occurred worldwide [5]. Gastric cancer rates are generally about twice as high in men as they are in women [6]. Most important, the incidence rates of gastric cancer vary widely across countries. Evidence has showed that incidence rates are highest in Eastern Asia, Central and Eastern Europe, and South America. In addition, more than half of newly diagnosed gastric cancer cases occurring in Eastern Asia [5, 7]. For example, in 2012, there were 3795 Taiwanese being diagnosed as gastric cancer and the gastric cancer was the fifth-most frequently diagnosed cancer with a age-standardized incidence rate of 15.03 per 100,000 people [8]. Moreover, gastric cancer has

* Correspondence: kvjang58@gmail.com
[1]Department of Psychiatry, Kaohsiung Veterans General Hospital, No.386, Dajhong 1st Rd., Zuoying Dist., Kaohsiung City 813, Taiwan

also a high mortality; for instance, in Taiwan, gastric cancer ranks as the sixth-highest cause of cancer-related deaths in 2012 with a standardized mortality rate of 6.4 per 100,000 people [7].

Cancer is a risk factor for developing emotional disturbances, especially depression [9]. Evidence has revealed that depressive disorders are associated with reduced quality of life and poorer outcomes in patients with cancer [10]. Several studies found an increased risk of suicide among patients with cancer compared with the general population [11–13]. Additionally, depression has also been associated with poor survival among gastric cancer patients in China [14].

Depression is the most prevalent psychiatric disorder among the various types of cancer patients. Massieet et al. reviewed previous studies regarding the prevalence of depression in patients with cancer and found that the reported prevalence (major depressive disorder: 0–38%; depression spectrum syndromes: 0–58%) varied significantly because of different conceptualizations of depression, criteria used to define depression, methodological approaches to the measurement of depression, and study populations [15]. Depression has been studied in patients with cancer using a range of assessment methods, such as self-report rating scales, brief screening instruments, and structured clinical interviews. The methods commonly used are the Hospital Anxiety and Depression Scale, Beck Depression Inventory, Hamilton Rating Scale for Depression questionnaire, and the Diagnostic and Statistical Manual of Mental Disorders criteria, published by the American Psychiatric Association. In general, the more narrowly the term is defined, the lower the reported prevalence of depression [15]. Bergquist et al. found that the rate of depression among those with esophagus or gastroesophageal junction cancer ranged from 27 to 44% [16]. Among these studies, diagnoses were usually not clinically defined and there have been few epidemiological studies specifically of depressive disorders among gastric cancer patients.

To reduce the evidence-to-practice gap and overcome the abovementioned shortage of previous studies and based on the fact that higher incidence and mortality rates of gastric cancer in Taiwan by annual government report and epidemiological studies, we designed a nationwide population-based retrospective cohort study, using a different definition for depressive disorders, to investigate the clinical pictures among the patients with gastric cancer and try to explore the differences on the incidence of subsequent depressive disorders compared with the matched cohort using the Taiwanese National Health Insurance Research Database (NHIRD). Also, independent predictive variables for subsequent depressive disorders following a gastric cancer diagnosis were also analyzed.

Methods

Data sources

The Taiwan National Health Insurance (NHI) program, which the government initiated in 1995, provides comprehensive health care for all Taiwanese residents. Enrollment in this program is mandatory, and the proportion of the population insured reached 99% in 2006 [17]. The NHIRD contains information regarding clinical visits, including prescription details and diagnostic codes based on the International Classification of Diseases, Ninth Revision, Clinical Modification (ICD-9-CM). The NHIRD is managed by the National Health Research Institutes (NHRI) and confidentiality is maintained according to the directives of the NHI Bureau. This database also provides comprehensive use of and enrollment information for all patients with "catastrophic illnesses." Catastrophic illnesses are a set of diseases, such as cancer, defined by the Taiwanese government; patients with catastrophic illness certificates are exempt from copayments under the NHI program. Application for catastrophic illness certificates requires sufficient medical records and an independent peer review process. Therefore, in our study, the diagnoses of gastric cancer were valid. Patients with gastric cancer and matched patients were identified from the NHI database. The Institutional Review Board of the Taipei Veterans General Hospital approved this study (2013-06-010 BC). Written consent from the study patients was not required because the NHI dataset consists of de-identified secondary data used for research purposes, and the Institutional Review Board of the Taipei Veterans General Hospital issued a formal written waiver regarding the need for consent.

Study population

Using the discharge codes (151.X) (Malignant neoplasm of stomach) of the ICD-9-CM in the Registry of Catastrophic Illness, we identified 28,753 patients who were newly diagnosed with gastric cancer between January 1, 2000, and December 31, 2011. We excluded patients under 20 years of age and those who were diagnosed with depressive disorders prior to the cancer diagnosis. Depressive disorders were defined according to the relevant ICD-9-CM codes (depressive disorders: 296.2×–296.3×, 300.4, 311.x) [18]. In addition, we collected information on the antidepressant prescriptions that could be used to treat depressive disorders. In order to ensure the validity of definition for depressive disorders in the study, the development of depressive disorders was based on the ICD-9-CM codes and the prescription of antidepressants by at least one qualified psychiatrist for at least 30 days [18, 19]. However, the definition of depressive disorders in the study should not be misinterpreted as to look upon antidepressants use or any other biological interventions as the major role in addressing depression among the patients with gastric cancer. For each gastric cancer patient included in the final cohort, one age-, sex-, common-comorbidity-, and enrollment-date-matched patient who was not diagnosed with gastric cancer was randomly selected from the same database.

Statistical analyses

The main dependent variable was the incidence of comorbid depressive disorders. The two cohorts were observed until the development of depressive disorders, death, withdrawal from the NHI system, or December 31, 2011. Each patient was followed for a maximum of 12 years. Incidence rates (per 1000 person-years) were analyzed. Formal comparisons between groups were performed using the chi-squared test for categorical variables and Mann-Whitney U test for continuous variables. Cumulative incidences of depressive disorders were calculated and stratified by gastric cancer and the matched cohort. The Kaplan-Meier method estimated the cumulative incidence and overall survival rate. A Cox proportional hazards model was used to identify risk factors for depressive disorders and patient death was included as an independent censor. Information about gastric cancer treatments, such as major surgery—including total gastrectomy, esophagogastrectomy, chemotherapy, and radiotherapy—and other control variables—such as age, sex, and comorbidities—were included in the model. Moreover, gastric cancer treatments were analyzed as a time-dependent covariate in order to avoid immortal time bias [20] and the Fine-Gray model was used for controlling the competing risk of death while calculating the incidence of newly-diagnosed depressive disorders. The data were extracted and computed using the Perl programming language (Version 5.12.2; Perl Foundation, Walnut, CA, USA). Microsoft SQL Server 2012 (Microsoft Corp., Redmond, WA, USA) was used for data linkage, processing, and sampling. SAS 9.2 software (SAS Institute Inc., Cary, NC, USA) or Stata statistical software (Version 11.0; Stata Corp, College Station, TX, USA) was used in the statistical analyses. A p value < .05 was considered statistically significant.

Results

Clinical characteristics of the study population

During the study period, 28,753 patients with gastric cancer were enrolled. The interquartile range for patient age was55–77 years (Median age = 69 years). The top three comorbidities were hypertension (49.7%), chronic obstructive pulmonary disease (COPD) (29.9%), and ischemic heart disease (29.7%). The demographic data and comorbidities of the patients with gastric cancer and the matched group are shown in Table 1. Age, sex, and all of the listed comorbid diseases were matched. The median follow-up period for the matched group was 4.75 years, which was significantly longer than the 1.23-year median follow-up period observed in the gastric cancer cohort ($P < .001$ according to the Mann-Whitney U test).

Incidence rates of depressive disorders

Of the 57,506 patients, 1545 patients (2.6%) were diagnosed with depressive disorders; 670 patients with depressive disorders belonged to the gastric cancer cohort (9.1 per 1000 person-years), and 875 belonged to the matched cohort (6.0 per 1000 person-years, $P < .001$). The results of the cumulative incidence of depressive disorders in the gastric cancer cohort and matched cohort are shown in Fig. 1. The cumulative incidence of depressive disorders was significantly higher in the gastric cancer patients compared to those in the matched cohort ($P < .001$, Log-rank test). In addition, the results of the Fine-Gray competing events model revealed that the observed risk of the depressive disorders among gastric cancer patients was still significantly higher than the matched cohort ($P < .001$, Gray's test).

The adjusted hazard ratio (HR) was 1.54 (95% confidence interval, CI = 1.39–1.70, $P < .001$) in the gastric cancer cohort compared with the matched cohort. As shown in Table 2, differences in the HR for depressive disorders were observed when the patients in both cohorts were stratified according to age and sex. The results showed that younger patients (age < 65 years old) (HR 2.05, 95% CI = 1.75–2.41, $P < .001$) had a higher HR for depressive disorders compared to those who were older (HR 1.27, 95% CI = 1.11–1.45, $P < .001$). When patients were stratified according to sex, female patients (HR 1.80, 95% CI = 1.53–2.12, $P < .001$) had a higher HR compared to the male patients (HR 1.40, 95% CI =1.23–1.59, $P < .001$).

Risk factors for depressive disorders in the gastric cancer cohort

In Table 3, we applied univariate analysis when trying to predict the development of depressive disorders in the gastric cancer cohort. The results indicated that female sex and some comorbidities—including diabetes mellitus, hypertension, heart failure, COPD, chronic kidney disease, cirrhosis, cerebrovascular disease, and ischemic heart disease—were possible risk factors ($P < .1$).The multivariate analysis confirmed that the following were independent risk factors for depressive disorders among patients with gastric cancer: female sex (HR = 1.46, 95% CI = 1.25–1.70, $P < .001$) and hypertension (HR = 1.27, 95% CI = 1.07–1.52, $p = .008$).

Discussion

The major finding of our study was that the risk of clinical depressive disorders requiring psychiatric intervention was higher among patients with gastric cancer compared to the matched cohort. In addition, female sex

Table 1 Baseline patient characteristics of patients with and without gastric cancer

Demographic data	Patients with gastric cancer *n* = 28,753		Matched cohort *n* = 28,753		*P* value
	n	%	*n*	%	
Age (years) (interquartile range)	69 (55–77)		69 (55–77)		
≥65	16,889	58.7	16,889	58.7	1.000
< 65	11,864	41.3	11,864	41.3	.
Sex					
Male	19,464	67.7	19,464	67.7	1.000
Female	9289	32.3	9289	32.3	.
Comorbidities					
Diabetes mellitus	7895	27.5	7894	27.5	0.993
Hypertension	14,302	49.7	14,304	49.7	0.987
Heart failure	3712	12.9	3711	12.9	0.990
COPD	8586	29.9	8584	29.9	0.985
Chronic kidney disease	4123	14.3	4122	14.3	0.991
Cirrhosis	1469	5.1	1420	4.9	0.350
Autoimmune diseases	1721	6	1719	6	0.972
Cerebrovascular disease	5565	19.4	5567	19.4	0.983
Ischemic heart disease	8549	29.7	8550	29.7	0.993
Follow-up years (median)	1.23 (0.41–3.68)		4.75 (2.19–7.89)		< 0.001

COPD chronic obstructive pulmonary disease

and hypertension were the risk factors for the development of subsequent depressive disorders following diagnoses of gastric cancer.

The current study design involved an unbiased participant selection process and used an age-, sex-, and comorbidity-matched cohort as the control group. Because participation in the NHI is mandatory, and nearly all Taiwanese residents can access healthcare with low copayments, referral bias is not a concern and follow-up compliance is high. Furthermore, to apply for a cancer catastrophic illness certificate, pathologic proof of malignancy is mandatory, and laboratory and imaging studies must be provided. Therefore, cancer diagnoses in this study were reliable. The strengths of this study were its large sample size, the long-term (12-year) follow-up period, and clinical depressive disorder diagnoses as

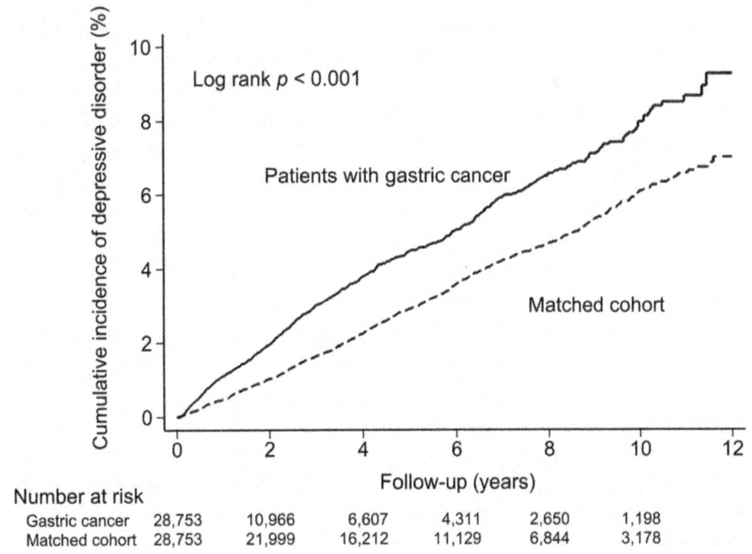

Fig. 1 Cumulative incidence of depressive disorders among patients with gastric cancer and matched cohort

Table 2 Incidence of depressive disorders occurrence in patients with and without gastric cancer

	Patients with gastric cancer		Matched cohort		Crude HR (95% CI)	*P* value	Adjusted HR[a] (95% CI)	*P* value
	Event No.	Per 1000 person-year	Event No.	Per 1000 person-year				
Depressive disorder								
Total	670	9.1	875	6.0	1.52 (1.38–1.69)	< 0.001	1.54 (1.39–1.70)	< 0.001
Age								
≥65	348	9.4	584	7.4	1.26 (1.10–1.44)	< 0.001	1.27 (1.11–1.45)	< 0.001
< 65	322	8.8	291	4.3	2.81 (1.76–2.43)	< 0.001	2.05 (1.75–2.41)	< 0.001
Sex								
Male	389	8.0	565	5.8	1.37 (1.21–1.56)	< 0.001	1.40 (1.23–1.59)	< 0.001
Female	281	11.2	310	6.2	1.79 (1.52–2.11)	< 0.001	1.80 (1.53–2.12)	< 0.001

HR incidence hazard ratio, *CI* indicates confidence interval
[a]Adjusted for age, sex, diabetes mellitus, hypertension, heart failure, chronic obstructive pulmonary disease, chronic kidney disease, cirrhosis, autoimmune diseases, cerebrovascular disease and ischemic heart disease

defined based on the ICD-9-CM codes and antidepressant prescriptions.

Consistent with the results of previous studies, we observed that the risk of depressive disorders in gastric cancer patients was higher than it was in the control patients. The result may be explained by several possible factors. First, gastric cancer is often diagnosed at a late stage and its outcome is often poor with a 5-year survival rate under 10% [21]; therefore, patients with gastric cancer may have a higher risk of experiencing emotional distress. Second, while the type of surgical procedure does not appear to impact quality of life (QOL), different types of gastric resection may affect eating behavior and physical and emotional functioning [22]. For example, dumping syndrome is more common with a distal gastrectomy, and reflux is more common if the gastroesophageal junction is included in the specimen. These problems may lead to depressive disorders and other QOL problems. Third, studies have shown that patients with gastric cancer exhibit higher levels of mixed depression and anxiety symptoms compared to those with other types of cancer, raising the question of whether

Table 3 Analyses of risk factors for depressive disorder in patients with gastric cancer

Predictive variables	Univariate analysis		Multivariate analysis[a]	
	HR (95% CI)	*P* value	HR (95% CI)	*P* value
Age ≥ 65	1.04 (0.89–1.21)	0.611		
Sex (female)	1.41 (1.21–1.64)	< 0.001	1.46 (1.25–1.70)	< 0.001
Comorbidities				
Diabetes mellitus	1.33 (1.12–1.57)	0.001	1.13 (0.94–1.35)	0.186
Hypertension	1.45 (1.24–1.68)	< 0.001	1.27 (1.07–1.52)	0.008
Heart failure	1.41 (1.12–1.77)	0.003	1.12 (0.87–1.43)	0.393
COPD	1.22 (1.03–1.44)	0.019	1.11 (0.93–1.32)	0.259
Chronic kidney disease	1.21 (0.97–1.51)	0.098	1.02 (0.81–1.28)	0.886
Cirrhosis	1.40 (0.99–1.98)	0.056	1.35 (0.95–1.91)	0.090
Autoimmune diseases	1.25 (0.92–1.68)	0.150		
Cerebrovascular disease	1.44 (1.19–1.75)	< 0.001	1.22 (1.00–1.50)	0.053
Ischemic heart disease	1.30 (1.10–1.53)	0.002	1.06 (0.88–1.28)	0.558
Treatment[b]				
Surgery alone	1.03 (0.89–1.21)	0.673		
Surgery with neoadjuvant and/or adjuvant chemoradiotherapy	1.11 (0.96–1.30)	0.167		
Chemoradiotherapy without surgery	0.79 (0.57–1.10)	0.164		

COPD chronic obstructive pulmonary disease
[a]All factors with $P < 0.1$ in univariate analyses were included in the Cox multivariate analysis
[b]Treatment was analyzed as a time-dependent covariate in the Cox regression model

gastric cancer is associated with more biological mechanisms of depression, such as cytokine release [23]. Consistent with this biological hypothesis, Koh et al. investigated the association between the brain-derived neurotrophic factor (BDNF) Val66Met polymorphism and stress coping response in patients diagnosed with gastric cancer and found that the BDNF Val66Met polymorphism may be involved in individual coping responses to cancer [24].

Previous studies have reported that depressive symptoms were frequently noted in gastric cancer patients [23, 25]. Although our results are consistent with such findings, the estimated incidence rate of depression among gastric cancer patients in these studies was approximately 20% [25]; this rate is much higher than the rate calculated in our study. There are two possible reasons for the discrepancy between these findings. First, in previous studies, rating scales—such as the HAMD-24 questionnaire—rather than clinical diagnostic interviews, were used to identify depression. Patients who were recorded as depressed may not have fulfilled the diagnostic criteria for depressive disorders from a psychiatric perspective. In our study, we focused on the patients with depressive disorders who were prescribed antidepressants for at least 30 days by clinical oncologists or psychiatrists. Therefore, our study may reflect the real conditions of the gastric cancer patients under the care of clinical conditions. Second, cultural differences may impact the reporting of depressive symptoms in cancer patients [26, 27]. Studies have shown that Asian patients focus more on their physical rather than their psychological symptoms [28]. Moreover, in addition to the difficulty evaluating the etiology of physical symptoms in diagnosing depressive disorders, oncology specialists may also be uncertain regarding the effectiveness of treatment for depressive disorder, limiting referrals for psychiatric interventions. Therefore, gastric cancer patients with depressive disorders may have been underestimated in our study.

In our analysis of the risk factors associated with subsequent depressive disorders among patients with gastric cancer, female sex and hypertension were independent risk factors. The prevalence of hypertension was about 27.2% in 2000 in Asia [29], and this has been increasing annually [30]. From a psychosomatic perspective, hypertension could be concomitant with depression [31]. Depression is closely associated with hypertension. Depression can promote the occurrence and development of hypertension [32]. Meanwhile, hypertension is prone to aggravate depression, and the increased prevalence of depression has been described among patients with hypertension. Rabkin et al. found a three-fold higher frequency of major depressive disorder in patients treated for hypertension [33]. These findings are in line with our study results, which indicated that hypertension may be a risk factor for subsequent depression among patients with gastric cancer. In addition, the female sex was at a greater risk for developing depressive disorders in the present study. This result is in line with previous studies in which the female sex was a risk factor for depression in patients with cancer [34]. Moreover, the results of the analysis of the risk factors showed that treatment regimens were not associated with the increased risk of depressive disorders among patients with gastric cancer; these results seem consistent with earlier research on esophageal cancer patients [16]. However, these results also highlight the complex life-life clinical situation and we should interpret the results carefully. For example, a gastric cancer patient who is eligible to receive curative surgery may have increased feelings of hope, possibly associated with the knowledge that the curative treatment implies a potential chance of a cure; however, the upcoming surgery and poor prognosis, despite undergoing curative treatment, may be reflected in heightened emotional distress. In addition, for those with gastric cancer that is diagnosed late and where surgical extirpation is unlikely, patients may focus on their physical illness needs and be reluctant or even hostile when asked about their psychological needs. These patients with later-stage gastric cancer were also expected to have a shorter life expectancy and, therefore, had fewer chances to receive psychiatric intervention.

Our study is one of the few nationwide studies to examine the association between gastric cancer and subsequent depressive disorders. Its strength is that it used a retrospective matched-cohort study design with a nationwide cohort of patients with gastric cancer and adequate controls for comorbidities. However, several limitations inherent to the use of medical care claims databases should be considered. First, depressive disorder causes are generally complex and vary depending on the patient. Many psychological and environmental factors can contribute to the development of these disorders. We acknowledge that several essential demographic variables—such as a family history of psychiatric disorders, stressful life situations, interpersonal relationships, and lifestyle—were unavailable in the medical care claims database. Second, the cancer stage could not be ascertained and, therefore, whether the severity of the gastric cancer influences the risk of developing depressive disorders warrants further study. Third, as mentioned previously, oncology specialists may view the depressive symptoms of gastric cancer patients as physical discomfort caused by gastric cancer and thus overlook these symptoms. The incidence of depressive disorders in our study may have been underestimated.

Conclusions

The study suggests that patients with gastric cancer may have more risk of developing subsequent depressive disorders compared with matched cohort. Although it was difficult to provide a clear mechanism to explain the possible role of female sex and hypertension on the association between the gastric cancer and subsequent depression, based on our data, we still suggest that additional attention should focus on both of them. Additional prospective clinical studies of the association between gastric cancer and depressive disorders are needed.

Abbreviations

aHR: Adjusted hazard ratio; BDNF: Brain-derived neurotrophic factor; CI: Confidence interval; COPD: Chronic obstructive pulmonary disease; HR: Hazard ratio; ICD-9-CM: The International Classification of Diseases, ninth revision, Clinical Modification; NHI: National Health Insurance; NHIRD: National Health Insurance Research Database

Acknowledgements

We thank the Economy Company Ltd. for their technical and English editing services. We are grateful for use of the National Health Insurance Research Database provided by Statistic Center of Department of Health and Welfare. The interpretations and conclusions contained herein do not represent those of the Bureau of Health Promotion, Taiwan.

Funding

This study was supported by Grants V103B-022, V103E10–001 from Taipei Veterans General Hospital and Grant VGHKS107-075 from Kaohsiung Veterans General Hospital, Taiwan.

Authors' contributions

LYH, CJL and CMY participated in the design of the study and analyzed the data. CHC and LYH contributed to the data analysis and wrote the manuscript. TL, YWH, TJC and PMC supervised the processes of data analysis and helped the interpretation of data. SCL contributed to the revision of the manuscript. All authors read and approved the final manuscript.

Consent for publication

Not applicable.

Competing interests

The authors declare that they have no competing interests.

Author details

[1]Department of Psychiatry, Kaohsiung Veterans General Hospital, No.386, Dajhong 1st Rd., Zuoying Dist., Kaohsiung City 813, Taiwan. [2]Department of Psychiatry, Taipei Veterans General Hospital, Taipei, Taiwan. [3]Center for Geriatrics and Gerontology, Kaohsiung Veterans General Hospital, Kaohsiung, Taiwan. [4]School of Medicine, National Yang-Ming University, Taipei, Taiwan. [5]Division of Hematology and Oncology, Department of Medicine Taipei Veterans General Hospital, Taipei, Taiwan. [6]Department of Family Medicine, Taipei Veterans General Hospital, Taipei, Taiwan. [7]Cancer Center, Taipei Veterans General Hospital, Taipei, Taiwan. [8]Department of Psychiatry, Yuanshan & Su-ao Branch, Taipei Veterans General Hospital, Yilan, Taiwan. [9]Department of Information Management, Chia Nan University of Pharmacy & Science, Tainan, Taiwan. [10]Department of Orthopedics, Chiayi Branch, Taichung Veterans General Hospital, Chiayi, Taiwan.

References

1. Haenszel W. Variation in incidence of and mortality from stomach cancer, with particular reference to the United States. J Natl Cancer Inst. 1958;21: 213–62.
2. Hirayama T. Epidemiology of cancer of the stomach with special reference to its recent decrease in Japan. Cancer Res. 1975;35:3460–3.
3. Fitzsimmons D, Osmond C, George S, Johnson CD. Trends in stomach and pancreatic cancer incidence and mortality in England and Wales, 1951-2000. Br J Surg. 2007;94:1162–71.
4. Jemal A, Siegel R, Ward E, Murray T, Xu J, Smigal C, et al. Cancer statistics, 2006. CA Cancer J Clin. 2006;56:106–30.
5. Torre LA, Bray F, Siegel RL, Ferlay J, Lortet-Tieulent J, Jemal A. Global cancer statistics, 2012. CA Cancer J Clin. 2015;65:87–108.
6. Jemal A, Bray F, Center MM, Ferlay J, Ward E, Forman D. Global cancer statistics. CA Cancer J Clin. 2011;61:69–90.
7. Ferlay J, Soerjomataram I, Dikshit R, Eser S, Mathers C, Rebelo M, et al. Cancer incidence and mortality worldwide: sources, methods and major patterns in GLOBOCAN 2012. Int J Cancer. 2015;136:E359–86.
8. Chiang C-J, Lo W-C, Yang Y-W, You S-L, Chen C-J, Lai M-S. Incidence and survival of adult cancer patients in Taiwan, 2002–2012. J Formos Med Asso. 2016;115:1076–88.
9. Smith HR. Depression in cancer patients: pathogenesis, implications and treatment (review). Oncol Lett. 2015;9:1509–14.
10. DiMatteo MR, Lepper HS, Croghan TW. Depression is a risk factor for noncompliance with medical treatment: meta-analysis of the effects of anxiety and depression on patient adherence. Arch Intern Med. 2000; 160:2101–7.
11. Misono S, Weiss NS, Fann JR, Redman M, Yueh B. Incidence of suicide in persons with cancer. J Clin Oncol. 2008;26:4731–8.
12. Allebeck P, Bolund C, Ringback G. Increased suicide rate in cancer patients: a cohort study based on the Swedish Cancer-environment register. J Clin Epidemiol. 1989;42:611–6.
13. Bjorkenstam C, Edberg A, Ayoubi S, Rosen M. Are cancer patients at higher suicide risk than the general population? Scand J Public Health. 2005;33:208–14.
14. Yu H, Wang Y, Ge X, Wu X, Mao X. Depression and survival in Chinese patients with gastric cancer: a prospective study. Asian Pac J Cancer Prev. 2012;13:391–4.
15. Massie MJ. Prevalence of depression in patients with cancer. J Natl Cancer Inst Monogr. 2004:57–71.
16. Bergquist H, Ruth M, Hammerlid E. Psychiatric morbidity among patients with cancer of the esophagus or the gastro-esophageal junction: a prospective, longitudinal evaluation. Dis Esophagus. 2007;20: 523–9.
17. Wu CY, Chen YJ, Ho HJ, Hsu YC, Kuo KN, Wu MS, et al. Association between nucleoside analogues and risk of hepatitis B virus-related hepatocellular carcinoma recurrence following liver resection. JAMA. 2012;308:1906–14.
18. Townsend L, Walkup JT, Crystal S, Olfson M. A systematic review of validated methods for identifying depression using administrative data. Pharmacoepidemiol Drug Saf. 2012;21(Suppl 1):163–73.
19. Huang KL, Su TP, Chen TJ, Chou YH, Bai YM. Comorbidity of cardiovascular diseases with mood and anxiety disorder: a population based 4-year study. Psychiatry Clin Neurosci. 2009;63:401–9.
20. Liu CJ, Hu YW. Immortal time bias in retrospective analysis: is there a survival benefit in patients with glioblastoma who received prolonged treatment of adjuvant valganciclovir? Int J Cancer. 2014;135:250–1.
21. Orditura M, Galizia G, Sforza V, Gambardella V, Fabozzi A, Laterza MM, et al. Treatment of gastric cancer. World J Gastroenterol. 2014;20:1635–49.
22. Karanicolas PJ, Graham D, Gonen M, Strong VE, Brennan MF, Coit DG. Quality of life after gastrectomy for adenocarcinoma: a prospective cohort study. Ann Surg. 2013;257:1039–46.
23. Brintzenhofe-Szoc KM, Levin TT, Li Y, Kissane DW, Zabora JR. Mixed anxiety/ depression symptoms in a large cancer cohort: prevalence by cancer type. Psychosomatics. 2009;50:383–91.
24. Koh MJ, Jeung HC, Namkoong K, Chung HC, Kang JI. Influence of the BDNF

Val66Met polymorphism on coping response to stress in patients with advanced gastric cancer. J Psychosom Res. 2014;77:76–80.
25. Tavoli A, Mohagheghi MA, Montazeri A, Roshan R, Tavoli Z, Omidvari S. Anxiety and depression in patients with gastrointestinal cancer: does knowledge of cancer diagnosis matter? BMC Gastroenterol. 2007;7:28.
26. Ell K, Sanchez K, Vourlekis B, Lee PJ, Dwight-Johnson M, Lagomasino I, et al. Depression, correlates of depression, and receipt of depression care among low-income women with breast or gynecologic cancer. J Clin Oncol. 2005; 23:3052–60.
27. Greenberg DB. Barriers to the treatment of depression in cancer patients. J Natl Cancer Inst Monogr. 2004:127–35.
28. Bailey RK, Geyen DJ, Scott-Gurnell K, Hipolito MM, Bailey TA, Beal JM. Understanding and treating depression among cancer patients. Int J Gynecol Cancer. 2005;15:203–8.
29. Wu Y, Huxley R, Li L, Anna V, Xie G, Yao C, et al. Prevalence, awareness, treatment, and control of hypertension in China: data from the China National Nutrition and health survey 2002. Circulation. 2008;118:2679–86.
30. Gao Y, Chen G, Tian H, Lin L, Lu J, Weng J, et al. Prevalence of hypertension in China: a cross-sectional study. PLoS One. 2013;8:e65938.
31. Scherrer JF, Xian H, Bucholz KK, Eisen SA, Lyons MJ, Goldberg J, et al. A twin study of depression symptoms, hypertension, and heart disease in middle-aged men. Psychosom Med. 2003;65:548–57.
32. Jonas BS, Franks P, Ingram DD. Are symptoms of anxiety and depression risk factors for hypertension? Longitudinal evidence from the National Health and nutrition examination survey I epidemiologic follow-up study. Arch Fam Med. 1997;6:43–9.
33. Rabkin JG, Charles E, Kass F. Hypertension and DSM-III depression in psychiatric outpatients. Am J Psychiatry. 1983;140:1072–4.
34. Hinz A, Krauss O, Hauss JP, Hockel M, Kortmann RD, Stolzenburg JU, et al. Anxiety and depression in cancer patients compared with the general population. Eur J Cancer Care (Engl). 2010;19:522–9.

Functional connectivity between the thalamus and the primary somatosensory cortex in major depressive disorder: a resting-state fMRI study

Lijun Kang[1,2], Aixia Zhang[1], Ning Sun[1], Penghong Liu[2], Chunxia Yang[1], Gaizhi Li[1], Zhifen Liu[1], Yanfang Wang[1] and Kerang Zhang[1*]

Abstract

Background: Studies have confirmed that the thalamus and the primary somatosensory cortex (SI) are associated with cognitive function. These two brain regions are closely related in structure and function. The interactions between SI and the thalamus are of crucial significance for the cognitive process. Patients with major depressive disorder (MDD) have significant cognitive impairment. Based on these observations, we used resting-state functional magnetic resonance imaging (rs-fMRI) to investigate whether there is an abnormality in the SI-thalamic functional connection in MDD. Furthermore, we explored the clinical symptoms related to this abnormality.

Methods: We included 31 patients with first-episode major depressive disorder and 28 age-, gender-, and education-matched healthy controls (HC). The SI-thalamic functional connectivity was compared between the MDD and HC groups. The correlation analyses were performed between areas with abnormal connectivity and clinical characteristics.

Results: Compared with healthy subjects, the MDD patients had enhanced functional connectivity between the thalamus and SI ($p < 0.05$, corrected). Brain areas with significantly different levels of connectivity had a negative correlation with the Assessment of Neuropsychological Status total score ($r = -0.383$, $p = 0.033$), delayed memory score ($r = -0.376$, $p = 0.037$) and two-digit continuous operation test score ($r = -0.369$, $p = 0.041$) in MDD patients.

Conclusions: These results demonstrate that SI-thalamic functional connectivity is abnormal and associated with the core clinical symptoms in MDD. The SI-thalamic functional connectivity functions as a neurobiological feature and potential biomarker for MDD.

Keywords: Major depressive disorder, Functional connectivity, Thalamus, Primary somatosensory cortex, SI-thalamic functional connectivity

Background

Major depressive disorder (MDD) is a prevalent psychiatric disorder [1]. MDD is characterized by affective disorder, vegetative symptoms, and cognitive function deficits. Clinicians and researchers have found that MDD patients are characterized by significantly poorer cognitive functions, including attention, executive functioning, episodic memory, and processing speed [2–4]. The evidence suggests that cognitive dysfunction is observed beyond the acute phase, and some of these impairments even persist during illness remission, which may lead to depressive relapse and dysfunction [5–7]. Researchers have proposed that functional and mood symptom recovery must include cognitive function recovery [8].

The thalamus is the hub of cortical-subcortical connections located deep in the brain and has been traditionally viewed as a simple relay station for neurons for all body sensations (except olfaction) to then project to

* Correspondence: atomsxmu@vip.163.com
[1]Department of Psychiatry, First Hospital of Shanxi Medical University, Taiyuan 030001, People's Republic of China

the cerebral cortex [9]. The thalamus works as a tightly connected "central core" of brain regions for multiple tasks and behaviours [10]. Some evidence suggests that the thalamus combined with the dorsal anterior cingulate cortex and anterior insular compose the salience network, which has been described as having a central role in cognitive control [11, 12]. Recent research has shown that the thalamus can amplify and sustain cortical representations, and a new framework acknowledging thalamus-frontal circuits in cognition has been defined [13]. In disease conditions, increased thalamic functional connectivity was related to decreased cognitive function [14–18]. These findings suggest that the importance of the thalamus in cognitive activity is gradually being recognized.

The primary somatosensory cortex (SI) is located in the postcentral gyrus and structurally and functionally connected to the thalamus [19, 20]. SI is viewed as an acquisition and transformation sensory signal structure; meanwhile, involvement in controlling and modulating associatively learned behaviors is becoming apparent [21–24]. SI participated in the non-painful stimulation encoding process, and furthermore, SI maintained task-related tactile information in the late maintenance stage and contributed to the memory trace of a pain sensation [25–28]. A researcher even suggested SI as an "embodied mind" that makes the unconscious self exist in concert with the embodied facet of the self [29].

All of this evidence provides promising opportunities for understanding the importance of the thalamus and SI in cognitive function. These two brain regions are closely related in structure and function. The interactions between SI and the thalamus are of crucial significance for the cognitive process. In MDD, patients have cognitive impairments. Therefore, we hypothesized that abnormal SI-thalamic functional connectivity might be a neurobiological feature of MDD that is closely related to these clinical symptoms. Resting-state functional magnetic resonance imaging (rs-fMRI) is a powerful neuroimaging technique that enables researchers to measure spontaneous fluctuations in activity among distinct brain regions [30]. The method of using rs-fMRI to explore the brain's intrinsic functional networks has been called resting-state functional connectivity (rs-FC) and has been used in numerous studies [31, 32]. Therefore, we used rs-FC as our experimental measure. This study may generate a new understanding of the underlying neurobiology depressive disorders.

Methods

Participants

Thirty-one patients with first-episode major depressive disorder were recruited from the First Hospital of Shanxi Medical University. At least two consultant psychiatrists diagnosed all patients according to the criteria for MDD in the "Diagnostic and Statistical Manual of Mental Disorders Fourth Edition (DSM-IV)" and the Chinese version of the Modified Structured Clinical Interview for DSM-IV TR Axis I Disorders Patient Edition (SCID-I/P). The patients were excluded if they met any of the following criteria: 1) had comorbid mental or neurological illnesses or personality disorders; 2) had used psychiatric drugs in the previous 2 weeks; 3) scored less than 17 on the 17-item Hamilton depressive scale (HAMD-17) administered by well-trained research assistants with backgrounds in psychology or psychiatry; 4) were pregnant; 5) were under 18 or over 60 years of age; 6) had a history of substance abuse or drug addiction; or 7) were left-handed or mixed-handed. We collected the patients' general information, including name, gender, age, education level, occupation and family history of psychotic diseases.

Twenty-eight age-, gender-, and education-matched healthy controls were recruited for comparison. Participants were excluded if they met any of the following criteria: 1) had mental or neurological illnesses or personality disorders; 2) had a history of substance abuse or drug addiction; 3) had a family history of mental disorders; 4) were pregnant; 5) were under 18 or over 60 years of age; or 6) were left-handed or mixed-handed.

The Ethical Committee for Medicine of the First Hospital of Shanxi Medical University approved this study. Written informed consent was received from all participants prior to inclusion.

Clinical assessment

An increasing number of studies have shown that depression cannot be observed from the single point of view of depression but must be observed from the multiple perspectives of affective and somatization symptoms and cognition [33]. We used the HAMD-17 and the Snaith-Hamilton Pleasure Scale (SHAPS) to assess affective experience. We used the fatigue severity scale (FSS) to assess somatization symptoms. Finally, we used the Repeatable Battery for the Assessment of Neuropsychological Status (RBANS) and Continuous Performance Test (CPT) to assess cognition features. Our senior psychologist evaluated all the scales in this study.

The HAMD-17 is the most commonly used scale for assessing the severity of MDD, and there is a good degree of confidence in the scale's validity and reliability [34].

The SHAPS is a 14-item scale, each item ranged from 0 to 3 ("strongly agree" to "disagree"), and it was filled out by the subject to evaluate the clinical absence of pleasure [35].

The FSS is a 9-item scale of fatigue severity, each item ranged from the lightest (i.e., 1) to the worst (i.e., 7), and evaluated clinically elevated fatigue [36].

The RBANS is a neuropsychological screening scale designed by Randolph in 1998 for ease of use and for rating neuropsychological function in 20 ~ 89-year-old people and has excellent reliability and validity [37]. The scale has 12 test items covering the five factors of immediate memory, visuospatial/constructional, language, attention, and delayed memory.

The CPT mainly examines the continuous attention level of the participants, the constant concentration on the response, and the level of arousal. For this task, different numbers are presented on the display screen in random order, asking the participants to identify when the same number appeared repeatedly and to react within a specified time. Based on the number of digits of the flashing figures, it is divided into two-digit, three-digit, and four-digit categories [38].

MRI acquisition and preprocessing of rs-fMRI data

MRI acquisition

A MAGNETOM Trio Tim 3.0 T scanner (Siemens Medical Solutions, Germany) with a 12-channel birdcage head coil located at the Shanxi Provincial People's Hospital was used to acquire rs-fMRI. rs-fMRI was performed using an echo planar imaging (EPI) sequence with the following parameters: TR = 2000 ms, TE = 30 ms, flip angle = 70°, FOV = 24 × 24 cm, matrix = 64 × 64, slice gap = 2 mm, slice thickness = 2 mm, 6 min acquisition. During the resting functional scan, participants were instructed to keep their eyes closed and let their minds wander and not to fall asleep; all participants reported that they did not fall asleep.

Preprocessing of rs-fMRI data

Data preprocessing was conducted using the DPARSFA toolbox version 3.2, which was based on statistical parametric mapping 8 (SPM8) and the Resting-State fMRI Data Analysis Toolkit (REST) [39, 40]. The first 10 volumes of functional time points were discarded to allow the participants to adapt to the scanning noise. The remaining 170 volumes were preprocessed, which included the following: 1) slice timing, 2) realigning to reduce head motion (all head movements exceeding 2 mm were excluded), 3) spatial normalizing to the Montreal Neurological Institute (MNI) coordinate space with 3 × 3 × 3 mm, 4) spatial smoothing with a 6 × 6 × 6 full-width at half maximum (FWHM) kernel, 5) linear detrending, 6) temporal bandpass filtering (0.01–0.08 Hz), and 7) white matter signal, cerebrospinal fluid signal, global mean signal and six head motion parameters were used as covariates.

Regions of interest (ROI) were obtained with the WFU Pick Atlas 3.0.5, which automatically generates segmented atlas ROI templates in MNI space [41, 42]. The thalamus was defined as both "Thalamus_L" and "Thalamus_R". SI was defined as "Brodmann areas 3, 1, 2". Then, the image was resliced to the dimension of our functional images (voxel dimension: 3x3x3).

Connectivity between the thalamus and SI was examined using DPARSFA. The mean time course for the thalamus ROI was calculated by averaging the time course for all voxels within the thalamus ROI [43]. Calculations of the functional connection of the thalamus to the whole brain were made. The resulting correlation coefficients were transformed into z scores by Fisher's z transform to create subject-specific maps [44]. Then, we performed a two-sample t-test across the two groups of subjects for the primary somatosensory cortex ROI.

Data analysis

All analyses were performed using IBM SPSS Statistics Version 23.0 (SPSS 23.0). Data are expressed as the means ± standard deviations (SD). Independent-sample t tests and χ^2 tests were used to analyse the demographic data of the two groups. A two-sample t-test was conducted to compare the clinical symptoms scores across groups. *P*-values of 0.05 were considered statistically significant (two-tailed).

The rs-FC of the HC and MDD groups was contrasted using the DPARSFA toolbox version 3.2. The two-sample t-test was used to identify abnormalities between the two groups. To ensure that effects were not accounted for by other factors, such as age, sex and years of education, these variables were included as regressors of no interest. Multiple comparison corrections were determined by Monte Carlo simulation (1000 iterations) using the REST AlphaSim program [45]. Voxels with $p < 0.01$ and cluster size ≥4 voxels (108 mm^3) were regarded as brain areas with a significant difference which confined within the SI mask, corresponding to corrected $p < 0.05$ [46]. From the preprocessed resting-state fMRI data, we extracted the mean time course of each of the statistically significant clusters.

Furthermore, we used Pearson's correlation coefficients to evaluate any relationships between abnormal clusters and clinical features of MDD patients by SPSS 23.0. The results were considered statistically significant at $p < 0.05$.

Results

Demographic data

As shown in Table 1, the mean age (mean ± SD) of the patients and the control group were 29.96 ± 9.73 and 26.79 ± 6.91 years, respectively. No differences in age, sex or years of education were observed between the patients and controls ($p < 0.05$). Table 1 also shows the HAMD-17, SHAPS, FSS, RBANS, and CPT scores for each group. All of these differences were significant between the patients and controls.

Table 1 Demographic and Clinical characteristics of participants

Characteristics (mean ± SD)	MDD patients($n = 31$)	Healthy controls($n = 28$)	p
Gender (male/female)	21/10	17/11	0.581
Age(years)	29.96 ± 9.73	26.79 ± 6.91	0.157
Educated(years)	13.74 ± 2.43	14.86 ± 2.43	0.084
HRSD17 score	20.26 ± 3.19	4.00 ± 1.09	< 0.001*
SHAPS total score	23.06 ± 5.97	4.59 ± 4.29	< 0.001*
FSS total score	45.83 ± 12.54	23.93 ± 5.58	< 0.001*
RBANS			
immediate memory	73.34 ± 15.43	95.48 ± 14.98	< 0.001*
visuospatial/constructional	88.78 ± 19.49	102.00 ± 14.71	0.009*
language	86.26 ± 17.06	97.52 ± 15.72	.0100*
attention	98.61 ± 15.79	119.56 ± 13.06	< 0.001*
delayed memory	83.13 ± 14.10	93.56 ± 10.68	0.013*
subpoint	82.30 ± 15.69	101.67 ± 11.99	< 0.001*
CPT			
two digits	2.38 ± 0.93	3.15 ± 0.82	0.002*
three digits	1.57 ± 0.94	2.74 ± 0.91	< 0.001*
four digits	0.94 ± 0.60	1.70 ± 0.76	< 0.001*
average	1.77 ± 1.08	2.53 ± 0.70	0.007*

*$p < 0.05$

Functional connectivity analysis results

Compared with the HC group, the MDD group showed significant decreases in rs-FC between the thalamus and SI in two clusters. As shown in Fig. 1 and Table 2, both clusters were in the right central posterior gyrus: the first cluster had the maximally intense voxel at MNI coordinates x = 27, y = − 33, z = 75 (8 voxels, about 216 mm^3, $T = 3.6162$, $p < 0.05$ AlphaSim correction), and the second cluster had the maximally intense voxel at MNI coordinates x = 45, y = − 30, z = 63 (8 voxels, about 216 mm^3, $T = 3.2803$, $p < 0.05$ AlphaSim correction).

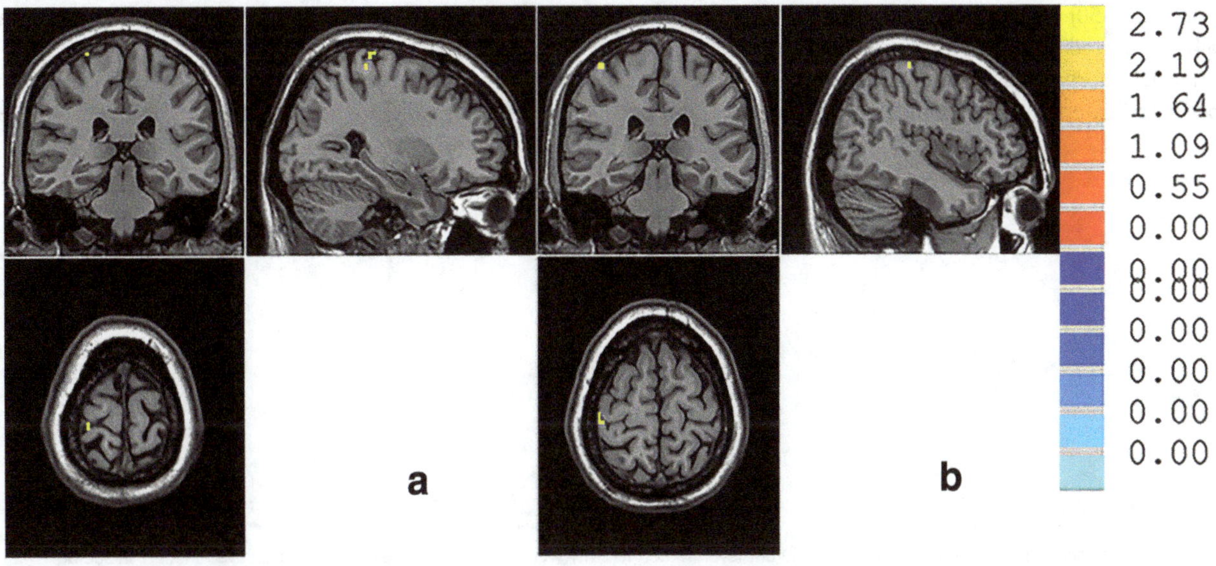

Fig. 1 The images display the regions in the right central posterior gyrus that show increased functional connectivity from the thalamus in major depressive disorder (MDD) compared to healthy controls (HC) at rest. The colour bar represents the range of T values

Table 2 Differences in SI-thalamic functional connectivity between MDD and HC (MDD > HC)

Area	L/R	Cluster size, mm^3	MNI coordinatesa			Tbvalues (peak)
			x	y	z	
central posterior gyrus	R	216	27	−33	75	3.6162*
central posterior gyrus	R	216	45	−30	63	3.2803*

*$p < 0.05$, single voxel threshold of $p < 0.01$ and cluster size ≥108 mm3, Alphasim correction

Correlational analysis

As shown in Fig. 2, significantly different brain regions and patient clinical symptoms in the SHAPS total score ($r = -0.383$, $p = 0.033$), delayed memory score ($r = -0.376$, $p = 0.037$), and two-digit continuous operation test score ($r = -0.369$, $p = 0.041$) showed significant negative correlations. The significantly different brain regions had no significant correlation with the other scores.

Discussion

Analysis of fMRI has been widely performed to study the dysfunction of brain systems in patients with psychiatric disorders. SI-thalamic functional connectivity in MDD patients has not been investigated. Our study found enhanced SI-thalamic functional connectivity, which was associated with affective experience and cognition function.

The rs-FC between the thalamus and the whole brain has been previously examined, and there were relatively consistent findings. MDD subjects had altered thalamocortical connectivity characterized by an intricate pattern in the region that was associated with clinical symptoms; indeed, one of them indicated the thalamus is hyper-connected with SI [47–50]. The importance of the SI has been gradually discovered in schizophrenia patients. For example, its abnormal internal activity predicted changes in processing speed, and external connections with the thalamus, as part of the thalamocortical-cerebellar dysconnectivity associated with schizophrenia, have become a reliable neurobiological marker [51, 52]. Our study does not emphasize the functional abnormalities of these two independent brain regions and their relationship to the development of MDD. We proposed that the differences in the SI-thalamic functional connectivity are the characteristic changes, as the central components of the experience of MDD.

Anhedonia is the most important clinical manifestation of MDD. Our study showed that abnormal connections between the thalamus and SI leads to the loss of pleasure. Numerous studies have reported that the role of SI has always been controversial with regards to the emergence of pleasure. Early studies showed that SI played an essential role in tactile pleasure perception, while studies that have used physical stimuli to modulate touch pleasantness have failed to control for differences in physical intensity and the perceived power of the overstimulation [53–55]. The research has shown that pleasant experience comes from outside of SI, but it is closely related to SI and brain activity, which may involve the thalamus [56, 57]. Our study confirmed that hyper-connection between the thalamus and SI is closely related to emotional experience, and to a certain degree, provides an explanation for the lack of pleasure experienced in MDD patients. However, further precision in identifying the role of these areas requires careful exploration of brain neuronal activity.

The starting point of our research was that cognitive function was an essential function, and our study emphasized that SI-thalamic functional connectivity is indeed closely related to attention and memory in MDD. In our research, we not only stressed the reliability of our previous theoretical basis but also provided a more detailed analysis of the cognitive items related to the SI-thalamic functional connectivity in MDD patients.

The research highlights the importance of SI for memory in different diseases or conditions [58, 59]. However,

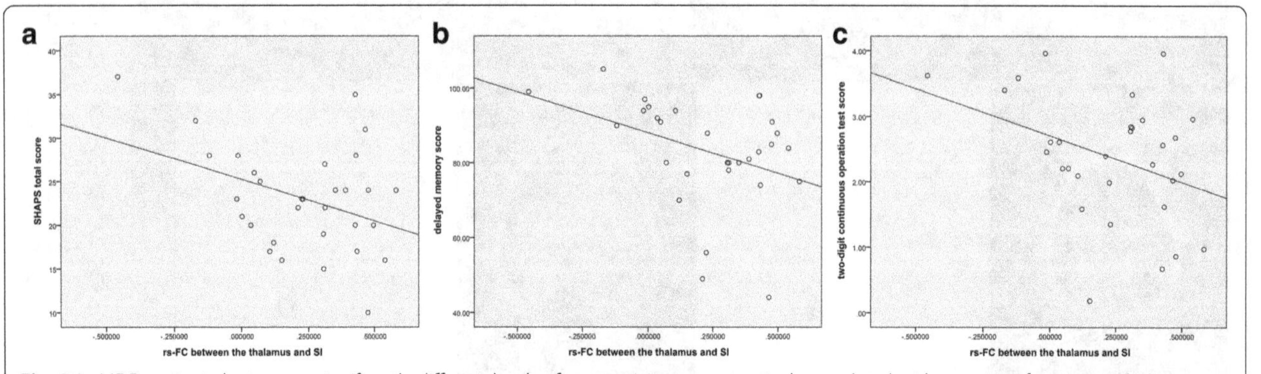

Fig. 2 In MDD patients, brain areas significantly different levels of connectivity were negatively correlated with cognitive function, including SHAPS total score ($r = -0.383$, $p = 0.033$), delayed memory score ($r = -0.376$, $p = 0.037$), and two-digit continuous operation test score ($r = -0.369$, $p = 0.041$) as shown in (**a**, **b**, and **c**), respectively

there are still some contradictory conclusions where researchers have proposed that SI did not affect the metacognitive accuracy of either temporal or spatial tactile working memory [60]. Unfortunately, the impact of thalamus and SI connections on cognition has been less explored. Research has demonstrated that in schizophrenia, hyper-connectivity with the thalamus correlated positively with working memory [61]. Our study also showed that similar changes occurred in MDD patients. The structural connection between the thalamus and SI may partially explain why the functional connections between the two are related to cognition. Thalamocortical responses provide input to SI for establishing context and storing sensory memories (e.g., slowly changing body memories stored in layer 4 and sensory memories rapidly stored in layer 2/3) [62]. However, the pathophysiological process for enhanced functional connectivity has not been elucidated.

The thalamus has a function of adjusting attention [63]. The thalamus functions as a master regulator of functional cortical connectivity. Therefore, the construction of a directed arousal state is useful for attention, impacting how a cognitive process such as attentional control unfolds over cortical space and time [64–66]. In MDD patients, we tentatively proposed that the hyper-connectivity between the thalamus and SI may disrupt the balance of this network, allowing the time for concentration to be prolonged. However, a new study shows that thalamus engagement in a delay is not to relay specific rule information but to sustain existing cortical representations [67]. These studies prompted us to carefully consider the role of thalamus inattention, and the mechanism for the inattention needs further investigation.

Our study has several limitations. First, our study design did not allow us to investigate causality or the role of change in functional connectivity between the thalamus and SI on the development of the MDD patients' cognitive impairment. Second, the thalamus could be divided into different subregions, but we did not subdivide when selecting regions of interest. Third, the heterogeneity of our patient population and a limited number of participants may lead to biased results. Fourth, long-term follow-up observations can lead to more profound experimental results. Fifth, we did not consider the impact of the length of the initial duration of the disease on brain function connectivity.

Conclusions

In conclusion, we have implicated enhanced SI-thalamic functional connectivity as a core feature of the pathophysiology underlying MDD. Furthermore, this abnormality is related to anhedonia, memory, and attention. The SI-thalamic functional connectivity may be a useful neural target for affective experience and cognitive interventions. Future research designed to track the effects of current treatments may develop more targeted pathophysiological therapies.

Abbreviations

CPT: Continuous performance test; DSM-IV: Diagnostic and Statistical Manual of Mental Disorders - Fourth Edition; HAMD-17: 17-item Hamilton depression rating scale; HC: Healthy controls; MDD: Major depressive disorder; MNI: Montreal Neurological Institute; RBANS: Assessment of Neuropsychological Status; ROI: Regions of interest; rs-FC: Resting-state functional connectivity; rs-fMRI: Resting-state functional magnetic resonance imaging; SCID-I/P: The Chinese version of the Modified Structured Clinical Interview for DSM-IV TR Axis I Disorders Patient Edition; SD: Standard deviation; SHAPS: Snaith-Hamilton Pleasure Scale; SI: Primary somatosensory cortex; SPSS 23.0: IBM SPSS Statistics Version 23.0

Acknowledgements

We would like to thank all the participants in this study.

Funding

Design and data collection of this work were supported by grants from the National Natural Science Foundation of China (81471379 and 81601193) and the National Clinical Research Center on Mental Disorders (2015BAI13B02). Data analysis and interpretation were supported by the National Natural Science Foundation of China (81701345) and the Shanxi Provincial Science Foundation for Youth (2015021204). Writing the manuscript was supported by the National Key R&D Program of China (2016YFC1307103). We sincerely thank the patients and the healthy volunteers for their participation and all the medical staff involved in the collection of cases.

Authors' contributions

ZKR designed the study and wrote the protocol. SN, WYF and ZAX were responsible for all aspects of patient recruitment and clinical diagnostic assessment. YCX, KLJ, LZF contributed to the collection of the data. ZAX, LPH, LGZ and KLJ performed the statistical analysis. KLJ and ZAX prepared the first draft. ZKR contributed to the conceptualization of the study and reviewed several manuscript drafts. All authors contributed to and approved the final manuscript.

Consent for publication

Not applicable.

Competing interests

The authors declare that they have no competing interests.

Author details

[1]Department of Psychiatry, First Hospital of Shanxi Medical University, Taiyuan 030001, People's Republic of China. [2]Shanxi Medical University, Taiyuan 030001, People's Republic of China.

References

1. Kessler RC, Berglund P, Demler O, et al. Lifetime prevalence and age-of-onset distributions of DSM-IV disorders in the National Comorbidity Survey Replication. Arch Gen Psychiatry. 2005;62(6):593–602.
2. Bora E, Harrison BJ, Yucel M, Pantelis C. Cognitive impairment in euthymic major depressive disorder: a meta-analysis. Psychol Med. 2013;43(10):2017–26. https://doi.org/10.1017/S0033291712002085.
3. Snyder HR. Major depressive disorder is associated with broad impairments on neuropsychological measures of executive function: a meta-analysis and review. Psychol Bull. 2013;139(1):81–132.
4. Mak ADP, Lau DTY, Chan AKW, So SH, Leung O, Wong SL, et al. Cognitive impairment in treatment-Naïve bipolar II and unipolar depression. Sci Rep. 2018;8(1):1905.
5. Polosa M, Lemogne C, Jardri R, Fossati P. Cognition-the core of major depressive disorder. L'Encephale. 2016;42(1 Suppl 1):1S3–11. https://doi.org/10.1016/S0013-7006(16)30014-8.
6. Ahern E, Semkovska M. Cognitive functioning in the first-episode of major depressive disorder: a systematic review and meta-analysis. Neuropsychology. 2017;31(1):52–72. https://doi.org/10.1037/neu0000319.
7. Nierenberg AA, Husain MM, Trivedi MH, Fava M, Warden D, Wisniewski SR, et al. Residual symptoms after remission of major depressive disorder with citalopram and risk of relapse: a STAR* D report. Psychol Med. 2010;40(1): 41–50.
8. Trivedi MH, Greer TL. Cognitive dysfunction in unipolar depression: implications for treatment. J Affect Disord. 2014;152-154:19–27. https://doi.org/10.1016/j.jad.2013.09.012.
9. Levin HS, Eisenberg HM, Benton AL. Frontal lobe function and dysfunction. Frontal lobe function and dysfunction. Oxford: Oxford University Press; 1991.
10. Modha DS, Mishkin M. Network architecture of the long-distance pathways in the macaque brain. Proc Natl Acad Sci U S A. 2010;107(30):13485–90.
11. Peters SK, Dunlop K, Downar J. Cortico-striatal-thalamic loop circuits of the salience network: a central pathway in psychiatric disease and treatment. Front Syst Neurosci. 2016;10:104.
12. Chang YT, Lu CH, Wu MK, Hsu SW, Huang CW, Chang WN, et al. Salience network and depressive severities in Parkinson's disease with mild cognitive impairment: a structural covariance network analysis. Front Aging Neurosci. 2018;9:417.
13. Parnaudeau S, Bolkan SS, Kellendonk C. The Mediodorsal thalamus: an essential partner of the prefrontal cortex for cognition. Biol Psychiatry. 2018; 83(8):648–56. https://doi.org/10.1016/j.biopsych.2017.11.008.
14. Schoonheim MM, Hulst HE, Brandt RB, Strik M, Wink AM, Uitdehaag BM, et al. Thalamus structure and function determine severity of cognitive impairment in multiple sclerosis. Neurology. 2015;84(8):776–83.
15. Tewarie P, Schoonheim MM, Schouten DI, Polman CH, Balk LJ, Uitdehaag BM, et al. Functional brain networks: linking thalamic atrophy to clinical disability in multiple sclerosis, a multimodal fMRI and MEG study. Hum Brain Mapp. 2015;36(2):603–18.
16. Bisecco A, Rocca MA, Pagani E, Mancini L, Enzinger C, Gallo A, et al. Connectivity-based parcellation of the thalamus in multiple sclerosis and its implications for cognitive impairment: a multicenter study. Hum Brain Mapp. 2015;36(7):2809–25.
17. Houtchens MK, Benedict RHB, Killiany R, Sharma J, Jaisani Z, Singh B, et al. Thalamic atrophy and cognition in multiple sclerosis. Neurology. 2007; 69(12):1213–23.
18. Koenig KA, Rao SM, Lowe MJ, Lin J, Sakaie KE, Stone L, et al. The role of the thalamus and hippocampus in episodic memory performance in patients with multiple sclerosis. Mult Scler J. 2018;1:1–11. https://doi.org/10.1177/1352458518760716.
19. Zhang D, Snyder AZ, Shimony JS, Fox MD, Raichle ME, et al. Noninvasive functional and structural connectivity mapping of the human Thalamocortical system. Cereb Cortex. 2010;20(5):1187–94.
20. Zhang D, Snyder AZ, Fox MD, Sansbury MW, Shimony JS, Raichle ME, et al. Intrinsic functional relations between human cerebral cortex and thalamus. J Neurophysiol. 2008;100(4):1740–8.
21. Penfield W, Boldrey E. Somatic motor and sensory representation in the cerebral cortex of man as studied by electrical stimulation. Brain. 1937;60(4): 389–443.
22. Simons D. Neuronal integration in the somatosensory whisker/barrel cortex. Cereb Cortex. 1995;11:263–97.
23. Galvez R, Weiss C, Weible AP, Disterhoft JF, et al. Vibrissa-signaled eyeblink conditioning induces somatosensory cortical plasticity. J Neurosci the Official Journal of the Society for Neuroscience. 2006;26(22):6062–8.
24. Chau LS, Davis AS, Galvez R. Neocortical synaptic proliferation following forebrain-dependent trace associative learning. Behav Neurosci. 2013;127(2): 285–92.
25. Tseng MT, Kong Y, Eippert F, Tracey I, et al. Determining the neural substrate for encoding a memory of human pain and the influence of anxiety. J Neurosci. 2017;37(49):11806–17.
26. Zhao D, Zhou YD, Bodner M, Ku Y, et al. The causal role of the prefrontal cortex and somatosensory cortex in tactile working memory. Cereb Cortex. 2017;28(10):1–10.
27. Hegner YL, Lutzenberger W, Leiberg S, Braun C, et al. The involvement of ipsilateral temporoparietal cortex in tactile pattern working memory as reflected in beta event-related desynchronization. NeuroImage. 2007; 37(4):1362–70.
28. Khoshnejad M, Roy M, Martinu K, Chen JI, Cohen-Adad J, Grondin S, et al. Brain processing of the temporal dimension of acute pain in short-term memory. Pain. 2017;158(10):2001–11.
29. Schaefer M, Northoff G. Who am I: the conscious and the unconscious self. Front Hum Neurosci. 2017;11:126.
30. Biswal B, Zerrin Yetkin F, Haughton VM, Hyde JS. Functional connectivity in the motor cortex of resting human brain using echo-planarmri. Magn Reson Med. 1995;34(4):537–41.
31. Zuo XN, Kelly C, Martino AD, Mennes M, Margulies DS, Bangaru S, et al. Growing together and growing apart: regional and sex differences in the lifespan developmental trajectories of functional homotopy. J Neurosci the Official Journal of the Society for Neuroscience. 2010; 30(45):15034–43.
32. Gorges M, Müller HP, Lulé D, Ludolph AC, Pinkhardt EH, Kassubek J, et al. Functional connectivity within the default mode network is associated with saccadic accuracy in Parkinson's disease: a resting-state FMRI and videooculographic study. Brain Connectivity. 2013;3(3):265–72. https://doi.org/10.1089/brain.2013.0146.
33. Harshaw C. Interoceptive dysfunction: toward an integrated framework for understanding somatic and affective disturbance in depression. Psychol Bull. 2015;141(2):311.
34. Hamilton M. A rating scale for depression. J Neurol Neurosurg Psychiatry. 1960;23(1):56.
35. Snaith RP, Hamilton M, Morley S, Humayan A, Hargreaves D, Trigwell P. A scale for the assessment of hedonic tone the snaith-Hamilton pleasure scale. Br J Psychiatry. 1995;167(1):99–103.
36. Krupp LB, LaRocca NG, Muir-Nash J, Steinberg AD, et al. The fatigue severity scale: application to patients with multiple sclerosis and systemic lupus erythematosus. Arch Neurol. 1989;46(10):1121–3.
37. Randolph C, Tierney MC, Mohr E, Chase TN, et al. The repeatable battery for the assessment of neuropsychological status (RBANS): preliminary clinical validity. J Clin Exp Neuropsychol. 1998;20(3):310–9.
38. Mur M, Portella MJ, Martínezarán A, Pifarre J, Vieta E, et al. Long-term stability of cognitive impairment in bipolar disorder: a 2-year follow-up study of lithium-treated euthymic bipolar patients. J Clin Psychiatry. 2008;69(5):712–9.
39. Yan C, Zang Y. DPARSF: a MATLAB toolbox for "pipeline" data analysis of resting-state fMRI. Front Syst Neurosci. 2010;4:13. https://doi.org/10.3389/fnsys.2010.00013.
40. Data Processing Assistant for Resting-State fMRI (DPARSF). http://rfmri.org/DPARSF. Accessed 20 May 2017.
41. Maldjian JA, Laurienti PJ, Kraft A, Burdette JH. An automated method for neuroanatomic and cytoarchitectonic atlas-based interrogation of fMRI data sets. NeuroImage. 2003;19(3):1233–39.
42. Software Packages that are currently available for download from the ANSIR Laboratory at Wake Forest University School of Medicine. www.fmri.wfubmc.edu/download.htm. Accessed 22 May 2017.
43. Salvador R, Suckling J, Schwarzbauer C, Bullmore E, et al. Undirected graphs of frequency-dependent functional connectivity in whole brain networks. Philos Trans R Soc Lond Ser B Biol Sci. 2005;360(1457):937–46. https://doi.org/10.1098/rstb.2005.1645.
44. Liu Y, Yu C, Liang M, Li J, Tian L, Zhou Y, et al. Whole brain functional connectivity in the early blind. Brain. 2007;130(8):2085–96.
45. Ledberg A, Åkerman S, Roland PE. Estimation of the probabilities of 3D clusters in functional brain images. NeuroImage. 1998;8(2):113–28.
46. Simultaneous Inference for FMRI Data. http://afni.nimh.nih.gov/pub/dist/doc/manual/AlphaSim.pdf. Accessed 20 May 2017.

47. Kong QM, Qiao H, Liu CZ, Zhang P, Li K, Wang L, et al. Aberrant intrinsic functional connectivity in thalamo-cortical networks in major depressive disorder. CNS Neurosci Ther. 2018;28:1–10. https://doi.org/10.1111/cns.12831.
48. Kim K, Kim SW, Myung W, Han CE, Fava M, Mischoulon D, et al. Reduced orbitofrontal-thalamic functional connectivity related to suicidal ideation in patients with major depressive disorder. Sci Rep. 2017;7(1):15772;1–11.
49. Zhu X, Helpman L, Papini S, Schneier F, Markowitz JC, Meter PE, et al. Altered resting state functional connectivity of fear and reward circuitry in comorbid PTSD and major depression. Depression and anxiety. 2017;34(7): 641–50.
50. Brown EC, Clark DL, Hassel S, MacQueen G, Ramasubbu R, et al. Thalamocortical connectivity in major depressive disorder. J Affect Disord. 2017;217:125–31.
51. Woodward ND, Karbasforoushan H, Heckers S. Thalamocortical dysconnectivity in schizophrenia. Am J Psychiatry. 2012;169(10):1092–9.
52. Krukow P, Jonak K, Karakuła-Juchnowicz H, Podkowiński A, Jonak K, Borys M, et al. Disturbed functional connectivity within the left prefrontal cortex and sensorimotor areas predicts impaired cognitive speed in patients with first-episode schizophrenia. Psychiatry Res Neuroimaging. 2018;275:28–35. https://doi.org/10.1016/j.pscychresns.2018.03.001.
53. Löken LS, Wessberg J, McGlone F, Morrison I, Olausson H, et al. Coding of pleasant touch by unmyelinated afferents in humans. Nat Neurosci. 2009; 12(5):547.
54. Sel A, Calvo-Merino B, Tuettenberg S, Forster B, et al. When you smile, the world smiles at you: ERP evidence for self-expression effects on face processing. Soc Cogn Affect Neurosci. 2015;10(10):1316–22.
55. Gazzola V, Spezio ML, Etzel JA, Castelli F, Adolphs R, Keysers C, et al. Primary somatosensory cortex discriminates affective significance in social touch. Proc Natl Acad Sci. 2012;109(25):E1657–66.
56. Case LK, Laubacher CM, Olausson H, Wang B, Spagnolo PA, Bushnell MC, et al. Encoding of touch intensity but not pleasantness in human primary somatosensory cortex. J Neurosci. 2016;36(21):5850–60.
57. McCabe C, Rolls ET, Bilderbeck A, Mcglone F, et al. Cognitive influences on the affective representation of touch and the sight of touch in the human brain. Soc Cogn Affect Neurosci. 2008;3(2):97–108.
58. Hara Y, Ago Y, Higuchi M, Hasebe S, Nakazawa T, Hashimoto H, et al. Oxytocin attenuates deficits in social interaction but not recognition memory in a prenatal valproic acid-induced mouse model of autism. Horm Behav. 2017;96:130–6.
59. Boutin A, Pinsard B, Boré A, Carrier FSM, Doyon J, et al. Transient synchronization of hippocampo-striato-thalamo-cortical networks during sleep spindle oscillations induces motor memory consolidation. NeuroImage. 2018; 169:419–30. https://doi.org/10.1016/j.neuroimage.2017.12.066.
60. Gogulski J, Zetter R, Nyrhinen M, Pertovaara A, Carlson S, et al. Neural substrate for metacognitive accuracy of tactile working memory. Cereb Cortex. 2017;27(11):5343–52.
61. Giraldo-Chica M, Rogers BP, Damon SM, Landman BA, Woodward ND, et al. Prefrontal-thalamic anatomical connectivity and executive cognitive function in schizophrenia. Biol Psychiatry. 2018;83(6):509–17.
62. Brecht M. The body model theory of somatosensory cortex. Neuron. 2017; 94(5):985–92.
63. Petersen SE, Robinson DL, Keys W. Pulvinar nuclei of the behaving rhesus monkey: visual responses and their modulation. J Neurophysiol. 1985;54(4): 867–86.
64. Nakajima M, Halassa MM. Thalamic control of functional cortical connectivity. Curr Opin Neurobiol. 2017;44:127–31.
65. Schmitt LI, Halassa MM. Interrogating the mouse thalamus to correct human neurodevelopmental disorders. Mol Psychiatry. 2017;22(2):183.
66. Duncan J. The structure of cognition: attentional episodes in mind and brain. Neuron. 2013;80(1):35–50.
67. Schmitt LI, Wimmer RD, Nakajima M, Happ M, Mofakham S, Halassa MM, et al. Thalamic amplification of cortical connectivity sustains attentional control. Nature. 2017;545(7653):219.

12

Association between hyperuricemia and metabolic syndrome in patients suffering from bipolar disorder

Jingxu Chen[1†], Hongmei Chen[1†], Junhui Feng[2], Ligang Zhang[1], Juyan Li[1], Ran Li[1], Shaoli Wang[1], Ian Wilson[3], Alison Jones[3], Yunlong Tan[1], Fude Yang[1*] and Xu-Feng Huang[3*]

Abstract

Background: Clinical studies have shown that bipolar patients have increased serum uric acid levels. High serum uric acid levels could play a role contributing to high prevalence of metabolic syndrome. Metabolic syndrome is known to increase the risk of developing a number of life threatening diseases including coronary heart disease, hypertension, and type 2 diabetes. This study investigated the association between hyperuricemia and metabolic syndrome and its components in individuals suffering from bipolar disorders.

Methods: This study recruited 318 inpatients suffering from bipolar disorders from Beijing Hui-Long-Guan Hospital in China and 160 healthy subjects from the same region as the controls. We used National Cholesterol Education Program Adult Treatment Panel III Adapted criteria (NCEP ATP-III A) for the diagnosis of metabolic syndrome. Hyperuricemia was determined as serum uric acid level above 420 μmol/L in men and 360 μmol/L in women (N Engl J Med 359(17):1811–1821, 2008).

Results: Among 318 bipolar patients, there was higher prevalence of metabolic syndrome (42.5%) and hyperuricemia (27.7%) than healthy controls (21.9 and 11.9%). Bipolar patients with metabolic syndrome had increased prevalence of hyperuricemia (OR = 3.0, CI95 [1.7–5.4]). Hypertriglyceridemia and larger waist circumference (WC) were associated with hyperunicemia (OR = 1.8, CI95 [1.1–3.1], OR = 1.9, CI95 [1.1–3.4]). Hyperuricemia was associated with metabolic syndrome in bipolar patients ($p < 0.001$) and especially with hypertriglyceridemia (OR = 1.9, CI95 [1.1–3.1] and increased WC (OR = 2.1 [1.2–4.0]). Bipolar patients over 50 years of age and hyperuricemia were highly prone to develop metabolic syndrome (OR = 14.0, CI95 [5.0–39.0]).

Conclusions: Hyperuricemia was highly associated with development of metabolic disorder particularly for aged patients suffering from bipolar disorders. Early prevention of hyperuricemia and metabolic syndrome may lead better life for bipolar patients when they get older.

Keywords: Bipolar, Hyperuricemia, Metabolic syndrome, Ageing

Background

Bipolar disorder is a chronic mental illness, which is associated with a potentially devastating long-term impact on the patient's health, as well as their job, social relationships and families [1–3]. The World Health Organization reported that bipolar disorder was the seventh among severe diseases in the year 2000 [4]. People suffering from bipolar disorders have high mortality, which could result in a 10–20 year shorter lifespan compared to the general population [5]. These patients have a high prevalence of cardiovascular disease to which 35–40% of deaths are attributable, which is associated with metabolic syndrome [6]. Increased ageing population leads to high burden of bipolar disorder patients [2]. Therefore, it is important to investigate possible contributing factors in order to prevent metabolic

* Correspondence: yangfd200@126.com; xhuang@uow.edu.au
†Jingxu Chen and Hongmei Chen contributed equally to this work.
[1]Beijing Hui-Long-Guan Hospital, Peking University, Beijing 100096, China
[3]Illawarra Health and Medical Research Institute and School of Medicine, University of Wollongong, Wollongong, NSW 2522, Australia

syndrome, reduce cardiovascular risk, and allocate health care resources to bipolar patients.

Metabolic syndrome is characterized by visceral obesity, altered lipid and glucose profiles and hypertension, all of which are known to increase the risk of developing cardiovascular diseases and type 2 diabetes [7]. Although the causal factors of developing metabolic syndrome in bipolar disorder patients are largely unknown, some contributing factors are proposed. For example, the risk factors may be due to the side effects of an unhealthy lifestyle including excessive food intake and reduced energy expenditure caused by mental illness or drug treatment, or inability to access appropriate health care [8–10].

Uric acid is the final oxidative product in the degradation of purine nucleotides. It has been evidenced by several studies that high serum uric acid levels were as a potential causal factor leading to high prevalence of metabolic syndrome and its components, including central obesity, hypertension, hyperlipidemia, diabetes, and insulin resistance [11–13]. Recently, clinical studies have confirmed that bipolar patients in all phases of the illness, especially manic episode, had increased serum uric acid levels [14–16]. Study also shows that the estimated effect between bipolar disorder and uric acid levels was partially mediated by metabolic abnormalities [17]. Therefore, the hyperuricemia and metabolic syndrome may reciprocally affect each other, which impairs glucose and lipid metabolism. This study investigated the relationship between hyperuricemia and metabolic syndrome and its components in individuals suffering from bipolar disorder.

Methods

Subjects

This study was carried out in Beijing Hui-Long-Guan hospital, a city-owned psychiatric hospital, China. A total of 318 patients (male/female = 150/168) were recruited from the inpatients suffering bipolar disorders. The study was conduction from July 2015 to June 2017. Patients were diagnosed as bipolar disorder based on DSM-IV diagnostic criteria for Bipolar Disorder I/II. Patients were referred by their psychiatrists to our research team. Patients were between 18 and 65 years of age and Han ethnic Chinese, agreed to participate in the study, and signed consent form either themselves or the first degree of their relative if the patient's condition did not allow him or her to do so. The research team evaluated the patients including their disease history, current symptoms, and general conditions. Those patients excluded were: 1) diagnosed with substance abuse within the previous 3 months, 2) pregnant or breast-feeding, and 3) those suffering from a neural degenerative disease including dementia and mental retardation.

One hundred and sixty healthy controls (male/female = 74/86) having no significant differences in age (± 1 year) and gender ratio to the patients were recruited from the same local community through the advertisement in media and pamphlets distributed to local residents (Table 1). We have performed psychiatric examination to all participants. Controls having a history of mental illness or substance abuse were excluded. The protocol of this study was approved by the Human Ethics Committee of Beijing Hui-Long-Guan Hospital and all patients were provided with a written informed consent in accordance with National Health and Medical Research Council Guidelines.

Assessment

The height and weight of all subjects were measured on the same calibrated weight scale standing barefoot with light clothes. Body mass index was calculated for all subjects. Patients with a BMI ≥25 kg/m^2 were considered overweight [18]. Waist circumference was measured at the mid-point level between the inferior costal margin and superior iliac crest at the time that the subject was at the end of his/her expiration while standing. A standard mercury manometer was used to measure blood pressure with the patient in a supine position. We recorded two readings with 5 min apart for blood pressure recordings. If one of the two blood pressure readings were greater than 130/85 mmHg, we took a third reading 30 min later. We then used the lowest of three readings in the analysis according to a previous study [19]. All subjects underwent venipuncture between 6:00 am and 7:00 am after overnight fasting (~ 12 h), and the blood samples were analyzed on the same day. Serum concentrations of blood glucose, triglycerides, high-density lipoprotein cholesterol, and uric acid were measured using commercial kits (Beckman Coulter, Brea, California, USA) and an OLYMPUS AU 2700 automatic biochemical analyzer.

The definition of metabolic syndrome and hyperuricemia

The present study used NCEP ATP-III-A for the diagnosis of metabolic syndrome [20]. This is because it has adjusted waist circumference for those of European descent to be more appropriate for Asian waist size [20] and sets a more stringent fasting glucose concentration to 5.6 mmol/L [21]. NCEP-ATP-III-A criteria requires the presence at least three of the following components: 1) increased waist circumference (WC): WC greater than 90 cm in men or 80 cm in women; 2) hypertriglyceridemia: triglycerides greater than 1.70 mmol/L (150 mg/dL); 3) high density lipoprotein cholesterol (HDL-C): HDL-C lower than 1.03 mmol/L (40 mg/dL) in men or 1.29 mmol/L (50 mg/dL) in women; 4) hypertension: blood pressure greater than 130 mmHg systolic or

Table 1 Socio-demographic and clinical characteristics of bipolar patient and health control groups

Variable	Patient Group (n = 318)	Control Group (n = 160)	X^2 /t	p
Age (years)	39.2 ± 13.1	38.5 ± 11.3	0.532	0.595
Male, n (%)	150 (47.2)	74 (46.3)	0.006	0.807
Education (years)	11.8 ± 3.5	11.7 ± 3.9	0.481	0.631
Married, n (%)	175 (55.0)	108 (67.5)	6.852	0.009
Smoker, n (%)	86 (27.0)	26 (16.3)	6.913	0.009
BMI(kg/m^2)	24.8 ± 3.3	23.3 ± 2.6	4.955	< 0.001
Overweight, n (%)	145 (45.6)	48 (30.0)	10.757	0.001
Diastolic BP (mm Hg)	75.2 ± 8.4	73.8 ± 8.1	1.793	0.074
Systolic BP (mm Hg)	114.6 ± 11.1	113.5 ± 11.1	1.046	0.296
Hypertension, n (%)	91 (28.6)	29 (18.1)	6.231	0.013
WC (cm)	87.5 ± 11.1	83.6 ± 8.9	3.844	< 0.001
Increased WC, n (%)	186 (58.5)	53 (33.8)	26.062	< 0.001
HDL-C (mmol/L)	1.2 ± 0.4	1.3 ± 0.4	3.331	0.001
Low HDL-C, n (%)	151 (47.5)	50 (31.3)	11.512	0.001
Triglyceride (mmol/L)	2.4 ± 1.5	1.4 ± 1.1	6.526	< 0.001
Hypertriglyceridemia, n (%)	118 (37.1)	37 (23.1)	9.497	0.002
FBG (mmol/L)	5.0 ± 1.2	4.8 ± 0.7	2.660	0.008
Hyperglycaemia, n (%)	75 (23.6)	22 (13.8)	6.365	0.012
MetS, n (%)	135 (42.5)	35 (21.9)	19.669	< 0.001
UA (mmol/L)	348.5 ± 91.8	300.2 ± 76.6	5.729	< 0.001
Hyperuricemia	88 (27.7)	19 (11.9)	15.290	< 0.001

Data were mean ± SD unless otherwise indicated. BMI: body mass index; *BP* blood pressure, *WC* waist circumference, *HDL-C* high density lipoprotein cholesterol, *FBG* fasting blood glucose, *MetS* metabolic syndrome, *UA* uric acid

greater than 85 mmHg diastolic; and 5) hyperglycemia: fasting glucose concentration greater than 5.6 mmol/L (100 mg/dL), or diagnosed as type 2 diabetes. In addition, treatment with specific drugs was also considered including triglyceride, cholesterol, and glucose lowering drugs and blood pressure lowering drugs. Hyperuricemia was defined as serum level of uric acid > 420 μmol/L (7.0 mg/dL) for men and > 360 μmol/L (6.0 mg/dL) for women [22, 23].

Statistical analysis

Statistical analysis was carried out using SPSS 15.0 for Windows (SPSS Inc., Chicago, USA). Demographics, clinical measures, and laboratory values were reported using measures of means and standard deviation. Group difference was compared using t-test for continuous variables having normal distribution and Mann-Whitney test for variables, which were not normal distribution including triglyceride, illness duration and CPZ equivalent dose. Chi-square test was used for categorical variable analyses. Univariate analysis was used to identify significant association between variables and metabolic syndrome. Simple binary logistic regression was used to establish correlation of metabolic syndrome and hyperuricemia as responding variable. Odds ratios and 95% confidence intervals for all independent variables were determined. Sample size calculation was set at an alpha value of 0.05, power 85% based on a previous study [24]. Marital status, illness duration, and illness episode were eliminated as confounding factors. All statistical tests were two-tailed, with alpha level set at 0.05.

Results

Demographic and clinical characteristics of subjects

A total of 362 inpatients suffering from bipolar disorders were enrolled in this study. Forty-four patients (12.2%) were excluded since there were no fasting blood and/or anthropometry data such as body weight, height, blood pressure, and waist circumference. Patients (n = 318) and control subjects (n = 160) had no significant differences in age and gender ratio ($p > 0.05$). Demographic and clinical characteristics of the study population were shown in Table 1.

The bipolar patient group had lower marriage rate ($p = 0.009$) and higher proportion of smokers ($p < 0.01$) than the control group. Patients suffering from bipolar disorders were overweight ($p = 0.001$), high BMI ($p < 0.001$), larger WC ($p = 0.013$), and low serum HDL-C

($p = 0.001$), increased triglyceride ($p < 0.001$), high fasting blood glucose ($p = 0.002$), and increased uric acid ($p < 0.001$) compared to control subjects without bipolar disorder. There were no statistical differences in systolic and diastolic blood pressures between patients and control subjects (both $p > 0.05$).

Bipolar patients had high prevalence of metabolic syndrome and hyperuricemia

The prevalence of both hyperuricemia and metabolic syndrome was higher in bipolar patients compared to control subjects (27.7% vs. 11.9%, $p < 0.001$ and 42.5% vs. 21.9%, $p < 0.001$). Patients having metabolic syndrome had increased WC (58.5%), hypertriglyceridemia (37.1%), hyperglycemia (23.6%), and hypertension (28.6%) and decreased HDL-C (47.5%) (Table 1). Bipolar patients had high prevalence of hyperuricemia than control subjects (27.7% vs 11.9%, $p < 0.001$).

Factors associated with metabolic syndrome and hyperuricemia

Hyperuricemia and metabolic syndrome in bipolar patients were associated with overweight, longer duration of the illness, and manic or mixed episodes (all $p < 0.05$). Metabolic syndrome was associated with ageing and uses of mood stabilizer and antipsychotics (all $p < 0.05$) (Table 2). Hyperuricemia was more common in male patients than female patients ($p < 0.05$). Bipolar patients with hyperuricemia had a high prevalence of metabolic syndrome than bipolar patients without hyperuricemia (Table 3). Hyperuricemia was associated with hypertriglyceridemia and hyperglycemia, but not with hypertension, in bipolar patients.

Association between metabolic syndrome and hyperuricemia

The factors that correlated with the presence of metabolic syndrome were ages including 30 and 49 years (OR = 2.2, CI95[1.1–4.2], > 50 years (OR = 8.6, CI95[4.1–18.0], overweight (OR = 3.0, CI95[1.8–5.5]), antipsychotic use (OR = 3.6, CI95[1.7–7.5]), mood stabilizer use (OR = 2.4, CI95[1.1–5.3]) and hyperuricemia (OR = 3.0, CI95[1.7–5.4]) (Table 4). The hyperuricemia were higher with increased WC (OR = 2.1, CI95[1.2–4.0]) and hypertriglyceridemia (OR = 1.9, CI95[1.1–3.1]) (Table 5). Bipolar patients having hyperuricemia and age greater than 50 years were more prone to develop metabolic syndrome (OR = 14.0, CI95[5.0–38.8]) (Fig. 1).

Discussion

The prevalence of metabolic syndrome in bipolar patients varies significantly from 8.5 to 67% from study to study reported in the literature [24–28]. A possible explanation for such large discrepancies may be due to different ethnicities, regions, dietary habits, and genetic backgrounds of patients investigated [29]. For example, high prevalence (67%) was reported in an Australian study and 53% prevalence in an Indian study in bipolar patients suffering metabolic syndrome [25, 27]. Low prevalence of metabolic syndrome in bipolar patients

Table 2 Characteristics of bipolar patients with metabolic syndrome and hyperuricemia

Variable	Metabolic syndrome			Hyperuricemia		
	Yes ($n = 135$)	No ($n = 183$)	p	Yes ($n = 86$)	No ($n = 232$)	p
Age (years)	44.1 (12.5)	35.4 (12.6)	< 0.001	40.5 (13.4)	38.6 (13.0)	0.265
Male, n (%)	67 (49.6)	83 (45.4)	0.450	50 (56.8)	100 (43.5)	0.033
Education (years)	11.5 (3.6)	12.10 (3.4)	0.104	11.4 (3.2)	12.0 (3.5)	0.150
Smoker, n (%)	42 (31.1)	44 (24.0)	0.161	26 (29.5)	60 (26.1)	0.534
Married, n (%)	83 (61.5)	92 (50.3)	0.047	47 (53.4)	128 (55.7)	0.719
Illness duration (year)	15.9 (11.3)	9.9 (9.3)	< 0.001	14.25 (10.6)	11.9 (10.6)	0.013
Over weight, n (%)	85 (63.0)	60 (32.8)	< 0.001	52 (59.1)	93 (40.4)	0.003
Illness episode, n (%)			0.012			0.001
Manic/hypomanic	91 (67.4)	104 (56.8)		68 (77.3)	127 (55.2)	
Depressive	31 (23.0)	69 (37.7)		14 (15.9)	86 (37.4)	
Mixed	5(3.7)	1 (0.5)		3 (3.4)	3 (1.3)	
Euthymic	8(5.9)	9(4.9)		3 (3.4)	14 (6.1)	
BPD type II, n (%)	9 (6.7)	12 (6.6)	0.969	6 (6.8)	15 (6.5)	0.924
Antipsychotics use, n (%)	120 (88.9)	135 (73.8)	0.001	72 (81.8)	183 (79.6)	0.652
CPZ equivalents (mg/d)	344.7 (205.9)	297.7 (248.1)	0.030	3602 (209.8)	307.0 (236.1)	0.081
Mood stabilizer use, n (%)	118 (87.4)	144 (78.7)	0.044	74 (84.1)	188 (81.7)	0.662

Data were mean ± SD unless otherwise indicated. *BPD* bipolar disorder, *CPZ* chlorpromazine

Table 3 Association between hyperuricemia and metabolic syndrome and its components

Variable	Hyperuricemia		X^2	p
	Yes(n = 86)	No(n = 232)		
MetS, n (%)	55 (62.5)	80 (34.8)	20.015	< 0.001
Increased WC, n (%)	63 (71.6)	123 (53.5)	8.600	0.003
Low HDL-C, n (%)	47 (53.4)	104 (45.2)	1.713	0.191
Hypertriglyceridemia, n (%)	44 (50.0)	74 (32.2)	8.666	0.003
Hypertension, n (%)	30 (34.1)	61 (26.5)	1.785	0.182
Hyperglycaemia, n (%)	29 (33.0)	46 (20.0)	5.927	0.015

MetS metabolic syndrome, *WC* waist circumference, *HDL-C* high density lipoprotein cholesterol

was reported in French (18.5%) and Spanish (22.4%) studies [24, 26]. There are two other Indian studies reports that the prevalence of metabolic syndrome in bipolar patients is about 40%, [20, 30], which is similar to 42% found in this study. On the other hand, the prevalence of metabolic syndrome in control subjects was 21.9% in the present study, which was similar to previous Chinese studies in normal population (24.5%) [31].

Visceral obesity should be closely monitored as the prevalence of larger WC was significantly higher in bipolar patients than control subjects (58.5% vs 33.8%). Visceral obesity is associated with metabolic syndrome, type 2 diabetes and coronary heart disease [32]. The prevalence of metabolic syndrome in bipolar patients was about eight times higher in the bipolar patients with age over 50 years than the bipolar patients with age less than 30 years. This could be due to increased uric acids, which worse insulin sensitivity in elderly patients. Patients having longer illness duration and experiencing manic or mixed episodes had higher rates of metabolic syndrome. The prevalence of gender difference having metabolic syndrome in bipolar patients is controversial. Some studies have reported that the prevalence of metabolic syndrome in male bipolar patients was about twice higher than female patients; but negative and opposite

Table 4 Associations between the various factors and the risk of having metabolic syndrome

Variable	OR	95%CI	p
< 30 years of age	1.000	Reference	–
30–49 years of age	2.149	1.122–4.177	0.021
≥50 years of age	8.587	4.087–18.044	< 0.001
BMI ≥25 kg/m2	3.005	1.767–5.110	< 0.001
Antipsychotics[a]	3.595	1.722–7.497	0.001
Mood stabilizer[b]	2.397	1.087–5.285	0.030
Hyperuricemia[c]	3.029	1.685–5.443	< 0.001

[a]: use of antipsychotic drug at clinical dose, [b]: use of mood stabilizer at clinical dose, [c]: serum uric acid > 420 μmol/l for men and > 360 μmol/l for women [21]

Table 5 Associations between WC and hypertriglyceridemia with the risk of having hyperuricemia

Variable	OR	95%CI	p
Increased WC	2.128	1.233–4.034	0.007
Hypertriglyceridemia	1.870	1.112–3.121	0.017

WC waist circumference

results were also reported in other studies [27, 33, 34]. The data presented in this study suggested no gender differences to develop metabolic syndrome in bipolar patients. About 80% of bipolar patients were prescribed atypical antipsychotic drugs and/or mood stabilizes, which were strongly linked to metabolic syndrome found in the current study.

Our results confirmed previous data that serum uric acid concentrations in bipolar patients were significantly higher than healthy controls [15, 17, 35]. Animal study shows that uric acid induces endothelial dysfunction and overproduction of reactive oxygen species, which has been considered as a major factor of insulin resistance [36]. In humans, hyperuricemia is also associated with insulin resistance and metabolic syndrome [37, 38]. It is possible that elevated uric acid worse insulin sensitivity and metabolic syndrome and vice versa. Both hyperuricemia and metabolic syndrome increase the risk of cardiovascular disease and dementia in elderly people [39]. Ageing is not necessarily associated increased blood uric acid [40]. This study showed that bipolar patient with hyperuricemia and over 50 years of age have very high prevalence for metabolic disorders and its components. Therefore, a special caution should be taken for preventing cardiovascular diseases when there is hyperuricemia in elderly bipolar patients.

Prevention and treatment of hyperuricemia are clearly important in terms of reducing the prevalence of metabolic syndrome in patients suffering from bipolar disorder. Since metabolic syndrome increases the risks of a number of life threatening diseases, reinstalling hyperuricemia back to normal level may help to reduce diabetes and kidney and cardiovascular diseases in these patients.

This study has some limitations. First, only inpatients with bipolar disorder were included, who tend to suffer more severely, have more comorbidities, and higher rates of pharmacological treatment than those of outpatients. Therefore, our data do not necessarily reflect the prevalence of metabolic syndrome of outpatients suffering from bipolar disorder. Second, antidepressant (eg: mirtazapine) uses were not obtained in this study, which could cause weight gain and metabolic disorders [41]. Finally, other possible confounding factors were not ruled out, which could play a role contributing to the development of metabolic syndrome including types and

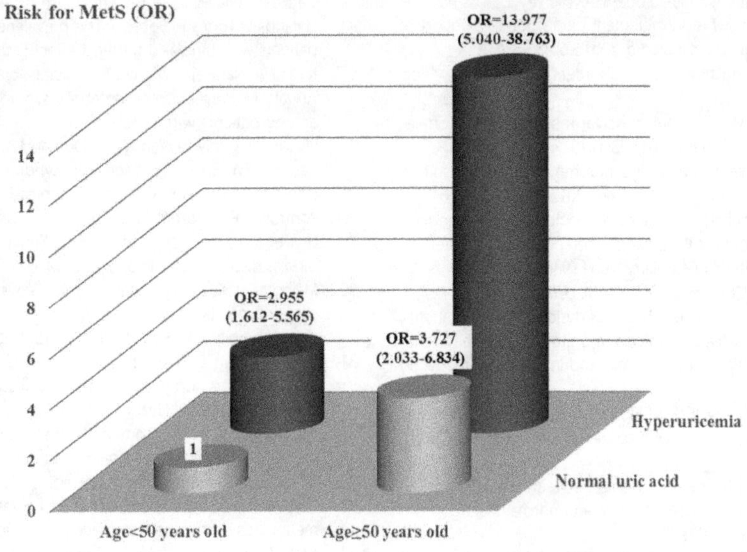

Fig. 1 Shows interaction between age ≥ 50 years of age or < 50 years of age and hyperuricemia for metabolic syndrome. Odd ratios are based on 95% confidence interval

duration of antipsychotic drugs used, diet, physical activity, socioeconomic status, and alcohol use.

Conclusions

Hyperuricemia is more common in bipolar patients with metabolic syndrome. The high prevalence of metabolic syndrome and hyperuricemia may be due to hyperglycemia, ageing, antipsychotic and mood stabilizer uses, illness duration, and visceral obesity. It is possible that elevated uric acid disrupts metabolic regulation and on the other hand, metabolic disorders could further worse hyperuricemia in bipolar patients. Bipolar patients with hyperuricemia and age greater than 50 years were highly prone to develop metabolic syndrome.

Abbreviations

BMI: body mass index; BP: blood pressure; BPD: bipolar disorder; CI: confidence interval; CPZ: chlorpromazine; DSM-IV: Diagnostic and Statistical Manual of Mental Disorders, 4th Edition; FBG: fasting blood glucose; HDL-C: high density lipoprotein cholesterol; MetS: metabolic syndrome; NCEP ATP-III A: National Cholesterol Education Program Adult Treatment Panel III Adapted criteria; OR: odds ratio; SPSS: Statistical Package for the Social Sciences; UA: uric acid; WC: waist circumference

Acknowledgements

The authors would like to thank Ning Wang, Yanxia Kang, Xia Du, Xuanwang, and Feng Yan for all of their hard work and contributions to this study.

Funding

This study was supported by the National Key Technologies R&D Program of China (2015BAI13B01)and the Special Foundation of Beijing Municipal Science & Technology Commission, China (grant no: Z131107002213099).

Authors' contributions

Conception of the study: XF Huang, JX Chen, FD Yang. JX Chen was the project manager. HM Chen, JH Feng, LG Zhang, JY Li, R Li, and SL Wang were responsible for recruiting the patients, performing the clinical rating, collecting all samples and helping with statistical analysis and manuscript preparation. XF Huang, JX Chen, FD Yang, YL Tan, A Jones and I Wilson were involved in interpreting the data and writing and editing the paper. All authors have read and approved the manuscript.

Consent for publication

Not applicable.

Competing interests

The authors have no conflicts of interest to disclose.

Author details

[1]Beijing Hui-Long-Guan Hospital, Peking University, Beijing 100096, China. [2]Jining Psychiatric Hospital, Jining 272051, China. [3]Illawarra Health and Medical Research Institute and School of Medicine, University of Wollongong, Wollongong, NSW 2522, Australia.

References

1. Revicki DA, Matza LS, Flood E, Lloyd A. Bipolar disorder and health-related quality of life : review of burden of disease and clinical trials. Pharmacoeconomics. 2005;23(6):583–94.
2. Ferrari AJ, Stockings E, Khoo JP, Erskine HE, Degenhardt L, Vos T, Whiteford HA. The prevalence and burden of bipolar disorder: findings from the global burden of disease study 2013. Bipolar Disord. 2016;18(5):440–50.
3. Vigo D, Thornicroft G, Atun R. Estimating the true global burden of mental illness. Lancet Psychiatry. 2016;3(2):171–8.

4. Morselli PL, Elgie R, Cesana BM. GAMIAN-Europe/BEAM survey II: cross-national analysis of unemployment, family history, treatment satisfaction and impact of the bipolar disorder on life style. Bipolar Disord. 2004;6(6):487–97.
5. Miller C, Bauer MS. Excess mortality in bipolar disorders. Curr Psychiatry Rep. 2014;16(11):499.
6. Weiner M, Warren L, Fiedorowicz JG. Cardiovascular morbidity and mortality in bipolar disorder. Ann Clin Psychiatry. 2011;23(1):40–7.
7. de Almeida KM, Moreira CL, Lafer B. Metabolic syndrome and bipolar disorder: what should psychiatrists know? CNS Neurosci Ther. 2012;18(2):160–6.
8. Mitchell AJ, Malone D, Doebbeling CC. Quality of medical care for people with and without comorbid mental illness and substance misuse: systematic review of comparative studies. Br J Psychiatry. 2009;194(6):491–9.
9. De Hert M, Cohen D, Bobes J, Cetkovich-Bakmas M, Leucht S, Ndetei DM, Newcomer JW, Uwakwe R, Asai I, Moller HJ, et al. Physical illness in patients with severe mental disorders. II. Barriers to care, monitoring and treatment guidelines, plus recommendations at the system and individual level. World Psychiatry. 2011;10(2):138–51.
10. Kilbourne AM, Rofey DL, McCarthy JF, Post EP, Welsh D, Blow FC. Nutrition and exercise behavior among patients with bipolar disorder. Bipolar Disord. 2007;9(5):443–52.
11. Meshkani R, Zargari M, Larijani B. The relationship between uric acid and metabolic syndrome in normal glucose tolerance and normal fasting glucose subjects. Acta Diabetol. 2011;48(1):79–88.
12. Robles-Cervantes JA, Ramos-Zavala MG, Gonzalez-Ortiz M, Martinez-Abundis E, Valencia-Sandoval C, Torres-Chavez A, Espinel-Bermudez C, Santiago-Hernandez NJ, Hernandez-Gonzalez SO. Relationship between serum concentration of uric acid and insulin secretion among adults with type 2 diabetes mellitus. Int J Endocrinol. 2011;2011:107904.
13. Kanbay M, Jensen T, Solak Y, Le M, Roncal-Jimenez C, Rivard C, Lanaspa MA, Nakagawa T, Johnson RJ. Uric acid in metabolic syndrome: from an innocent bystander to a central player. Eur J Intern Med. 2016;29:3–8.
14. Albert U, De Cori D, Aguglia A, Barbaro F, Bogetto F, Maina G. Increased uric acid levels in bipolar disorder subjects during different phases of illness. J Affect Disord. 2015;173:170–5.
15. Kesebir S, Suner O, Yaylaci ET, Bayrak A, Turan C. Increased uric acid levels in bipolar disorder: is it trait or state? J Biol Regul Homeost Agents. 2013;27(4):981–8.
16. Bartoli F, Crocamo C, Mazza MG, Clerici M, Carra G. Uric acid levels in subjects with bipolar disorder: a comparative meta-analysis. J Psychiatr Res. 2016;81:133–9.
17. Bartoli F, Crocamo C, Gennaro GM, Castagna G, Trotta G, Clerici M, Carra G. Exploring the association between bipolar disorder and uric acid: a mediation analysis. J Psychosom Res. 2016;84:56–9.
18. WHO-Expert-Consultation. Appropriate body-mass index for Asian populations and its implications for policy and intervention strategies. Lancet. 2004;363(9403):157–63.
19. Grover S, Aggarwal M, Chakrabarti S, Dutt A, Avasthi A, Kulhara P, Malhotra N, Somaiya M, Chauhan N. Prevalence of metabolic syndrome in bipolar disorder: an exploratory study from North India. Prog Neuro-Psychopharmacol Biol Psychiatry. 2012;36(1):141–6.
20. Tan CE, Ma S, Wai D, Chew SK, Tai ES. Can we apply the National Cholesterol Education Program Adult Treatment Panel definition of the metabolic syndrome to Asians? Diabetes Care. 2004;27(5):1182–6.
21. Grundy SM, Cleeman JI, Daniels SR, Donato KA, Eckel RH, Franklin BA, Gordon DJ, Krauss RM, Savage PJ, Smith SC Jr, et al. Diagnosis and management of the metabolic syndrome: an American Heart Association/ National Heart, Lung, and Blood Institute scientific statement. Circulation. 2005;112(17):2735–52.
22. Feig DI, Kang DH, Johnson RJ. Uric acid and cardiovascular risk. N Engl J Med. 2008;359(17):1811–21.
23. Yu FN, Shi YX, Cheng HY, Huang XL, Liu SS. An observational study on the relationship between serum uric acid and hypertension in a northern Chinese population aged 45 to 59 years. Medicine (Baltimore). 2017;96(17):e6773.
24. Godin O, Etain B, Henry C, Bougerol T, Courtet P, Mayliss L, Passerieux C, Azorin JM, Kahn JP, Gard S, et al. Metabolic syndrome in a French cohort of patients with bipolar disorder: results from the FACE-BD cohort. J Clin Psychiatry. 2014;75(10):1078–85 quiz 1085.
25. John AP, Koloth R, Dragovic M, Lim SC. Prevalence of metabolic syndrome among Australians with severe mental illness. Med J Aust. 2009;190(4):176–9.
26. Garcia-Portilla MP, Saiz PA, Benabarre A, Sierra P, Perez J, Rodriguez A, Livianos L, Torres P, Bobes J. The prevalence of metabolic syndrome in patients with bipolar disorder. J Affect Disord. 2008;106(1–2):197–201.
27. Kumar A, Narayanaswamy JC, Venkatasubramanian G, Raguram R, Grover S, Aswath M. Prevalence of metabolic syndrome and its clinical correlates among patients with bipolar disorder. Asian J Psychiatr. 2017;26:109–14.
28. Silarova B, Giltay EJ, Van Reedt Dortland A, Van Rossum EF, Hoencamp E, Penninx BW, Spijker AT. Metabolic syndrome in patients with bipolar disorder: comparison with major depressive disorder and non-psychiatric controls. J Psychosom Res. 2015;78(4):391–8.
29. Grover S, Malhotra N, Chakrabarti S, Kulhara P. Metabolic syndrome in bipolar disorders. Indian J Psychol Med. 2012;34(2):110–8.
30. Malhotra N, Kulhara P, Chakrabarti S, Grover S. A prospective, longitudinal study of metabolic syndrome in patients with bipolar disorder and schizophrenia. J Affect Disord. 2013;150(2):653–8.
31. Li R, Li W, Lun Z, Zhang H, Sun Z, Kanu JS, Qiu S, Cheng Y, Liu Y. Prevalence of metabolic syndrome in mainland China: a meta-analysis of published studies. BMC Public Health. 2016;16:296.
32. Kato MM, Currier MB, Gomez CM, Hall L, Gonzalez-Blanco M. Prevalence of metabolic syndrome in Hispanic and non-Hispanic patients with schizophrenia. Prim Care Companion J Clin Psychiatry. 2004;6(2):74–7.
33. Czepielewski L, Daruy Filho L, Brietzke E, Grassi-Oliveira R. Bipolar disorder and metabolic syndrome: a systematic review. Rev Bras Psiquiatr. 2013;35(1):88–93.
34. Nayerifard R, Bureng MA, Zahiroddin A, Namjoo M, Rajezi S. Comparison of metabolic syndrome prevalence in patients with schizophrenia and bipolar I disorder. Diabetes Metab Syndr. 2017;11(Suppl 1):S411–6.
35. Muti M, Del Grande C, Musetti L, Marazziti D, Turri M, Cirronis M, Pergentini I, Corsi M, Dell'Osso L, Corsini GU. Serum uric acid levels and different phases of illness in bipolar I patients treated with lithium. Psychiatry Res. 2015;225(3):604–8.
36. Soltani Z, Rasheed K, Kapusta DR, Reisin E. Potential role of uric acid in metabolic syndrome, hypertension, kidney injury, and cardiovascular diseases: is it time for reappraisal? Curr Hypertens Rep. 2013;15(3):175–81.
37. Li C, Hsieh MC, Chang SJ. Metabolic syndrome, diabetes, and hyperuricemia. Curr Opin Rheumatol. 2013;25(2):210–6.
38. Osgood K, Krakoff J, Thearle M. Serum uric acid predicts both current and future components of the metabolic syndrome. Metab Syndr Relat Disord. 2013;11(3):157–62.
39. Latourte A, Soumare A, Bardin T, Perez-Ruiz F, Debette S, Richette P. Uric acid and incident dementia over 12 years of follow-up: a population-based cohort study. Ann Rheum Dis. 2018;77(3):328–35.
40. Gephardt MC, Hanlon TJ, Matson CF. Blood uric acid values as related to sex and age. JAMA. 1964;189:1028–9.
41. Carvalho AF, Sharma MS, Brunoni AR, Vieta E, Fava GA. The safety, tolerability and risks associated with the use of newer generation antidepressant drugs: a critical review of the literature. Psychother Psychosom. 2016;85(5):270–88.

13

Abnormal resting state activity of left middle occipital gyrus and its functional connectivity in female patients with major depressive disorder

Changjun Teng[1], Jing Zhou[2], Hui Ma[1], Yarong Tan[1], Xin Wu[1], Chengbin Guan[1], Huifen Qiao[1], Jijun Li[1], Yuan Zhong[3], Chun Wang[1*] and Ning Zhang[1]

Abstract

Background: Women are more susceptible to major depressive disorder (MDD). A possible explanation is that women have a trait tendency to engage in a ruminative response style. Depending on cognitive model of depression, attention bias, memory bias and self-referential bias were closely related among depressed patients. Previous studies have explored the neural mechanism of the cognitive biases by using amplitude of low frequency fluctuations (ALFF) or functional connectivity (FC), and few combined these two metrics, especially focusing on female patients.

Methods: We assessed 25 female patients diagnosed with MDD and 13 well matched healthy controls (HCs) using Rs-fMRI. Two metrics ALFF and FC based on abnormal ALFF were explored and made comparisons.

Results: Compared with HCs, female patients with MDD showed that one cluster with significantly decreased ALFF in the left middle occipital gyrus(L-MOG). Furtherly we founded depressed female subjects showed significantly lower FC between the L-MOG seed and left orbitofrontal cortex, and significantly higher FC between the L-MOG seed and left medial prefrontal gyrus and left hippocampus.

Conclusions: Our results showed L-MOG may act as a connection, which involved in the processing of cognitive biases of MDD by connected with limbic-cortical regions in resting state. These findings may enhance the understanding of the neurobiological mechanism in female patients with MDD.

Keywords: Major depressive disorder, Female, Resting-state fMRI, Amplitude of low frequency fluctuations, Functional connectivity, Left middle occipital gyrus

Background

Major depressive disorder (MDD) is a very common heterogeneous mental disorder characterized by depressed affective and cognitive disturbances, especially for women, with an incidence and prevalence twice that of men [1]. An availably possible explanation is that women have a trait tendency to engage in a ruminative response style characterized by a repetitive pattern of self-referent cognitions [2]. Some studies furtherly posited that rumination is clearly related to attentional bias. Review found that participants who primarily respond to a negative mood by ruminating showed difficulty disengaging from negative material even after controlling for depression severity [3]. Researchers consider that female's tendency to habitually ruminate in response to a negative mood suggests that gender will evidence greater attentional biases for negative information, because they will exhibit difficulties inhibiting negative stimuli, and that females may be more vulnerable to attentional manipulations for negative stimuli than males [4].

According to cognitive model of depression, attention, memory, thoughts and rumination biases are stable

* Correspondence: fm51109@163.com
[1]Nanjing Brain Hospital Affiliated to Nanjing Medical University, Nanjing 210029, People's Republic of China

abnormalities of depressed patients. Negative bias in the processing of information plays a critical role in influencing the onset, maintenance and recurrence of depressive episodes [5, 6]. Although the causative link between attention bias and mood disorder is not completely clear, some studies have found that attentional bias modification had been used to reduce anxiety and depressive symptoms [7–9]. A meta-analysis has found reducing negative bias could decrease depressive symptoms and increasing negative bias could increase depressive symptoms [9]. These findings indicated that attentional bias may contribute directly to depressive symptoms and not a consequence of depression [10]. Some studies also suggest that attention bias arise prior to the onset of a disorder, representing a risk factor [11–13].

Attention bias have been reported to be particularly prominent of emotional face, and these findings are all from specific task state studies like identifying emotional face [14]. Task stimuli help to explore the specific stimuli process, and could not delineate a comprehensive process in common daily life. MDD is a pervasive disorder and has an impact on very realm of daily life. Biased cognitive processes play a crucial role in social function including interpersonal problems. "Resting-state hypothesis" of MDD considered neural predisposition at rest as a fundamental neural mechanism of MDD. So, study using resting state combining with functional magnetic resonance imaging (Rs-fMRI) without any task stimulus also may provide some insight for neural mechanism of pervasive abnormal cognition patterns [15].

Rs-fMRI has been widely explored in patients with the neuropsychiatric disorder, including MDD. The amplitude of low-frequency fluctuation (ALFF) is to examine low frequency fluctuation at Rs-fMRI. ALFF is confirmed to be reliable and sensitive measure in the study of both healthy and clinical populations [16–18]. Functional connectivity (FC) measures the correlation of low frequency fluctuation between spatially independent regions. MDD is considered a disease from localist models to the circuit or network models [19–21]. Numbers of studies have provided lots of findings in MDD using these two metrics. Yao and his colleagues found that male MDD patients showed higher ALFF values in the left postcentral gyrus, the left inferior parietal lobule and right precuneus and lower ALFF values in left superior temporal pole, right superior/middle frontal gyrus and bilateral crus 1 of the cerebellum for main effects of gender compared with females [22]. Buchanan investigated whole brain FC in MDD and found that depressed female patients showed significantly decreased FC in the right/left frontoparietal regions and language networks compared to healthy control subjects [23]. Another study founded that high-risk female adolescents had decrease FC between right inferior prefrontal cortex and other critical nodes of attention control network compared with low-risk ones, and they concluded that adolescent daughters might inherit depression vulnerability from their depressed patients [24]. Previous studies have also described sex difference in brain structure and function. Morphometric study in normal adults found that differences of some indices of corpus callosum and ventricles in female and male populations [25]. Amygdala volumes in adolescents showed sex differences, smaller left amygdala volumes were associated with better parental reports of emotional controls in girls and larger left amygdala volumes in boys [26]. Using fMRI, McRae explored the gender differences in cognitive reappraisal strategy of emotional regulation, and found women showed larger increases activation in prefrontal regions, smaller decreases activation in the amygdala and larger engagement of ventral striatal regions compared with men [27]. A recent multimodal meta-analysis identified abnormalities in regional cerebral blood flow and ALFF in the left insula in depressed individuals and founded that the percentage of female participants was negatively associated with the regional cerebral blood flow [28]. All of these studies showed us that gender factor should be taken into consideration in the study of fMRI. Consequently, study directly focusing on women may help to investigate potentially additional insight into the neural mechanisms in MDD.

Depending on the current most consistent theories of limbic-cortical dysfunction in MDD, MDD is accompanied by functional and structural abnormalities in many regions including the prefrontal cortex (lateral and medial) and limbic areas (such as hippocampus and amygdala) [29]. Regions in medial prefrontal cortex (mPFC) [5, 30–32] and hippocampus [5, 33–36] are believed to be the neural correlate of self-referential thoughts, rumination and biased memory, and orbitofrontal cortex (OFC) [37–39]is believed to involve in the inhibitory control and selective attention.

We are aware of few studies combining these two methods to examine resting-state differences in depressed female patients directly. Previous studies of FC usually took region of interest selection based on accumulated priori knowledge of disorder. This method has a certain subjectivity and artificial. Thus, combining ALFF and FC based on the abnormal ALFF maybe provide some insights into the neural basis of disease in term of fMRI signal of low-frequency fluctuation. We aimed to test the hypotheses that 1) female MDD would have altered ALFF activity in cortical regions related to attentional bias which acted as a connection and 2) abnormal ALFF-based FC with hippocampus and mPFC which involved in cognitive bias of depression.

Methods

Participants

Thirty-eight subjects participated in the present study. Twenty-five female depressed patients were recruited from the Department of Medical Psychology, Nanjing Brain Hospital Affiliated to Nanjing Medical University. Two experienced psychiatrists made a diagnosis of current depressive episode according to the structured clinical interview for DSM-IV Axis I Disorder (SCID). The patient must meet the inclusion criteria of the first episode depression, drug-naive, duration of depression less than a year, 20 < age < 50 years old, right-handed and no history of unstable cardiac or neurological disease. The exclusion criteria included schizophrenia, bipolar and any psychotic disorder, history of head injury or loss of consciousness, history of substance abuse, contraindications to MRI and 24-item Hamilton Depression Rating Scale (HAMD) score less than 18.

Thirteen right-handed aged-matched and education-matched healthy controls (HCs) with HAMD less than 8 were enrolled from the community through advertisements. The HCs group was interviewed by SCID non-patient edition to confirm without any neurological disease, mental illness, or family history of psychiatric disorders, contraindications to MRI.

Data acquisition

All Rs-fMRI data were obtained with a 3.0 T Siemens MR scanner (Erlangen, Germany). Before scanning, a foam pad was used to minimize the head motion of all participants. Participants were instructed to keep head motionless, keep their eyes closed and not think anything till the end. Firstly, T1-weighted images were acquired to make sure that there are no brain structural changes. The parameters of three-dimensional T1-weighted sequence: repetition time 1900 ms with echo time 2.48 ms, flip angle 9°, 176 slices, 256*256 image matrix, the field of view 256*256, slice thick 1 mm with slice gap 0.5 mm. Total acquire time is 4 min 18 s. Secondly, Rs-fMRI data were acquired with single shot echo planner imaging (EPI) sequence using the parameters: repetition time 3000 ms with echo time 40 ms, flip angle 90°, 32 slices, 64*64 image matrix, the field of view 24*24 cm2, slice thick 4 mm with slice gap 4 mm. Total scan time is 5 min 06 s.

fMRI data preprocessing

Special fMRI software Data Processing Assistant for Resting-State fMRI (DPARSF, v2.2, http://www.restfmri.net) was used to preprocess Rs-fMRI data. First six volumes were discarded to establish steady-state signal equilibrium and account for participants' adaptation to circumstance. The remaining volumes were sliced timing and realigned head motion correction. Two HC were excluded due to excessive head motion (more than 1.5 mm or 1.5° during scanning). Furtherly, there was no significant difference between group (two sample t test, $t = 0.625$, $P = 0.536$ for translation, and $t = 0.452$, $P = 0.653$ for rotation) based on the formula [40]. The imaging was then spatially normalized to the standard Montreal Neurological Institute (MNI) EPI template. Spatial smoothed with 4 mm full width at half maximum Gaussian filter were done. Finally, linear trend subtraction and temporal bandpass filtering (0.01–0.08HZ) were performed to remove low-frequency drifts and physiological noise.

ALFF calculation

ALFF was calculated and compared by the Resting State fMRI Data Analysis Toolkit (REST, V1.8, http://www.restfmri.net). Briefly, the time series was converted to the frequency domain using a fast Fourier Transformation, the square root of measures power spectrum was computed and then the mean was calculated across 0.01–0.08 Hz for each voxel. The mean square root was referred to ALFF. Each voxel was further standardized by divided by the global mean value for subsequent statistical analysis.

FC analysis

Seed-based FC analysis was also calculated with REST. The clusters of ALFF that appeared in group differences were used as regions of interest for the FC analysis based on literature [41]. The mean time series of abnormal ALFF region was calculated as the reference time course. Then we conducted a correlation analysis between seed reference time course and the rest voxels in the whole brain. Finally, the correlation coefficients were transformed to z-value by applying Fisher's r-to-z conversion to improve their Gaussian distribution for subsequent FC group comparisons.

Statistical analysis

Independent sample t-test was used to compare demographic and HAMD scores in SPSS. Then we first do one-sample t-tests in MDD and HCs group using standardized ALFF that was significantly greater than 1 in RESR to make a mask for subsequent two-sample t test for ALFF, because of the processing of standardized by the global mean value. Differences in ALFF were assessed used two- sample t-tests with REST within the mask. Differences in FC were also assessed as the same with ALFF within the whole brain mask. In all the analysis, Monte Carlo simulation was applied to correct for multiple comparisons using the REST Alphasim program [42, 43], and the significance threshold of $p < 0.05$ was set by using a combination of each voxel threshold $p < 0.05$ and cluster size of 42 voxels for ALFF and 85 voxels for FC calculation.

Results

Demographics

Compared to HCs, there was no significant difference between the two group in terms of age or level of education. As expected, patients with MDD had significantly higher HAMD scores (Table 1).

The ALFF group results of the two group from one sample *t*-tests

One sample t-tests reveal that bilateral frontal lobe, bilateral temporal lobe, bilateral parietal lobe, bilateral occipital lobe, anterior cingulate cortex, posterior cingulate cortex/ precuneus had a standardized ALFF value that was significantly greater than 1 in the two groups (Fig. 1).

ALFF differences between groups from two sample *t*-tests

Female with MDD group had only one cluster with significantly lower ALFF in left middle occipital gyrus (L-MOG) compared to HCs. There was no significantly higher ALFF cluster in MDD group (Table 2 and Fig. 2).

FC differences between groups from two sample *t*-tests

The L-MOG was selected as a seed for FC analysis as it appeared between-group differences. Female MDD group showed significantly increased FC between L-MOG and left medial prefrontal gyrus (L-mPFG) and left hippocampus compared with HCs. They also showed significantly decreased FC between L-MOG and left OFC (L-OFC) compared with HCs (Table 2, Fig. 3).

Discussion

The current study aimed to explore the neural basis of MDD in first-episode untreated female patients. We combined ALFF with FC analysis methods based on brain coactivation mechanisms among the different regions. Specifically, we sought to examine FC pattern of a region which had abnormal ALFF activation. We found that a unique decreased abnormal activation in L-MOG in depressed female patients. Moreover, significantly increased FC of L-MOG with L-mPFG and left hippocampus, and significantly decreased FC between L-MOG and L-OFC were also showed in depressed female patients.

We found significantly decrease ALFF in L-MOG which was consistent with our hypothesis. The occipital lobe contains most of the anatomical region of the visual cortex and contributes to visual information processing and communication with the cerebral cortex, and plays a role in the perception of facial emotion. Cerullo noticed that patients with bipolar-I showed decreased activation in the bilateral MOG compared with HC and MDD, while MDD only showed decreased activation in L-MOG compared to bipolar-I patients under the emotional imaging stimulus [44]. Furey found baseline activation of MOG may predict treatment response to scopolamine [45]. Many resting state studies and recent meta-analysis of Rs-fMRI also found decreased activation in L-MOG [46–49]. Structural research showed that occipital bending might be characteristic of MDD [50]. Guo and his colleagues have founded decreased ALFF in occipital cortex and considered it relevant to MDD and implicated disrupted visual processing in MDD [46]. One study demonstrated the role of MOG in category-selective attention modulating unconscious face/tool processing and found decreased activation in MOG under the face-selective attention during unconscious face processing [51]. Consistent with these studies, the decreased ALFF in L-MOG may provide a neural basis for disrupted visual processing in female MDD. A common cognitive feature of MDD is mood congruent processing bias that is a preference for negative emotional information [6, 52]. Some researches considered the model of selective bias in processing and interpretation for emotional information to be one of the risk factors of MDD for young people [13, 53] and that attention to negative information may maintain depression [5, 54]. Consequently, our finding may suggest that processing bias in MDD may be initiated as a perceptual visual bias, which may cause a series of cognitive and affective symptoms of MDD.

Furthermore, we found significantly increased FC between L-MOG and L-mPFG and hippocampus. The

Table 1 Demographic, clinical characteristics

	HCs (n = 13)	MDD(n = 25)	t values	P values
Age (years)	38.23 ± 10.12	35.80 ± 8.08	0.84	0.41[a]
Education (years)	13.92 ± 3.40	13.10 ± 2.80	0.83	0.41[a]
HAMD	1.93 ± 0.96	25.67 ± 5.31	−15.92	0.00[a]
During of disorder (months)	–	6.33 ± 3.45	–	–

Abbreviation: *HCs* healthy controls, *MDD* major depressive disorder, *HAMD* Hamilton Rating Scale for Depression
[a]The *P* values were obtained by two sample *t*-test

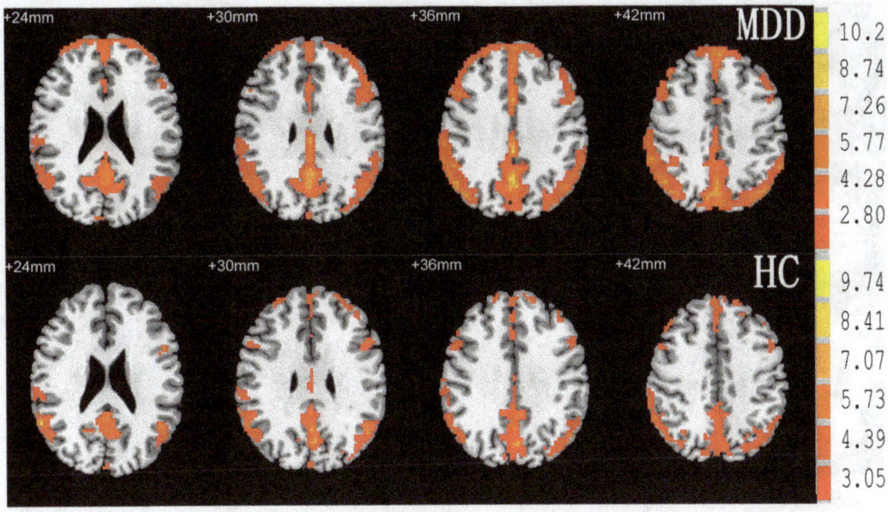

Fig. 1 Maps of within condition patterns of resting state amplitude of low-frequency fluctuation in group MDD and HCs. The numbers above the imaging refer to the MNI z coordinate. The color bar on the right side refers to the range of *T* values

mPFG and its adjacent areas play a crucial role in depression symptomatology [46, 47, 55]. It has been confirmed that mPFG was involved in self-referential thought [30] and depressive rumination [30, 32]. Yoshimura showed that patients with depression displayed hyperactivity in mPFC during the self-referential processing of negative valence personality trait words [56] and negative emotional words [57]. Delaveau also found that antidepressant medicine in females depressed patients could bring the hyperactivity of mPFC during self-referential processing back to normal [58]. A visual search task study showed increased FC between mPFC and lateral occipital cortex, and observed white matter tracts between mPFC and lateral occipital cortex using imaging-guided diffusion tensor imaging [59]. In previous resting state studies, we have not found FC between mPFC and occipital cortex. The different findings may be related to differences in samples and medications status [60]. We speculate that the increase FC between L-MOG and L-mPFG may be related to exaggerated self-referential processing bias and depressive rumination in MDD.

Hippocampus is also a vital region in the pathogenesis of MDD [34, 61]. As a key structure of limbic circuit involved in memory formation, emotional learning and emotional regulation [62]. In particular, memory biases of negative information rely heavily on it [35, 36]. An associative and item recognition memory fMRI study showed that association recognition memory for object-color relationship led to bilateral hippocampus and parahippocampus activation and L-MOG, while old item recognition of objects showed activation in L-MOG and L-middle temporal gyrus. New item recognition of objects just showed activation in the bilateral hippocampus [63]. Emotional memory recollection involved in the hippocampus and mPFC [64]. Studies showed that sleeping could help to consolidate emotional memory by enhancing the FC between the hippocampus and mPFC [64] and promote the neural reorganization of remote emotional memory by enhancing the FC between mPFC and precuneus and occipital cortex [65]. Increasing FC between L-MOG and L-hippocampus in this study may be related to memory impairment and sleep disturbance in MDD.

Table 2 Area of decreased amplitude of low frequency fluctuation (ALFF) and altered functional connectivity (FC) in female subjects with major depressive disorder compared to healthy controls

Metrics	Brain region (BA area)	Cluster size	MNI coordinates			*T* values
			X	Y	Z	
ALFF	Left Middle Occipital Gyrus (BA37)(L-MOG)	159	−30	−93	3	−2.90
L-MOG seed FC	Left Medial Prefrontal Gyrus(BA9/10)(L-mPFG)	115	−6	57	18	3.44
	Left Hippocampus (BA21)	112	−33	−33	−9	5.09
	Left Orbitofrontal cortex (BA11/47) (L-OFC)	85	−12	33	−27	−4.14

Abbreviations: *BA* Brodmann area, *MNI* Montreal Neurologic Institute

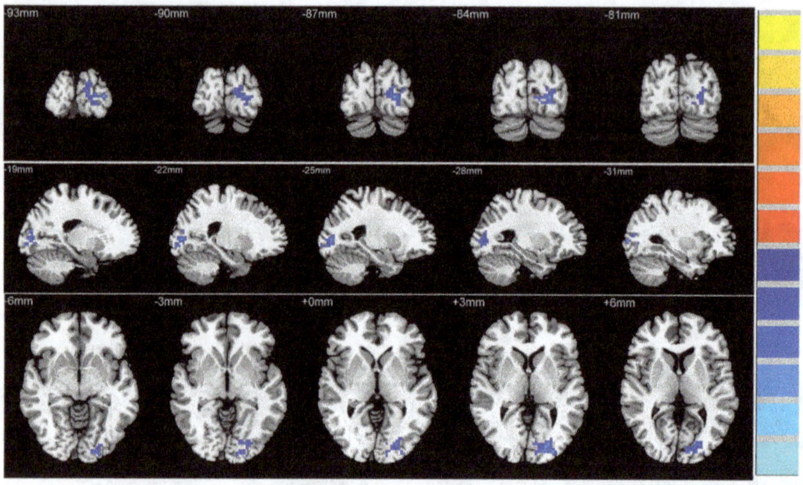

Fig. 2 T-statistical map region showing decreased (blue) amplitude of low-frequency fluctuation(ALFF) in female patients with major depressive disorder MDD compared with healthy controls. Significant clusters of bigger than 42 voxels with correction for multiple comparison applied at $p<0.05$ (cluster-corrected with alphasim). The Numbers above the imaging refer to the MNI z coordinate. The color bar on the right side refers to the range of *T* values

Hippocampus and mPFG are also key nodes of default mode network (DMN) [66, 67]. Although DMN has been linked to episodic memory and memory consolidation in some studies [68], a study paid more attention to its function in self-generated thought and rumination during rest, especially in depression [66]. In this current study, we found increase FC between L-MOG and hippocampus and mPFG may be relevant to bias attention, bias memory and biased thought and rumination in MDD [5].

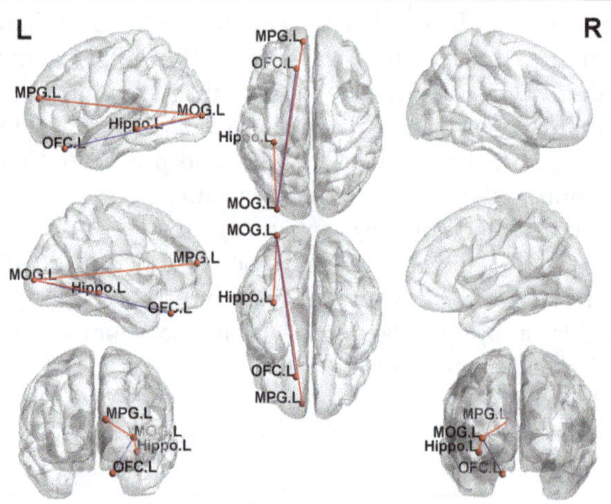

Fig. 3 Graph visualization of functional connectivity comparison differences. Compared with healthy controls, female major depressive disorder patients show significantly increased FC of left middle occipital gyrus (MOG.L) with left medial prefrontal gyrus (MPG.L) and left hippocampus (Hippo.L) and significantly decreased FC between L-MOG and left orbitofrontal cortex (OFC.L) L, Left. The red line refers to higher FC, and the blue line refers to lower FC

At last, we found decreased FC between L-MOG and L-OFC. OFC is regarded as a region in integrating sensory and emotional information through white matter connections with visual, auditory and limbic structures [39], and play a vital role in mood regulation, response inhibition, selective attention and reward processing in the pathophysiology of MDD [29, 37–39]. Previous study revealed decreased ALFF in OFC in patients with MDD and suggested hypofunction of emotion regulation [69]. Dynamic causal modeling was applied to explored neural mechanisms of a bottom-up and top-down process for emotional facial expression during memory formation. Xiu and his collogues found that emotion information could affect bottom-up connections from the occipital visual cortex to the OFC [70]. Lateral OFC act an important role in facilitating selective attention to modulate irrelevant emotional materials from the environment [37]. MDD patients showed increased OFC activity in attentional task asking to ignore sad words with attending to happy ones compared with ignoring happy with attending to sad [52]. In this sense, decrease FC between L-MOG and L-OFC may indicate impairment inhibited capability in response to visual information and related to dysfunctional mood regulation in female depression.

It is worth noting that we found left-lateralized cortical regions in female MDD. This finding was also in consistent with previous findings. Jiang has founded that differences in predominated lateralization of ALFF alteration between MDD and bipolar depression which meant left hemisphere for MDD and bilateral of bipolar depression [71]. Of course, these findings may be related to gender difference. In brain study, sex-related hemisphere lateralization was founded in healthy young Chinese adults. This study suggested that regional difference of gray matter density between men and women, and that functional regional homogeneity (ReHo) difference with higher ReHo in the right hemisphere for men and in left for women [72]. Our findings were also compatible with previous study. Recently, an event-related potential study suggested that female depression may be more vulnerable that male during emotional face processing with the unconscious negative cognitive bias, and considered that unconscious cognitive bias may be modulated by sex effects [73].

Some limitations should be addressed. First, the small number of participants and the imbalance in HCs might be insufficient to summarize the results to a larger population. Second, the data are cross-sectional; we cannot ensure the clinical diagnosis consistency of MDD patients because of the risk of switching to bipolar disorder. Third, although ALFF was used wildly, the true neurophysiological mechanism is still not clear. Future studies should include a larger number of participants with a longer observation period.

Conclusions

In summary, the present study revealed that female subjects with MDD had decreased ALFF in L-MOG and increased FC between L-MOG with L-mPFG, and left hippocampus and decreased FC between L-MOG and L-OFC. Importantly, these findings indicated L-MOG act as a connection, and abnormal FC may be potentially related to cognition biases of MDD and may help to advance our understanding of the neurobiological mechanism underlying female depressed patients.

Abbreviations

ALFF: Amplitude of low-frequency fluctuation; FC: Functional connectivity; HCs: Healthy controls; L-MOG: Left middle occipital gyrus; L-mPFG: Left medial prefrontal gyrus; L-OFC: Left orbitofrontal cortex; MDD: Major depressive disorder; mPFC: Medial prefrontal cortex; OFC: Orbitofrontal cortex; Rs-fMRI: Resting state functional magnetic resonance imaging

Acknowledgments

The authors are grateful to all the patients and the healthy volunteers for their participation and cooperation in our study. We also sincerely thank Professor Chaoyong Xiao, Jun Hu and Zonghong Li for assistance with fMRI data collection, Department of Radiology, The Affiliated Brain Hospital with Nanjing Medical University. We also thank Shuai Gao and Honglei Li for their assistant in subject recruiting.

Funding

The study was supported by National Natural Science Foundation of China (81571344, 81201064); Natural Science Foundation of Jiangsu Province (BK20161109); Key research and Development program (Social Development) project of Jiangsu province (BE20156092015); Nanjing Medical Science and Technique Development Foundation, Outstanding Youth Project (JQX14008). The funders had no direct involvement in the design of the study and collection, analysis, and interpretation of data and in writing the manuscript.

Authors' contributions

CW designed the study along with NZ. CT, JZ, HM, YT, CG, HQ and JL collected and provided patients. CT and XW managed and analyzed the imaging data. YZ gave the guidance in data analysis. CT wrote the first draft of the manuscript. CW revised the draft. All authors contributed to and had approved the final manuscript.

Consent for publication

Not applicable.

Competing interests

The authors declare that the research was conducted in the absence of any commercial or financial relationships and they have no competing interests.

Author details

[1]Nanjing Brain Hospital Affiliated to Nanjing Medical University, Nanjing 210029, People's Republic of China. [2]Nanjing PuKou Central Hospital, Nanjing 211800, People's Republic of China. [3]School of Psychology, Nanjing Normal University, Nanjing 210024, People's Republic of China.

References

1. Holsen LM, Spaeth SB, Lee JH, Ogden LA, Klibanski A, Whitfield-Gabrieli S, Goldstein JM. Stress response circuitry hypoactivation related to hormonal dysfunction in women with major depression. J Affect Disord. 2011;131(1–3):379–87.
2. Bagby RM, Rector NA, Bacchiochi JR, McBride C. The stability of the response styles questionnaire rumination scale in a sample of patients with major depression. Cogn Ther Res. 2004;28(4):527–38.
3. Whitmer AJ, Gotlib IH. An attentional scope model of rumination. Psychol Bull. 2013;139(5):1036–61.
4. Beshai S, Prentice JL, Dobson KS, Nicpon K. Gender and attention in depression: examining the role of modified attention in shifting mood and cognitions. Cogn Ther Res. 2014;38(6):621–33.
5. Disner SG, Beevers CG, Haigh EA, Beck AT. Neural mechanisms of the cognitive model of depression. Nat Rev Neurosci. 2011;12(8):467–77.
6. Foland-Ross LC, Gotlib IH. Cognitive and neural aspects of information processing in major depressive disorder: an integrative perspective. Front Psychol. 2012;3:489.
7. Beevers CG, Clasen PC, Enock PM, Schnyer DM. Attention bias modification for major depressive disorder: effects on attention bias, resting state connectivity, and symptom change. J Abnorm Psychol. 2015;124(3):463–75.
8. Kuckertz JM, Amir N. Attention bias modification for anxiety and phobias: current status and future directions. Curr Psychiatry Rep. 2015;17(2):9.
9. Hallion LS, Ruscio AM. A meta-analysis of the effect of cognitive bias modification on anxiety and depression. Psychol Bull. 2011;137(6):940–58.
10. Koster EH, Fox E, MacLeod C. Introduction to the special section on cognitive bias modification in emotional disorders. J Abnorm Psychol. 2009;118(1):1–4.
11. Ajilchi B, Nejati V. Attention Bias to sad faces and images: which is better for predicting depression? Open J Depend. 2013;02(03):19–23.
12. Albert K, Gau V, Taylor WD, Newhouse PA. Attention bias in older women with remitted depression is associated with enhanced amygdala activity and functional connectivity. J Affect Disord. 2017;210:49–56.
13. Joormann J, Talbot L, Gotlib IH. Biased processing of emotional information in girls at risk for depression. J Abnorm Psychol. 2007;116(1):135–43.

14. Stuhrmann A, Suslow T, Dannlowski U. Facial emotion processing in major depression: a systematic review of neuroimaging findings. Biol Mood Anxiety Disord. 2011;1(1):10.
15. Northoff G, Wiebking C, Feinberg T, Panksepp J. The 'resting-state hypothesis' of major depressive disorder-a translational subcortical-cortical framework for a system disorder. Neurosci Biobehav Rev. 2011;35(9):1929–45.
16. Kublbock M, Woletz M, Hoflich A, Sladky R, Kranz GS, Hoffmann A, Lanzenberger R, Windischberger C. Stability of low-frequency fluctuation amplitudes in prolonged resting-state fMRI. Neuroimage. 2014;103:249–57.
17. Zang YF, He Y, Zhu CZ, Cao QJ, Sui MQ, Liang M, Tian LX, Jiang TZ, Wang YF. Altered baseline brain activity in children with ADHD revealed by resting-state functional MRI. Brain and Development. 2007;29(2):83–91.
18. Zhou M, Hu X, Lu L, Zhang L, Chen L, Gong Q, Huang X. Intrinsic cerebral activity at resting state in adults with major depressive disorder: a meta-analysis. Prog Neuro-Psychopharmacol Biol Psychiatry. 2017;75:157–64.
19. Treadway MT, Pizzagalli DA. Imaging the pathophysiology of major depressive disorder - from localist models to circuit-based analysis. Biol Mood Anxiety Disord. 2014;4(1):5.
20. Veer IM, Beckmann CF, van Tol MJ, Ferrarini L, Milles J, Veltman DJ, Aleman A, van Buchem MA, van der Wee NJ, Rombouts SA. Whole brain resting-state analysis reveals decreased functional connectivity in major depression. Front Syst Neurosci. 2010;4:41.
21. Dutta A, McKie S, Deakin JF. Resting state networks in major depressive disorder. Psychiatry Res. 2014;224(3):139–51.
22. Yao Z, Yan R, Wei M, Tang H, Qin J, Lu Q. Gender differences in brain activity and the relationship between brain activity and differences in prevalence rates between male and female major depressive disorder patients: a resting-state fMRI study. Clin Neurophysiol. 2014;125(11):2232–9.
23. Buchanan A, Wang X, Gollan JK. Resting-state functional connectivity in women with major depressive disorder. J Psychiatr Res. 2014;59:38–44.
24. Clasen PC, Beevers CG, Mumford JA, Schnyer DM. Cognitive control network connectivity in adolescent women with and without a parental history of depression. Dev Cogn Neurosci. 2014;7:13–22.
25. Karakas P, Koc Z, Koc F, Gulhal Bozkir M. Morphometric MRI evaluation of corpus callosum and ventricles in normal adults. Neurol Res. 2011;33(10):1044–9.
26. Blanton RE, Chaplin TM, Sinha R. Sex differences in the correlation of emotional control and amygdala volumes in adolescents. Neuroreport. 2010;21(14):953–7.
27. McRae K, Ochsner KN, Mauss IB, Gabrieli JJD, Gross JJ. Gender differences in emotion regulation: an fMRI study of cognitive reappraisal. Group Process Intergroup Relat. 2008;11(2):143–62.
28. Li W, Chen Z, Wu M, Zhu H, Gu L, Zhao Y, Kuang W, Bi F, Kemp GJ, Gong Q. Characterization of brain blood flow and the amplitude of low-frequency fluctuations in major depressive disorder: a multimodal meta-analysis. J Affect Disord. 2017;210:303–11.
29. Seminowicz DA, Mayberg HS, McIntosh AR, Goldapple K, Kennedy S, Segal Z, Rafi-Tari S. Limbic-frontal circuitry in major depression: a path modeling metanalysis. Neuroimage. 2004;22(1):409–18.
30. Gusnard DA, Akbudak E, Shulman GL, Raichle ME. Medial prefrontal cortex and self-referential mental activity: relation to a default mode of brain function. Proc Natl Acad Sci U S A. 2001;98(7):4259–64.
31. Ridderinkhof KR, Ullsperger M, Crone EA, Nieuwenhuis S. The role of the medial frontal cortex in cognitive control. Science. 2004;306(5695):443–7.
32. Cooney RE, Joormann J, Eugene F, Dennis EL, Gotlib IH. Neural correlates of rumination in depression. Cogn Affect Behav Neurosci. 2010;10(4):470–8.
33. Frodl T, Meisenzahl EM, Zetzsche T, Born C, Groll C, Jager M, Leinsinger G, Bottlender R, Hahn K, Moller HJ. Hippocampal changes in patients with a first episode of major depression. Am J Psychiatry. 2002;159(7):1112–8.
34. Sheline YI. Depression and the hippocampus: cause or effect? Biol Psychiatry. 2011;70(4):308–9.
35. Koster EH, De Raedt R, Leyman L, De Lissnyder E. Mood-congruent attention and memory bias in dysphoria: exploring the coherence among information-processing biases. Behav Res Ther. 2010;48(3):219–25.
36. Hamilton JP, Gotlib IH. Neural substrates of increased memory sensitivity for negative stimuli in major depression. Biol Psychiatry. 2008;63(12):1155–62.
37. Hartikainen KM, Ogawa KH, Knight RT. Orbitofrontal cortex biases attention to emotional events. J Clin Exp Neuropsychol. 2012;34(6):588–97.
38. Kramer UM, Solbakk AK, Funderud I, Lovstad M, Endestad T, Knight RT. The role of the lateral prefrontal cortex in inhibitory motor control. Cortex. 2013;49(3):837–49.
39. Rolls ET. The functions of the orbitofrontal cortex. Brain Cogn. 2004;55(1):11–29.
40. Chen Y, Wang C, Zhu X, Tan Y, Zhong Y. Aberrant connectivity within the default mode network in first-episode, treatment-naive major depressive disorder. J Affect Disord. 2015;183:49–56.
41. Tadayonnejad R, Yang S, Kumar A, Ajilore O. Clinical, cognitive, and functional connectivity correlations of resting-state intrinsic brain activity alterations in unmedicated depression. J Affect Disord. 2015;172:241–50.
42. Ledberg A, Akerman S, Roland PE. Estimation of the probabilities of 3D clusters in functional brain images. Neuroimage. 1998;8(2):113–28.
43. Song XW, Dong ZY, Long XY, Li SF, Zuo XN, Zhu CZ, He Y, Yan CG, Zang YF. REST: a toolkit for resting-state functional magnetic resonance imaging data processing. PLoS One. 2011;6(9):e25031.
44. Cerullo MA, Eliassen JC, Smith CT, Fleck DE, Nelson EB, Strawn JR, Lamy M, DelBello MP, Adler CM, Strakowski SM. Bipolar I disorder and major depressive disorder show similar brain activation during depression. Bipolar Disord. 2014;16(7):703–12.
45. Furey ML, Drevets WC, Hoffman EM, Frankel E, Speer AM, Zarate CA Jr. Potential of pretreatment neural activity in the visual cortex during emotional processing to predict treatment response to scopolamine in major depressive disorder. JAMA Psychiat. 2013;70(3):280–90.
46. Guo WB, Liu F, Xue ZM, Xu XJ, Wu RR, Ma CQ, Wooderson SC, Tan CL, Sun XL, Chen JD, et al. Alterations of the amplitude of low-frequency fluctuations in treatment-resistant and treatment-response depression: a resting-state fMRI study. Prog Neuro-Psychopharmacol Biol Psychiatry. 2012;37(1):153–60.
47. Liu J, Ren L, Womer FY, Wang J, Fan G, Jiang W, Blumberg HP, Tang Y, Xu K, Wang F. Alterations in amplitude of low frequency fluctuation in treatment-naive major depressive disorder measured with resting-state fMRI. Hum Brain Mapp. 2014;35(10):4979–88.
48. Fan T, Wu X, Yao L, Dong J. Abnormal baseline brain activity in suicidal and non-suicidal patients with major depressive disorder. Neurosci Lett. 2013;534:35–40.
49. Zhong X, Pu W, Yao S. Functional alterations of fronto-limbic circuit and default mode network systems in first-episode, drug-naive patients with major depressive disorder: a meta-analysis of resting-state fMRI data. J Affect Disord. 2016;206:280–6.
50. Maller JJ, Thomson RH, Rosenfeld JV, Anderson R, Daskalakis ZJ, Fitzgerald PB. Occipital bending in depression. Brain. 2014;137(Pt 6):1830–7.
51. Tu S, Qiu J, Martens U, Zhang Q. Category-selective attention modulates unconscious processes in the middle occipital gyrus. Conscious Cogn. 2013;22(2):479–85.
52. Elliott R, Rubinsztein JS, Sahakian BJ, Dolan RJ. The neural basis of mood-congruent processing biases in depression. Arch Gen Psychiatry. 2002;59(7):597–604.
53. Montagner R, Mogg K, Bradley BP, Pine DS, Czykiel MS, Miguel EC, Rohde LA, Manfro GG, Salum GA. Attentional bias to threat in children at-risk for emotional disorders: role of gender and type of maternal emotional disorder. Eur Child Adolesc Psychiatry. 2016;25(7):735–42.
54. Clasen PC, Wells TT, Ellis AJ, Beevers CG. Attentional biases and the persistence of sad mood in major depressive disorder. J Abnorm Psychol. 2013;122(1):74–85.
55. Liu CH, Ma X, Yuan Z, Song LP, Jing B, Lu HY, Tang LR, Fan J, Walter M, Liu CZ, et al. Decreased resting-state activity in the Precuneus is associated with depressive episodes in recurrent depression. J Clin Psychiatry. 2017;78(4):e372–82.
56. Yoshimura S, Okamoto Y, Onoda K, Matsunaga M, Ueda K, Suzuki S, Shigetoyamawaki. Rostral anterior cingulate cortex activity mediates the relationship between the depressive symptoms and the medial prefrontal cortex activity. J Affect Disord. 2010;122(1–2):76–85.
57. Yoshimura S, Ueda K, Suzuki S, Onoda K, Okamoto Y, Yamawaki S. Self-referential processing of negative stimuli within the ventral anterior cingulate gyrus and right amygdala. Brain Cogn. 2009;69(1):218–25.
58. Delaveau P, Jabourian M, Lemogne C, Allaili N, Choucha W, Girault N, Lehericy S, Laredo J, Fossati P. Antidepressant short-term and long-term brain effects during self-referential processing in major depression. Psychiatry Res Neuroimaging. 2016;247:17–24.
59. Pantazatos SP, Yanagihara TK, Zhang X, Meitzler T, Hirsch J. Frontal-occipital connectivity during visual search. Brain Connect. 2012;2(3):164–75.

60. Mulders PC, van Eijndhoven PF, Schene AH, Beckmann CF, Tendolkar I. Resting-state functional connectivity in major depressive disorder: a review. Neurosci Biobehav Rev. 2015;56:330–44.
61. Rao U, Chen LA, Bidesi AS, Shad MU, Thomas MA, Hammen CL. Hippocampal changes associated with early-life adversity and vulnerability to depression. Biol Psychiatry. 2010;67(4):357–64.
62. MacQueen G, Frodl T. The hippocampus in major depression: evidence for the convergence of the bench and bedside in psychiatric research? Mol Psychiatry. 2011;16(3):252–64.
63. Yonelinas AP, Hopfinger JB, Buonocore MH, Kroll NE, Baynes K. Hippocampal, parahippocampal and occipital-temporal contributions to associative and item recognition memory: an fMRI study. Neuroreport. 2001; 12(2):359–63.
64. Sterpenich V, Albouy G, Boly M, Vandewalle G, Darsaud A, Balteau E, Dang-Vu TT, Desseilles M, D'Argembeau A, Gais S, et al. Sleep-related hippocampo-cortical interplay during emotional memory recollection. PLoS Biol. 2007;5(11):e282.
65. Sterpenich V, Albouy G, Darsaud A, Schmidt C, Vandewalle G, Dang Vu TT, Desseilles M, Phillips C, Degueldre C, Balteau E, et al. Sleep promotes the neural reorganization of remote emotional memory. J Neurosci. 2009;29(16):5143–52.
66. Sheline YI, Barch DM, Price JL, Rundle MM, Vaishnavi SN, Snyder AZ, Mintun MA, Wang S, Coalson RS, Raichle ME. The default mode network and self-referential processes in depression. Proc Natl Acad Sci U S A. 2009;106(6):1942–7.
67. Hamilton JP, Furman DJ, Chang C, Thomason ME, Dennis E, Gotlib IH. Default-mode and task-positive network activity in major depressive disorder: implications for adaptive and maladaptive rumination. Biol Psychiatry. 2011;70(4):327–33.
68. Chai XJ, Ofen N, Gabrieli JD, Whitfield-Gabrieli S. Development of deactivation of the default-mode network during episodic memory formation. Neuroimage. 2014;84:932–8.
69. Zhang X, Zhu X, Wang X, Zhu X, Zhong M, Yi J, Rao H, Yao S. First-episode medication-naive major depressive disorder is associated with altered resting brain function in the affective network. PLoS One. 2014;9(1):e85241.
70. Xiu D, Geiger MJ, Klaver P. Emotional face expression modulates occipital-frontal effective connectivity during memory formation in a bottom-up fashion. Front Behav Neurosci. 2015;9:90.
71. Jiang X, Dai X, Kale Edmiston E, Zhou Q, Xu K, Zhou Y, Wu F, Kong L, Wei S, Zhou Y, et al. Alteration of cortico-limbic-striatal neural system in major depressive disorder and bipolar disorder. J Affect Disord. 2017;221:297–303.
72. Wang L, Shen H, Tang F, Zang Y, Hu D. Combined structural and resting-state functional MRI analysis of sexual dimorphism in the young adult human brain: an MVPA approach. Neuroimage. 2012;61(4):931–40.
73. Wu X, Chen J, Jia T, Ma W, Zhang Y, Deng Z, Yang L. Cognitive Bias by gender interaction on N170 response to emotional facial expressions in major and minor depression. Brain Topogr. 2016;29(2):232–42.

14

Meaning and medication: a thematic analysis of depressed adolescents' views and experiences of SSRI antidepressants alongside psychological therapies

Rita A. Maroun[1,2], Lisa A. Thackeray[1,2] and Nick Midgley[3*]

Abstract

Background: Adolescence is a key period of risk for the emergence of Major Depressive Disorder (MDD). The prescription of selective serotonin re-uptake inhibitors (SSRIs) for the treatment of depression in adolescents is an issue of worldwide controversy, and evidence regarding their safety and efficacy is inconclusive. In the UK, NICE guidelines have recently recommended offering SSRIs to adolescents alongside psychological therapy or on their own if therapy is refused. Thus, SSRIs are increasingly becoming a major component of treatment for adolescents. This study qualitatively explored adolescents' views and experiences of SSRIs within their accounts of engaging in a psychological therapy for depression, particularly focusing on meanings they attached to medication-use.

Methods: The qualitative study reports data from semi-structured interviews conducted 12-months post-treatment with 12 adolescents who were clinically referred and treated for depression as part of the IMPACT trial. The interviews were analysed using Thematic Analysis.

Results: Four themes were identified: 'a perceived threat to autonomy', 'a sign of severity', 'a support, not a solution', and 'an ongoing process of trial and error'.

Conclusions: This study highlights the value of bringing adolescents' voices into the broader debate on the use of antidepressants in their age group and in the development of future guidelines. Future implications for research and clinical practice are discussed.

Keywords: Depression, Antidepressants, SSRIs, Adolescents, Patient perspectives, Medication use, Qualitative

Background

The safety and efficacy of antidepressants for adolescents is an issue of ongoing worldwide controversy due to concerns about elevated risk of self-harm and suicidal behavior [1, 2]. For over a decade, numerous studies have examined the safety and efficacy of Selective Serotonin Re-Uptake Inhibitors (SSRIs) in adolescents, but results have been conflicting [see 1]. A recent systematic review and meta-analysis of clinical trials for several SSRIs found that serious risks, including suicide and aggression, were underreported and the extent of potential harm is not always discernable [3]. Still, prescription of antidepressants for under 19's increased worldwide from 2005 to 2012 [4]. In the UK, first-ever prescriptions of antidepressants for 3–17-year-olds approximately doubled between 2006 and 2015 [5].

The National Institute for Health Care and Excellence (NICE) makes recommendations for treatment in the UK based on systematic reviews of best available evidence [6]. For adolescents presenting with moderate-to-severe depression, previous guidelines recommended an evidence-based psychological therapy as first line treatment and cautioned against prescribing antidepressants unless the adolescent is unresponsive to psychological therapy, in which case they recommended

* Correspondence: nick.midgley@annafreud.org
[3]The Child Attachment and Psychological Therapies Research Unit (ChAPTRe), University College London and Anna Freud National Centre for Children and Families, London, UK

Fluoxetine, a Selective-Serotonin Re-Uptake Inhibitor (SSRI), in addition to psychological therapy [6]. The 2015 amendment recommended offering combined psychological therapy and Fluoxetine as an alternative first line of treatment. SSRIs can also be offered on their own if psychological therapies are declined, albeit with close monitoring. These amendments could mean that more adolescents in the UK will be offered antidepressants and potentially at an earlier stage of treatment. A recent study suggests that SSRIs are being prescribed in the absence of psychological therapies, contrary to NICE recommendations; at least 19% of 465 adolescents were prescribed SSRIs prior to beginning psychological treatment [7].

The rising prescribing trends, aforementioned prescribing practices, and the amendment in guidance all suggest that antidepressants are increasingly becoming a major component of treatment for adolescents. Further, the inconclusive evidence regarding safety and efficacy of antidepressants highlights the need to better understand the impact of these medications on adolescents. Developing an understanding of the impact of antidepressants that is grounded in adolescents' perspectives and narratives can offer new insight into current prescribing practices and the broader debate around antidepressant use, especially given that they are the main stakeholders in treatment.

Antidepressant use in adolescents has been extensively researched (e.g.[1, 8, 9]). However, only a small number of studies have focused on adolescents' own understanding and interpretation of antidepressants as well as their subjective experience of the effects [10–13]. The available literature on antidepressants, and psychiatric medication more broadly, suggests that adolescents attribute different meanings to medication, which could coincide with developmental issues pertinent to adolescence, such as identity formation, autonomy, and social acceptance [10–16]. For instance, adolescents in one study describe hiding their medication use due to feelings of shame and differentiation from peers, stating that it marked them as 'defective' [15]. In other studies, adolescents have reported that they view medication use as contradictory to their identity as 'normal' and 'autonomous' teenagers, and that this can act as a barrier to accepting and adhering to treatment [10, 12, 15]. One study found that adolescents felt resistant to even seeking help for depression due to fear of being prescribed medication [10].

Together, these studies highlight the importance of exploring personal meanings that adolescents may attribute to antidepressant medication throughout the treatment process, and how these meanings impact not only their acceptance and adherence to the treatment, but also their developing sense of self. Further, for adolescents who choose to take it, medication is a daily and possibly important part of the experience of depression and treatment. This study therefore aimed to qualitatively explore adolescents' views and experiences of SSRI medication within in their accounts of overcoming depression; specifically, to identify patterns of meaning that these adolescents attribute to medication within their broader experience of depression and treatment.

Methods

Setting

This study drew on interviews with adolescents who participated in Improving Moods with Psychoanalytic and Cognitive Therapies (IMPACT), a randomized controlled superiority trial which compared the effectiveness of three psychological therapies for adolescent depression (see [17, 18]). The study recruited 470 adolescents aged 11–17 years with a diagnosis of Major Depressive Disorder (MDD) from 15 Child and Adolescent Mental Health Services (CAMHS) across three UK regions. Adolescents were randomly allocated to one of three manualized treatments: Cognitive Behavioral Therapy (CBT), Short Term Psychodynamic Psychotherapy (STPP), and Brief Psychosocial Intervention (BPI). Adolescents were offered SSRIs during and post-treatment in combination with the allocated therapy as recommended by NICE guidelines. IMPACT-My Experience (IMPACT-ME), a qualitative, longitudinal study, took place alongside IMPACT. Interviews were conducted with adolescents participating in the trial before therapy (baseline), at the end of therapy, and one year after (follow-up) see [19].

Data collection and sampling

The current study drew on follow-up data from the 'Thinking back about therapy' interview, a semi-structured schedule which invites adolescents to reflect on their experience of overcoming depression soon after therapy ended. Interviews were carried out by research psychologists with additional training in in-depth interviewing and lasted between 30 and 90 min. However, medication was not the primary focus of the interview. Therefore, any mention of medication was either in response to a specific question related to medication, 'was medication ever discussed with you?' or volunteered by the adolescent.

Interviews with all 70 adolescents who took part in the IMPACT-ME study were first reviewed. As per the current study's aim to identify patterns of meaning that are attributed to medication, adolescents who gave a yes / no answer to the interviewer's question but did not expand the discussion beyond a single statement or did not elaborate beyond logistical information (e.g. when medication was suggested, which medication they took, dosages) were excluded. This resulted in a sample of 12 interviews in which adolescents spoke about their views and experiences of being offered medication and/or of taking medication. Given that this is a relatively under-explored topic, the accounts of both adolescents who had and had not taken medication were included in the sample.

Participants

The 12 adolescents (10 female, 2 male) were 13–18 years old at baseline. All sought and received treatment as part of IMPACT and met diagnostic criteria for moderate-to-severe unipolar depression at time of recruitment, as assessed by Kiddie-SADs [20]. Exclusion criteria were generalized learning difficulties, pregnancy, primary diagnosis of bipolar Type 1, schizophrenia, pervasive developmental disorder, and eating disorders. Two had received treatment in the STPP arm, five in the BPI arm, and five in the CBT arm. Three adolescents expressed their views about medication despite not having been offered it, three had refused to take medication when offered, and six had taken medication – four of whom had stopped. Of the adolescents who took medication, three of the adolescents had been prescribed prior to being recruited and receiving psychological treatment in the study. When examining their baseline characteristics, no differences were identified between this sub-group and the complete set of participants in the IMPACT-ME study, other than a slightly lower proportion of young people in the STPP arm of the study.

Study design

The current study employed a qualitative design to explore the sections of the interviews in which adolescents discussed medication with the aim of obtaining an in-depth, nuanced account, emphasizing adolescents' personal views and/or experiences of medication whilst also drawing broader patterns of meaning across interviews. To facilitate this, interviews were analyzed using thematic analysis (TA), a flexible method of qualitative analysis that allows researchers to actively identify, analyze, and report patterns of meaning in data, while providing a detailed and rich account of themes [21]. Following Braune and Clarke's [21] six-phase approach to TA, 'familiarization' with the data was achieved by listening to audio-recordings and reading entire transcripts to grasp contextual details of adolescents' broader narratives, noting initial ideas about the data. In phase two, the first author coded areas that discussed medication by systematically identifying and highlighting interesting features and labelling them according to their content. Each extract was coded with as many codes as possible until a list of codes had been generated. In phase three, the author identified patterns in the codes across the whole dataset and grouped them into potential themes via mind-map, whereby different combinations of codes were arranged and re-arranged until candidate themes and their sub-themes had been devised. Phase four involved refining identified themes in a recursive process; coded data extracts were tabulated under themes and were then read together under each theme to determine whether they adequately and coherently captured data patterns and to ascertain whether themes were sufficiently supported. Afterwards, the author re-read the interviews to determine whether themes reflected the data and captured an overall picture of meanings adolescents attributed to medication. At each stage the first author discussed and refined overarching themes and sub-themes with the co-authors. Extracts were re-coded again and any data missed in previous phases were added under identified themes. In phase five, a detailed analysis identified the over-arching message for each individual theme in relation to research aims, with attention to nuances while still highlighting broader 'story' that the combined themes tell about the data. Finally, each theme was named and given a concise definition describing its content.

Trustworthiness and credibility of the analysis

Braune and Clarke's [21] 15-point-criteria for conducting 'good' thematic analysis were followed, with a particular emphasis on trustworthiness, credibility, transferability, dependability, and confirmability [22]. Throughout the process, the research team took a position of reflexivity [23], continuously acknowledging and evaluating the impact of their own perceptions, experiences, interests, and background. Interpretations of data were discussed with co-authors and examined by peers and necessary changes were made. Further, the data was iteratively coded three times. A journal was used to document and review thought progression, decisions, and discussions. An audit trail documented how data was coded and grouped into themes. The research team attempted to 'stay close to the data' during analysis and used direct quotes from adolescents when reporting findings to allow readers to check the analysis against original accounts. Additionally, information about the study setting and adolescents' individual contexts were incorporated into write-up to aid transferability.

Results

Four interrelated themes were identified in relation to the study aim. Three of these themes were central across the entire dataset: 'a perceived threat to autonomy', 'a sign of severity', 'a support, not a solution'. One theme was specifically salient to adolescents who had taken medication: 'an ongoing process of trial and error'. These themes are reported along with their respective sub-themes (see Fig. 1).

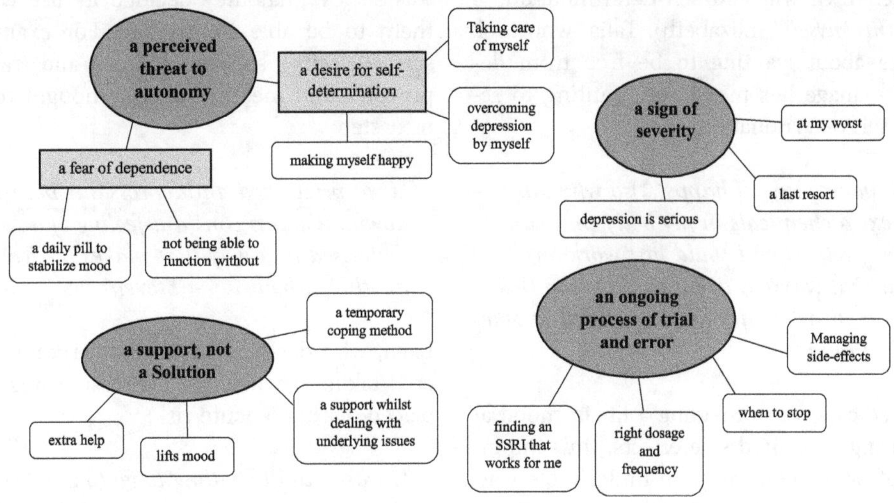

Fig. 1 Final thematic map: themes, sub-themes, and features

Theme 1: 'A perceived threat to autonomy'

For some adolescents, medication seemed to be a threat to their sense of autonomy. Taking medication appeared to challenge their view of themselves as independent and free from external control. This theme was characterized by two interconnected sub-themes: 'a fear of dependency' and 'a desire for self-determination'. These adolescents either never sought medication, refused to take it when offered, or took it and stopped. For all these adolescents, this perception had implications for whether they took medication as well as adhered to it.

'A fear of dependency'

A fear of dependency was present in many adolescents' narratives—whereby taking medication seemed to demarcate a forfeit of their independent functioning to an 'added chemical' in order to regulate mood and manage depression.

Adolescents spoke about how taking a daily pill to manage their depression can be daunting. Talia, who took medication, described how relying on medication every day to keep her mood stabilized was simultaneously a source of anxiety and confusion:

> *"It's annoying I have to take these pills every day…if I forget it could be bad(...)It's unnerving when you're feeling happy and having a side thought going yeah but are you happy or is it just added chemicals making you feel happy?" - (Talia)*

For Talia, taking medication led her to question her ability to function without it and interfered with her perception of her emotions as being her own. She recalled her decision to stop taking medication because she felt it was a risk worth taking in exchange for being free from having to rely on it daily, even if this meant ending up in hospital:

> *"It wouldn't be worth having to take pills every single day just to stop that one day coming around every now and again(...)so I was like I might as well stop, see what happens(...)worst comes to worse I might end up in hospital again" - (Talia)*

Adolescents also described a fear of being physically dependent on anti-depressants. For example, for Mathilda, this seemed to be associated with a fear of experiencing a difficult withdrawal, making her hesitant to stop taking medication:

> *"I didn't wanna depend on it too much …but at the same time I was worried about coming off it, especially doing A-levels cos it's a stressful time" - (Mathilda)*

Whereas, for Elizabeth, these fears, which arose from family experience, contributed to her decision not to take medication:

> *"My Mum's been on the medications and I don't really wanna go on it cause I've seen her try and come off it. It's taken her three or four attempts before she could come off it, so I said 'I don't wanna be dependent on it'." - (Elizabeth)*

'A desire for self-determination'

This sub-theme delineates a simultaneous desire to manage depression via one's own will, whereby change has to be self-induced and on one's own terms.

Many adolescents who talked about their fear of dependency also expressed a desire to overcome their depression by their own will and self-determination: *"I want to get over this myself"* (Elizabeth). Talia, who took medication, spoke about wanting to be free from depending on it to manage her mood and wanting to regain her sense of self-determination:

> *"I'm capable of making myself happy(...)so why am I having to take extra chemicals in my body that can cause these side effects when I could just work on myself and do it that way?(...) like I need to stop this. I was getting to a point where it's like I can kind of take care of myself." - (Talia)*

Talia describes medication as providing a lift in mood at the price of enduring unwanted side effects, thus impinging on a sense of bodily control in an undesirable way. For Talia, this seemed to elicit a desire to regain a sense of control over her body, which, together with her belief that she can make herself happy, contributed to her decision to stop medication. For Callum, his preference to overcome his depression by his own means led to his decision not to take medication at all:

> *"I wouldn't even wanna take medication. I'd rather just deal with it my way." - (Callum).*

Overall, the need for medication is understood here as a sign of an inability to cope with depression via self-determination. Further, adolescents seemed to have a shared perception that taking medication would take away a degree of control over their bodies and impinge on their ability to take care of themselves.

Theme 2: 'A sign of severity'

Almost all adolescents identified a particular point at which they deemed or would deem medication to be necessary, referring to how low they perceived their mood to be and its impact on their functioning.

Medication was seen as necessary when depression was experienced as particularly severe. The adolescents who had never considered or had declined taking medication spoke of how they were not at a point in their depression that warranted its use, *"I don't think my depression was that serious, so I didn't take medication"* (Priya). Further, medication seemed to be reserved for a level of severity that adolescents were able to recognize:

> *"I think that should be the last resort, I don't think you should put everyone on meds because sometimes it's not serious for them to be on meds. For me, it was not that serious" - (Natasha)*

Similarly, adolescents who had taken medication referred to a certain point at which they felt their mood was so low that they decided its use was necessary for them to be able to manage. For example, Steven described feeling so overwhelmed and trapped by his depression that medication was thought to be a necessary next step:

> *"I got prescribed antidepressants because I felt really down...like this constant feeling of down(...)I'm depressed in a way that makes me feel like I can't do anything about it." - (Steven)*

Lana, who declined medication, recalls that she considered taking it when her depression was so severe that it placed her at an acute risk:

> *"I was actually willing to go to medication for the first time ever because I was so bad. I was like okay I might go on an antidepressant(...)That one time I went to A&E was the only time I was actually resorting--- for me to actually accept that okay I might actually take medication I was in a very bad place." - (Lana)*

To Lana, taking medication was only conceivable when she had to make use of emergency services, denoting it as an option that is 'resorted' to at a time of utmost severity. Thus, for all these adolescents, medication was viewed as a resource that can be drawn on when depression was particularly severe and chronic; when they were feeling particularly at their worst and no longer able to manage their depression.

However, for some adolescents, medication featured as a resource only to be drawn on when other options have been exhausted. For example, Charlotte mentioned that medication was only warranted at a time when other treatments have failed, and it was the last option available:

> *"I thought try therapy cause then you see if that works and if it does it might help me long-term and if that didn't work I could always resort to medication"- (Charlotte)*

However, other options were not always described as accessible because of depression severity. For example, Leila described experiencing such chronic low mood and feelings of helplessness that she was unable to manage on her own or engage with help from professionals, at which point she was willing to try medication despite feeling uncertain:

> *"I mean I think it was just because I was so low that I couldn't like benefit from therapy. I was too upset to even like put anything into action or help myself." - (Leila)*

Medication seemed to be a necessary precursor to being able to access other forms of help. Therefore, these adolescents described medication as the next step when depression felt overpowering and/or nonresponsive to other forms of help. As such, the perceived need for medication acted as a point of reference for adolescents whereby they could gauge not only how severe their depression was, but also how well they were able to manage it.

Theme 3: 'A support, not a solution'

The majority of adolescents shared the belief that medication can play a beneficial role whilst overcoming depression. However, its role was deemed to be facilitative, whereby adolescents described medication as a form of additional rather than a solution in its own right. This theme applied to those who had and had not taken medication.

Adolescents who had taken medication described it as playing a key role in their recovery during a time of stagnation, by helping them engage in treatment, regain functioning, and resume pleasurable activities they had stopped due to depression. However, it was seen as offering something additional alongside therapy rather than a standalone treatment—described by Leila as *"extra help from something else"* and by Steven as *"something to lift mood"*. Similarly, Mathilda saw medication as having a supportive role in recovery, whereby it stabilized mood so that it felt manageable.:

> *"Therapy was really good, and it helped and probably medication as well, but that was more about the lack of safety blanket until I was feeling better. But I think the main thing was the therapy...just different methods for coping (...) I knew that if things did go downhill again I could just go back on medication I suppose." -(Mathilda)*

For Mathilda, medication served as a temporary extra component and an option that she could fall back on if needed—particularly at a point of relapse. Further, therapy and medication were seen here as distinct ways of coping, although both were described as contributing to recovery. Similarly, Kayleigh stated that medication allowed her to better engage in therapy and experience a sense of hope despite it initially being a difficult decision:

> *"I was getting better but I needed a final push (...)it was a tough decision cause I didn't like taking tablets but I think looking back now it was the right decision to go on it (...)I started crawling out of the hole but then once the medication kicked in it was just like I can actually see the light at the end." - (Kayleigh)*

For Kayleigh, combining medication with therapy was described as a turning point in her treatment, whereby medication offered a different kind of support that she experienced as essential to her recovery.

Similarly, to those who did take medication, those who did not talked about how medication might help ease the burden of depression. However, they expressed a desire to deal with underlying issues, which contributed to their decision to refuse medication:

> *"Medication doesn't solve the problem it just helps you deal with it a bit more cause at the end of the day you're still gonna have to deal with it yourself. Even if medication takes a bit off the edge...it just kind of covers the problem" - (Lana)*

As such, they tended to see medication as a temporary way of managing their depression and preferred to enhance their own ability to cope, describing this as more sustainable in the long-term:

> *"The medications not always gonna be there so I would just come to terms with myself and stuff." - (Callum)*

These adolescents also expressed a preference for therapy: *"if you just take a tablet, you can't just expect to get better straight away. It's better to talk things out" (Priya)*, appearing to believe that it was a more long-term solution than medication. Natasha, who was offered medication, but declined, cited this preference as her reason. Moreover, she expressed a belief that medication could not help her resolve her difficulties, despite acknowledging that it might temporarily help her manage her symptoms:

> *"If I got straight away offered medication without dealing with the real issues, I would have just refused(...)Medication would make me feel okay, but it wouldn't deal with my deeper demons. I think if we just give someone medication and not give them opportunity to try and explore and work with their issues within themselves...It's just gonna deal with the problem there and then but it's not going to help in the long-term" - (Natasha)*

For Natasha, her belief that her depression was linked to relational difficulties seemed to be a key reason for her refusal of medication and preference for therapy:

> *"Me having therapy has helped my life in so much ways, it's gonna help my future in the long run. But if you gave me medication, I would still be battling with my past, my Dad's relation, and I would just be kind of a neutral person, coping with pills." - (Natasha)*

Here, medication was described as a temporary method of coping with low mood, whereby the perceived cause of depression remains unaddressed.

Thus, adolescents appeared to denote medication as having the specific role of alleviating low mood, while therapy was seen as addressing underlying issues. Although all adolescents assigned some value to medication, whether they took it seemed to be related to what they felt was the most pertinent to overcoming their depression. Specifically, adolescents who took medication described experiencing low mood as overpowering and debilitating, and thus felt that medication was a necessary step to take to enable them to address underlying issues in therapy. Whereas, adolescents who did not take medication, felt they were functioning well enough and could manage their depression without medication, preferring to deal with underlying issues in the first instance. Still, they did see medication as being available to help them cope with low mood if necessary.

Theme 4: 'An ongoing process of trial and error'

This theme relates solely to adolescents who had taken medication. To these adolescents, taking medication was not a straightforward process, rather, it was an ongoing, recursive process of trial and error during which they struggled to find the right type, dosage, frequency, and length of treatment. For example,

> *"I was taking anti-depressants for six, seven months, and then eventually I got to a point, before the psychiatrist said I could... I came off medication, but in October I went back onto medication" – (Ada).*

Adolescents also described their struggle to cope with side effects, sometimes having to experiment with different types of medication and understand how they affected their bodies:

> *"we went through different antidepressants then I chose one I haven't taken before (...) Dunno I hope they help but with every anti-depressant there's a different side-effect...so interesting to see what the side-effects of these are (...)Oh [medication 1]...I just slept constantly(...) and the other ones I just felt completely numb that's why I stopped taking them..."– (Steven)*

Adolescents also described the difficulty of gaging whether to stop taking medication, which induced a level of anxiety about withdrawal effects. Talia recalled how her decision to suddenly stop medication caused concern from her parents and professionals, resulting in a period of careful monitoring afterwards:

> *"I was on fluoxetine twice. I was on it for like a year and then it stopped working and then we tried it again, like a year or so later and it didn't have the same effect as when I started the first time so we stopped that (...) then I was on citalopram and then spring this year I was like I don't wanna take these anymore so I stopped (...)Mum and dad were worried, they're like 'you 'can't just stop taking your medications"- (Talia)*

Thus, for these adolescents, the experience of taking medication was more than merely receiving a prescription and taking it. Rather, it was an ongoing process whereby adolescents wrestled with tough questions relating to the meaning and potential consequences of medication use.

Discussion

The current study explored the meanings that adolescents attached to SSRI medication within their narratives of overcoming depression. Four main themes were identified: 'a perceived threat to autonomy', 'a sign of severity', 'a support, not a solution', and 'an ongoing process of trial and error'.

The first theme, 'a perceived threat to autonomy' is consistent with previous studies that have shown that adolescents who are resistant to medication tend to describe taking it as inconsistent with being 'autonomous' [10, 12, 15]. Adolescence is recognised as a key period for identity formation whereby individuals strive for autonomy, thus adolescents may view medication as a further impingement on their identity as autonomous individuals [24]. Moreover, some adolescents in this study associated antidepressant use with being 'dependent' and referred to medication as 'added chemicals' that are an undesirable means of obtaining happiness, expressing their wish to do so by their own means. This could indicate some anxiety about what medication does to their body, but also that medication use could be perceived as a loss of control over their bodies, especially at a time when they may be experiencing significant biological changes [25]. Furthermore, this theme was salient for adolescents who had refused to take medication and those who accepted it then decided to stop. Thus, this could have implications for whether adolescents seek or accept medication as part of treatment and whether they adhere to it. Even if antidepressant treatment is effective, it has limited value if adolescents do not seek it and adhere to it [1]. A systematic review found that adolescents' positive beliefs about their treatment was associated with improved adherence [26].

The second theme, 'a sign of severity' showed that medication was deemed necessary when depression was perceived and experienced as severe. This aligns with the NICE recommendations' stepped care model, which indicates that antidepressants should only be prescribed for adolescents presenting with moderate-to-severe depression [6]. However, all adolescents in this study had a diagnosis of moderate-to-severe depression, indicating there may be qualitative differences in 'severity'. Adolescents captured this difference, describing a level of 'severity' that warrants antidepressant use, associated with the experience of depression as too overwhelming and debilitating, having extremely low mood, and feeling they could no longer manage on their own. These descriptions have been reported by other adolescents in previous qualitative research [27, 28], where this 'overwhelming' quality to depression was also prominent.

Moreover, adolescents' descriptions of feeling too low to benefit from therapy, feeling trapped by depression, and being at a dangerous low point are consistent with previous findings that suggest adolescents are prescribed antidepressants as a first line treatment when they present with severe depression or are too reluctant to initially engage with therapy [29]. Therefore, introducing antidepressants at an earlier stage in treatment may be beneficial to some adolescents. This is supported by the latest NICE guidelines which suggest antidepressants as a first line treatment in combination with psychological therapy or on their own if the adolescents do not engage with psychological therapy [6].

Adolescents' understanding of the need to take medication also seemed related to how they perceived their ability to cope. This ties in with the first theme, which suggests medication is perceived as a sign of being incapable of managing depression via their self-determination. These two themes may indicate that taking a daily pill to cope with depression could be perceived by adolescents as a concrete statement that they are at a particularly low point, unable to manage without it. As such, these themes echo the findings of other studies in which adolescents described psychiatric medication as a marker of their 'defectiveness' and or a sign that they are 'not autonomous' [10, 12, 15]. Underlying beliefs of being 'defective' and 'dependent' are also characteristic of depression more generally [30]. When these meanings are associated with medication, it is possible that the suggestion of medication may trigger, or heighten, these beliefs. Given that adolescence is recognized as a developmental stage in which issues of identity and autonomy are particularly salient, these beliefs may impact adolescents' views of themselves and have longer term consequences if not addressed [14]. This highlights the need for further research and careful consideration when prescribing antidepressant medication, specifically in relation to how adolescents' personal meanings might interact with relevant developmental issues.

The third theme, 'a support, not a solution' is consistent with previous qualitative research with adults where antidepressants were described as helpful to cope with and improve low mood, but only a partial or temporary fix [31, 32] or as not addressing social and psychological issues that were perceived as causes of depression [33]. However, the current findings indicate that while adolescents seem to assign SSRIs and psychological therapy distinct roles in treatment, they do not discount medication as an option. Whether and when adolescents believe SSRIs to be beneficial to their treatment could be related to whether they believe alleviating symptoms or addressing other psychological or social issues was most pertinent to their recovery. This also links to the previous theme, where adolescents felt that medication could play a beneficial role in treatment when depressive symptoms did not allow them to address underlying issues in therapy. Subsequently, the value adolescents place on the role of antidepressants in their treatment could be related to their beliefs about their depression. Although both adolescents who had and had not taken medication seemed to share the view that the act of taking antidepressants implies that they are not autonomous or that their depression is particularly severe, they simultaneously maintained that medication can play a facilitative role in treatment. These results are consistent with those reported in studies with adults, which show that they to struggle with ambivalent views about antidepressant medication [32, 34, 35]. These simultaneous beliefs could create a dilemma for adolescents who are deciding whether to take medication for the first time, or for those who are taking medication, whether to stop.

The fourth theme, 'an ongoing process of trial and error' highlights that taking antidepressants can be a difficult process marked by a continuous struggle to enhance benefits and reduce adverse effects. This supports NICE guidelines' emphasis on close and continuous monitoring of adolescents taking antidepressants [6]. However, this theme highlights how frustrating and disillusioning this process can be, potentially heightening feelings of hopelessness, which are associated with depression [36]. Thus, more holistic support is required in addition to routine monitoring, holding implications for both treatment effectiveness and adherence. Additionally, it emphasizes that adolescents may have concerns about when to stop their medication, what it means to function without it, or difficult withdrawals—a significant issue for adolescents discontinuing antidepressants [37]. Qualitative studies have found that adults may choose to remain on antidepressants despite perceiving that they no longer need them due to fears of withdrawal, relapse, or lack of support [38, 39].

Together, these four themes highlight how antidepressant treatment can hold complex meanings for adolescents throughout their experience of overcoming depression and may have implications for their views of themselves and the way they conceptualize their depression. This aligns with adult literature showing that experiences with antidepressant use are complex and dynamic, characterized by a temporal process of 'decision-making' and 'meaning-making' where treatment decisions are interlinked with the emergence of new self-concepts [32, 40].

Clinical implications

This study holds implications regarding antidepressant treatment with adolescents. Particularly, it re-emphasizes that practitioners should involve adolescents in the discussion about risks and benefits of SSRIs and provide them with the latest information to help them make informed choices and that antidepressant treatment should be monitored continuously [6]. These findings also emphasize that in addition to addressing issues of symptom control, physical tolerability, adherence, and side effects, clinicians should continuously and actively elicit, address and reflect on the impact of medication on adolescents' perceptions of themselves, their depression, and their quality of life with consideration to their developmental context. Further, this study supports the need for better implementing models of shared decision making (SDM) and involving adolescents as active partners their antidepressant treatment advocated by others [41–46].

Strengths and limitations

The current study elucidated meanings grounded in adolescents' perspectives on antidepressant use, which have scarcely been explored. Further, it captured specific nuances of meaning and potential commonalities in adolescents' views and experiences. However, as all the adolescents sought out, engaged with, and completed psychological therapy by the time of interview, these findings may not be representative of those who do not seek help, drop out of treatment, or do not engage with therapy and opt for solely taking antidepressant medication. Adolescents were also interviewed at the final time point of the IMPACT-ME study and the interviews were selected only if they spoke about their experience or feelings about medication—which was not the interviews' primary focus. Therefore, these findings may only be representative of adolescents who had strong opinions on medication and were invested in expressing their views and experiences and cannot be extrapolated to all depressed adolescents. Additionally, meanings were derived from adolescents' retrospective accounts. Thus, it is difficult to discern whether and how these meanings may have shifted over time from initial discussions.

Conclusions

Overall, the current study highlights the value of bringing adolescents' voices into the broader debate on the use of antidepressants in their age group and in the development of future guidelines. The findings showed how adolescents' may attribute highly personal meanings to antidepressant use, which hold implications for their view of themselves and their depression, and in turn, may impact on their treatment decision, their adherence, their response to medication if it is taken. Hence, the current study also emphasizes the importance of collaboratively exploring these meanings with adolescents throughout the treatment process in order to enhance their treatment experience.

The findings of this study also echo previous literature advocating a shift from questioning whether antidepressants work to questioning whom they work for [44, 47]. They highlight the value of incorporating qualitative research from an adolescent-centered perspective into future NICE guidelines as is already the case in relation to guidelines on ADHD medication use [48]. Future research should explore adolescents' perspectives of SSRIs at different stages of treatment, which may provide insight into how to better support adolescents during the course of their treatment. Over time it may be possible to create a valuable body of literature that can be referred to when making life-changing decisions about whether to initiate, continue, or discontinue antidepressant treatment with adolescents.

Abbreviations

BPI: Brief psychosocial intervention; CAMHS: Child and adolescence mental health services (CAMHS); CBT: Cognitive behavioral therapy; IMPACT: Improving moods with psychoanalytic and cognitive therapies; IMPACT-ME: Impact my experience; MDD: Major depressive disorder; NICE: National Institute for Health Care and Excellence; SSRIs: Selective serotonin reuptake inhibitors; STPP: Short-term psychodynamic psychotherapy; TA: Thematic analysis

Acknowledgements

The authors would like to thank the young people who took part in the IMPACT-ME study for sharing their stories. The authors would also like to thank Dr. Liz McDonnell for her guidance and support during the early stages of this research.

Funding

The IMPACT-ME study was funded by the Monument Trust. The current study did not receive any additional funding; the first author was an MSc student at UCL and AFNCCF and carried out this study as part of her academic program. The funding body did not have a role in the design of the study, data collection, analysis, interpretation of data, or writing of the manuscript.

Authors' contributions

RM planned and executed the design of the study, conducted the qualitative analysis of the data, and wrote the draft of the paper. LT cross-coded the data. LT and NM also participated in the design process and provided comment on paper drafts. NM is Principal Investigator on the IMPACT-ME study, which the data reported in this paper is derived from. All authors read, commented on, and approved the final manuscript.

Authors' information
Not Applicable.

Consent for publication
Not applicable.

Competing interests
The authors declare that they have no competing interests.

Author details
[1]Faculty of Brain and Language Sciences, University College London, London, UK. [2]Anna Freud National Centre for Children and Families (AFNCCF), London, UK. [3]The Child Attachment and Psychological Therapies Research Unit (ChAPTRe), University College London and Anna Freud National Centre for Children and Families, London, UK.

References

1. Fonagy P, Cottrell D, Phillips J, Bevington D, Glaser D, Allison E. Chapter 3: Depressive disorders. In: Fonagy P, Cottrell D, Phillips J, Bevington D, Glaser D, Allison E, editors. What works for whom? A critical review of treatments for children and adolescents (2nd ed.). New York: The Guilford Press; 2015. p. 74–119. https://doi.org/10.1111/camh.12090.
2. Seedat S. Editorial: Controversies in the use of antidepressants in children and adolescents: a decade since the storm and where do we stand now? J Child Adolesc Ment Health. 2014;26(2):iii–v. https://doi.org/10.2989/17280583.2014.938497.
3. Sharma T, Guski LS, Freund N, Gotzsche P. Suicidality and aggression during antidepressant treatment: systematic review and meta-analyses based on clinical study reports. BMJ. 2016;1-10. https://doi.org/10.1136/bmj.i65.
4. Bachmann CJ, Aagaard L, Burcu M, Glaeske G, Kalverdijk LJ, Hoffmann F, et al. Trends and patterns of antidepressant use in children and adolescents from five western countries, 2005-2012. Eur Neuropsychopharmacol. 2016;26:411–9. https://doi.org/10.1016/j.euroneuro.2016.02.001.
5. Sarginson J, Webb TR, Stocks JS, Esmail A, Garg S. Temporal trends in antidepressant prescribing to children in UK primary care, 2000-2015. J Affect Disord. 2016;210:312–8. https://doi.org/10.1016/j.jad.2016.12.047.
6. NICE. Depression in children and young people: identification and management: Clinical guideline [CG28] 2015 update . NICE Guidance. https://www.nice.org.uk/guidance/cg28. Accessed 2 Jul 2017.
7. Cousins L, Whitaker KJ, Widmer B, Midgley N, Byford S, Dubicka B, Goodyer IM, et al. Clinical characteristics associated with the prescribing of SSRI medication in adolescents with major unipolar depression. Eur Child Adolesc Psychiatry. 2016;25(12):1287–95. https://doi.org/10.1007/s00787-016-0849-y.
8. Cheung AH, Levitt AJ, Szalai JP. Impact of antidepressant side effects on adolescent quality of life. Can J Psychiatr. 2003;48(11):727–33. https://doi.org/10.1177/070674370304801104.
9. Cousins L, Goodyer I. Antidepressants and the adolescent brain. J Psychopharmacol. 2015;29(5):545–55. https://doi.org/10.1177/0269881115573542.
10. Wisdom J, Clarke G, Green C. What teens want: barriers to seeking Care for Depression. Admin Pol Ment Health. 2006;33:133. https://doi.org/10.1007/s10488-006-0036-4.
11. Floesrch J, Townsend L, Longhofer J, Munson M, Winbush V, Kranke D, Findling R, et al. Adolescent experience of psychotropic treatment. Transcult Psychiatry. 2009;46(1):157–78. https://doi.org/10.1177/1363461509102202.
12. Meredith L, Stein B, Paddock S, Jaycox L, Quinn V, Chandra A, Burnam A. Perceived barriers to treatment for adolescent depression. Med Care. 2009;47(6):677–84. https://doi.org/10.1097/MLR.0b013e318190d46b.
13. Kranke D, Floersch J, Townsend L, Munson M. Stigma experience among adolescents taking psychiatric medication. Child Serv Rev. 2010;32:496–505. https://doi.org/10.1177/1473325013510545.
14. Floersch J. The subjective experience of youth psychotropic treatment. Soc Work Ment Health. 2003;1(4):51–69. https://doi.org/10.1300/J200v01n04_04.
15. Kranke D, Floersch J, Kranke B, Munson M. A qualitative investigation of self-stigma among adolescents taking psychiatric medication. Psychiatr Serv. 2011;62(8):893–9. https://doi.org/10.1176/ps.62.8.pss6208_0893.
16. Rappaport N, Chubinsky P. The meaning of psychotropic medications for children, adolescents, and their families. J Am Acad Child Psychiatry. 2000;39(9):1198–200 0890-8567/00/3909.
17. Goodyer IM, Tsancheva S, Byford S, Dubicka B, Hill J, Kelvin R, Fonagy P, et al. Improving mood with psychoanalytic and cognitive therapies (IMPACT): a pragmatic effectiveness superiority trial to investigate whether specialised psychological treatment reduces the risk for relapse in adolescents with moderate to severe unipolar depres. Trials. 2011;12(175). https://doi.org/10.1186/1745-6215-12-175.
18. Goodyer IM, Reynolds S, Barrett B, Byford S, Dubicka B, Hill J, Fonagy P, et al. Cognitive behavioral therapy and short-term psychoanalytical psychotherapy versus a brief psychosocial intervention in adolescents with unipolar major depressive disorder (IMPACT): a multi-centre, pragmatic, observer-blind, randomised controlled superiori. Lancet Psychiatry. 2017;4:109–19. https://doi.org/10.1016/S2215-0366(16)30378-9.
19. Midgley N, Ansaldo F, Target M. The meaningful assessment of therapy outcomes: incorporating a qualitative study into a randomized controlled trial evaluating the treatment of adolescent depression. Psychotherapy. 2014;51(1):128–37. https://doi.org/10.1037/a0034179.
20. Kautman J, Blrmaher B, Brent D, Rao U, Flynn C, Moreci P, Ryan N, et al. Schedule for affective disorders and schizophrenia for school-age children-present and life version (K-SADS-PL): initial reliability and validity data. J Am Acad Child Adolesc Psychiatry. 1997;36(7):980–8. https://doi.org/10.1097/00004583-199707000-00021.
21. Braune V, Clarke V. Using thematic analysis in psychology. Qual Res Psychol. 2006;3:77–101. https://doi.org/10.1191/1478088706qp063oa.
22. Lincoln YS, Guba EG. Naturalistic Inquiry. Newbury Park: Sage Publications; 1985.
23. Johnson S, Rasulova S. Qualitative research and the evaluation of development impact: incorporating authenticity into the assessment of rigour. J Dev Effect. 2017;9(2):263–76.
24. Son SE, Kirchner JT. Depression in children and adolescents. Am Fam Physician. 2000;62(10):2297–308.
25. Carr A. Mood Disorders. In: Carr A, editor. The handbook of child and adolescent clinical psychology: a contextual approach. London: Routledge; 2015. p. 615–67. https://doi.org/10.4324/9781315744230.
26. Timlin U, Hakko H, Heino R, Kyngas H. Factors that affect adolescent adherence to mental health and psychiatric treatment: a systematic integrative reveiw of the literature. Scand J Child Adolesc Psychiatr Psychol. 2015;3(2):99–107.
27. Lachal J, Speranza M, Schmitt A, Spodenkiewicz M, Falissard B, Moro M-R, Revah-Levy A. Depression in Adolesence: from qualitative research to measurement. Adolesc Psychiatry. 2012;2:296–308. https://doi.org/10.2174/2210676611202040296.
28. Midgley N, Parkinson S, Holmes J, Stapley E, Eatough V, Target M. Beyond a diagnosis: the experience of depression among clinically-referred adolescents. J Adolesc. 2015;44:269–79. https://doi.org/10.1016/j.adolescence.2015.08.007.
29. Herick S, Simmons M, Thompson A, Parker AG. What are specialist mental health clinician attitudes to guideline recommendations for the treatment of depression in young people? Aust N Z J Psychiatry. 2011;45(11):993–1001. https://doi.org/10.3109/00048674.2011.619161.
30. Hawke LD, Provencher MD. Schema theory and Schema therapy in mood and anxiety disorders: a review. J Cogn Psychother. 2011;25(4):257–76. https://doi.org/10.1891/0889-8391.25.4.257.
31. Bogner HR, Cahill E, Frauenhoffer C, Barg FK. Older primary care patient views regarding antidepressants: a mixed-methods approach. J Mental Health. 2009;18(1):57–64. https://doi.org/10.1080/09638230701677795.
32. Gibson K, Cartwright C, Read J. In my life antidepressants have been a qualitative analysis of users' diverse experiences with antidepressants. BMC Pscyhiatry. 2016;16:135. https://doi.org/10.1186/s12888-016-0844-3.
33. Hoencamp E, Stevens A, Haffmans J. Patients' attitude toward antidepressants. Psychiatr Serv. 2002;53(9):1180–1. https://doi.org/10.1176/appi.ps.53.9.1180-a

34. Garfield S, Smith F, Francis SA. The paradoxical role of antidepressant medication- returning to normal functioning while losing the sense of being normal. J Ment Health. 2003;12(5):521–35. https://doi.org/10.1080/09638230310001603582.
35. Grime J, Pollock K. Patients' ambivalence about taking antidepressants: a qualitative study. Pharm J. 2003;271(7270):516–9.
36. Hankin B, Abramson H, Siler M. A prospective test of the hopelessness theory of depression in adolesence. Cognit Ther Res. 2001;25(5):607–32. https://doi.org/10.1023/A:1005561616506.
37. Hosenbocus S, Chahal RSSRI. SNRIs: a review of the discontinuation sydnrome in children and adolesscents. J Can Acad Child Adolesc Psychiatry. 2011;20(1):60–7.
38. Leydon GM, Rodgers L, Kendrick T. A qualitative study of patient views on discontinuing long-term selective serotonin reuptake inhibitors. Fam Prac. 2007;24(6):570–5. https://doi.org/10.1093/fampra/cmm069.
39. Verbeek-Heida PM, Mathot EF. Better safe than sorry--why patients prefer to stop using selective serotonin reuptake inhibitor (SSRI) antidepressants but are afraid to do so: results of a qualitative study. Chronic Ill. 2006;2:133–42.
40. Malpass A, Shaw A, Sharp D, Walter F, Feder G, Ridd M, Kessler D. "Medication career" or "moral career"? The two sides of managing antidepressants: a meta-ethnography of patient's experiencing antidepressants. Soc Sci Med. 2009;68(1):154–68. https://doi.org/10.1016/j.socscimed.2008.09.068.
41. Deegann P, Drake R. Shared decision making and medication Management in the Recovery Process. Psychiatr Serv. 2006;57:1636–9. https://doi.org/10.1176/ps.2006.57.11.1636.
42. Department of Health. The expert patient: a new approach to chronic disease management for the 21st century. London: The Stationary Office; 2011. Accessed 1 Jul 2017
43. Healthcare Commission. Talking about medication: the management of medicines in trusts providing mental health services. London: Commision for Healthcare, Audit, and Inspection; 2007.
44. Lawrence HR, Nangle DW, Schwartz-Mette RA, Erdley C. Medication for child and adolescent depression: questions, answers, clarifications, and caveats. Pract Innov. 2017;2(1):39–53.
45. NICE. Medicines adherence: involving patients in decisions about prescribed medicines and supporting adherences. London: NICE. 2009. Retrieved from https://www.nice.org.uk/Guidance/CG76. Accessed 1 Jul 2017.
46. NIMHE. Medicines management: everybody's business: a guide for service users, carers, and health and social care practitioners. London: Department of Health; 2008. Accessed May 29 2017
47. Gibson K, Cartwright C, Read J. Patient-centered perspectives on antidepressant use. Int J Ment Health. 2014;43(1):81–99. https://doi.org/10.2753/IMH0020-7411430105.
48. Brinkman W, Sherman S, Zmitrovich A, Visscher M, Crosby L, Phelan K, Donovan E. In their own words: adolescent views on ADHD and their evolving role managing medication. Acad Pediatr. 2012;12:53–61. https://doi.org/10.1016/j.acap.2011.10.003.

15

Hypochondriac concerns and correlates of personality styles and affective states in bipolar I and II disorders

Bing Pan[1,2], Qing Zhang[1], Huitzong Tsai[1], Bingren Zhang[2] and Wei Wang[2*]

Abstract

Background: Hypochondriac concerns are associated with the treatment-difficulty of bipolar disorder, which might be due to the personality styles and affective states.

Methods: We invited outpatients with bipolar I disorder (BD I, $n = 87$), bipolar II disorder (BD II, $n = 92$) and healthy volunteers ($n = 129$) to undergo the Illness Attitude Scales and Parker Personality Measure tests, and measurements of concurrent affective states.

Results: Compared to healthy volunteers, BD I and BD II patients scored significantly higher on mania, hypomania and depression. BD I and BD II patients also scored significantly higher on Symptom Effect and Treatment Seeking, and BD II patients scored higher on Patho-thanatophobia and Hypochondriacal Belief. BD II in addition scored higher on Patho-thanatophobia than BD I did. In controls, the Dependent style predicted Patho-thanatophobia and Symptom Effect, Schizoid with Hypochondriacal Belief; in BD I, Narcissistic (–) with Hypochondriacal Belief, Histrionic with Patho-thanatophobia and Hypochondriacal Belief, depression with Hypochondriacal Belief, and hypomania with Symptom Effect and Hypochondriacal Belief; in BD II, depression with Symptom Effect and Hypochondriacal Belief, mania with Symptom Effect.

Conclusions: Bipolar disorder, especially BD II, is associated with greater hypochondriac concerns, which relates to personality disorder functioning styles and concurrent affective states.

Keywords: Affective states, Bipolar I and II disorders, Hypochondriasis, Illness attitude scales, Personality disorder functioning styles

Introduction

Bipolar disorder has two major types, i.e., bipolar I (BD I) and II (BD II) disorders. Both are devastating and are characterized by recurrent episodes of mania/ hypomania and depression [1], with frequent relapse, lingering residual symptoms, impaired cognition, and diminished wellbeing [2]. In particular, the BD II exhibits more serious symptoms [3], more chronicity [4], and more comorbidity with physical illness, anxiety, and personality disorders than BD I [5]. The poor prognoses of BD I and BD II are related to the poor adherences to treatment, the anxious attitudes and beliefs towards health [6].

The hypochondriasis is a preoccupation of having or acquiring a serious illness, which is frequently defined as a chronic condition distinctive from affective disorders [7] or is referred as health anxiety disorder [8], illness anxiety disorder, or somatic symptom disorder [9]. Specifically, there are several aspects of hypochondriasis as measured with the Illness Attitude Scales (IAS), which is considered one of the most suitable instruments for hypochondriasis screening and to discriminate hypochondriac patients from healthy volunteers [10, 11]. Recently, Luo et al. [12] have validated the IAS structures into four factors: Patho-thanatophobia reflecting the fears of serious illness or death, Symptom Effect describing the effects of symptoms on everyday life and work, Treatment Seeking

* Correspondence: drwangwei@zju.edu.cn; wangmufan@msn.com
[2]Department of Clinical Psychology and Psychiatry/ School of Public Health, Zhejiang University College of Medicine, Zhejiang 310058, Hangzhou, China
Full list of author information is available at the end of the article

reflecting the action of disease treatment and prevention, and Hypochondriacal Beliefs representing the doubting of being healthy despite medical reassurance.

However, the exact role of the hypochondriasis played in BD I and BD II etiopathology is unknown. The implicit theories might offer some explanation for the hypochondriasis in the disorder. According to the theories, the belief is connected with cognition and behavior in psychological processes, while the maladapted belief is related to the onset and maintenance of anxiety and depression in psychiatric patients in particular [13, 14]. In clinics, some patients with major depressive disorder also met the diagnosis of hypochondriasis [15]. Compared to patients without hypochondriasis, depressed patients who are comorbid with hypochondriasis display more somatic symptoms, higher suicidal attempts, and more treatment-seeking [16–18]. Increased manic episodes during a lifetime are associated with an elevated hypochondriasis score in BD I [19]. In bipolar spectrum patients, the perception of their overall physical health can predict mania/ hypomania and depression severity levels, and life satisfaction at concurrent and future visits [20]. Meanwhile, as an ego defense, hypochondriasis was reported to often signal an imminently affective change in bipolar disorder patients, especially when the switch out of mania was started [21]. Moreover, BD II displays more depressive symptoms than BD I [3]. However, whether different affective states affect the hypochondriasis differently in BD I and BD II remains uncertain.

Again according to the implicit theories, personality trait plays an important role in regulating decision-making and behavioral reactions of an individual [13], and it might also be related to the etiopathology of hypochondriasis. For instance, one study reported that 76.5% patients with hypochondriasis had one or more personality disorders, with common disorders being obsessive-compulsive and avoidant types [22]. Another study indicated that patients with hypochondriasis presented characteristics of paranoid, borderline, avoidant, and dependent personality disorders [23]. Interestingly, bipolar disorder patients display some unique personality traits or personality disorders. For example, the neuroticism and borderline personality disorder functioning style (trait) were reportedly higher in BD II than those in BD I [23, 24], and the impulsive sensation seeking trait was lower in BD II than in BD I [25]. The borderline style predicted depression and mania in BD I and BD II, antisocial predicted hypomania in BD I, and passive-aggressive predicted hypomania in BD II [24]. Nonetheless, it is unclear whether the involvements of antisocial, borderline, histrionic, narcissistic, or other disordered personality symptoms in hypochondriasis are different in BD I and BD II.

Therefore, it is reasonable to speculate that both affective states and personality disorder functioning styles affect hypochondriasis in both BD I and BD II. In the current study, we hypothesized that: (1) the bipolar disorder patients score higher than healthy volunteers do on the psychopathological variables, and BD II patients score higher than BD I patients do on most aspects of hypochondriasis; and (2) the associations between the hypochondriac concerns and depression and mania, or the antisocial, borderline, histrionic, and narcissistic personality disorder styles are different in the two types of bipolar disorder. Thus, we used the Chinese version of IAS [12] to measure different aspects of hypochondriasis, besides applying the measurements for personality disorder functioning styles and concurrent affective states in our participants.

Methods

Participants

We enrolled 129 healthy participants (58 men; mean age, 24.55 ± 3.48 years; age range, 16 ~ 49 years), who were physically healthy and had no history of psychiatric or neurological abnormalities. We also invited 241 outpatients with bipolar disorder, but later 27 patients comorbid with personality disorder(s), and 35 with the complex somatic symptom disorder/ illness anxiety disorder, were excluded. Finally, 87 with BD I (41 men; mean age, 25.15 ± 7.95 years; range, 16 ~ 45 years) and 92 with BD II (33 men; mean age, 25.27 ± 6.83 years; range, 16 ~ 49 years) were enrolled, who were diagnosed according to the Diagnostic and Statistical Manual of Mental Disorders, Version 5 (DSM-5) [9], by two experienced psychiatrists (PB and WW). In BD I, 25 patients were in depression state, 21 in mania state, one in mixed state, and 40 in remission; In BD II, 30 were in depression state, 24 in hypomania state, and 48 in remission.

A recent computed tomography or magnetic resonance imaging scan was available to ensure that all patients were free from any organic brain lesions. All patients were also confirmed to have no other confounding factors including schizophrenia, schizoaffective disorder, or prior history of head injury, alcohol, or tobacco abuse, psychoactive substance abuse, central nervous system inflammation, or neurocognitive or other disorders influencing their decisional capacity (understanding, appreciation, reasoning, and expression of action choice) through the semistructured clinical interview. Moreover, all participants completed their 9 years of education. No significant differences were found among the three groups regarding gender ($\chi^2 = 2.71$, $p = .26$) or age (F [2, 308] = .46, $p = .64$, mean square effect (MSE) = 16.76) distributions. Participants had to be free from alcohol and other substances for at least 72 h prior to testing. The study protocol was approved by the Medical Ethics Committee of School of Public Health, Zhejiang University. All participants provided their written informed consent, and guardians signed the written informed consent for the adolescents or bipolar disorder patients.

Measures

Illness Attitude Scale (IAS)

The IAS is a scale measuring medically unexplained physical symptoms relating to hypochondriasis [10, 26]. Its Chinese version is comprised of 27 items rated on a five-point scale (0 - no, 1 - rarely, 2 - sometimes, 3 - often, 4 - most of the time) that measuring four factors of hypochondriasis. Patho-thanatophobia (internal alpha, .82), Symptom Effect (.82), Treatment Seeking (.74), And factor 4, Hypochondriacal Beliefs (.68) [12].

Parker Personality Measure (PERM)

The PERM is a self-report questionnaire helping identify types of personality disorder. It consists of 92 items each with a five-point Likert scale (1 - very unlike me, 2 - moderately unlike me, 3 - somewhat unlike and like me, 4 - moderately like me and 5 - very like me) [27]. The questionnaire assesses 11 personality disorders: paranoid (internal alpha, .70), schizoid (.35), schizotypal (.62), antisocial (.68), borderline (.78), histrionic (.55), narcissistic (.70), avoidant (.75), dependent (.72), obsessive-compulsive (.50), and passive-aggressive (.68) types [28].

Mood Disorder Questionnaire (MDQ)

The MDQ consists of three parts comprising13 forced-choice (yes or no) questions [29]. It assesses the presence of symptoms and behaviors related to mania or hypomania, one question to determine whether two or more symptoms have been experienced at the same time, and one question to determine the extent to which symptoms have caused functional impairment on a scale ranging from "no problems" to "serious problems". Its internal reliability was .79 in a Chinese sample [30].

Hypomania Checklist-32 (HCL-32)

The HCL-32 consists of 32 items [31]. Individuals were instructed to answer the forced-choice (yes or no) questions about emotions, thoughts, or behaviors, and to answer questions regarding the duration, the impact on family, social and work life, or people's reactions. Its internal reliability was .88 in a Chinese sample [32].

Plutchik - van Praag Depression Inventory (PVP)

The PVP is a self-assessment instrument including 34 items for detecting depressive symptoms [33]. Each item has three scale points (0, 1, and 2) corresponding with increasing depressive tendencies. Participants have "possible depression" if they score between 20 and 25, or "depression" if they score above 25. The internal reliability of the inventory was .94 in a Chinese sample [34].

Statistical analyses

Two-way ANOVA was applied to the mean IAS and PERM scale scores, and one-way ANOVA to the mean scores of PVP, MDQ, and HCL-32 in the three groups of participants. Later, the effect sizes (the eta squared values) of ANOVA were calculated. Whenever a significant main effect was found, post-hoc analysis by the Bonferroni test was employed to evaluate between-group differences. In addition, we applied the stepwise multiple linear regression analysis (backward method) to search for the relationships between the IAS, PERM, PVP, MDQ, and HCL-32 scales, taking PERM styles and affective states as potential predictors for IAS factors. A p-value < .05 (in ANOVA) or .01 (in prediction, to prevent false positives) was considered significant.

Results

Group differences of illness attitudes (hypothesis 1) and personality styles

The mean IAS scores were significantly different among the three groups (F [2, 304] = 13.84, $p < .001$, MSE = 730.75, $\eta^2 = .08$). Post-hoc analyses showed that BD I scored significantly higher than controls did on Symptom Effect and Treatment Seeking; BD II scored significantly higher than controls did on Patho-thanatophobia, Symptom Effect, Treatment Seeking and Hypochondriacal Belief. In addition, BD II scored significantly higher than BD I did on Patho-thanatophobia (Table 1). The mean PERM scale scores were significantly different among the three groups (F [2, 305] 1 = 44.98, $p < .001$, MSE = 8039.75, $\eta^2 = .23$). Post-hoc analyses showed that BD I and BD II scored significantly higher than the controls did on most scales. BD II also scored significantly higher than controls did on Schizoid. BD II scored significantly higher on Borderline, Schizotypal and Dependent scales than BD I did (Table 2).

Group differences of affective states

The mean PVP scores were significantly different among the three groups (F [2, 306] = 31.70, $p < .001$, MSE = 3993.90, $\eta^2 = .08$). The scores in BD II were higher than those in BD I and the controls, and BD I scored higher than that in controls. Mean MDQ scores were significantly different among the three groups (F [2, 306] = 127.19, $p < .001$, MSE = 948.61, $\eta^2 = .46$); with that in BD I higher than those in BD II and the controls, and BD II scored higher than controls did. The mean HCL-32 scores were also significantly different among the three groups (F [2, 306] = 62.05, $p < .001$, MSE = 1756.77, $\eta^2 = .29$), with those in BD I and BD II higher than that in controls (also see Table 2).

Table 1 Scores (mean ± S.D.) of the Illness Attitude Scales in healthy volunteers (controls, $n = 129$), and patients with bipolar I (BD I, $n = 87$) and II (BD II, $n = 92$) disorders

	Controls	BD I	95% Confidence Interval	BD II	95% Confidence Interval
Patho-thanatophobia	13.95 ± 8.05	12.19 ± 6.99	−3.39~1.83 vs. controls	16.86 ± 9.58a,b	1.43~6.55 vs. controls 1.96 ~ 7.58 vs. BD I
Symptom Effect	5.25 ± 3.15	7.62 ± 4.10a	1.12 ~ 3.61 vs. controls	8.36 ± 4.05a	1.91 ~ 4.35 vs. controls
Treatment Seeking	11.62 ± 3.45	13.31 ± 4.90a	.30 ~ 3.08 vs. controls	13.35 ± 4.22a	.38 ~ 3.10 vs. controls
Hypochondriacal Belief	7.23 ± 2.88	8.05 ± 3.66	−.36~1.98 vs. controls	8.74 ± 4.15a	.42 ~ 2.72 vs. controls

Note: a, $p < .05$ vs. controls; b, $p < .05$ vs. BD I

Associations between illness attitudes, personality and affective states (hypothesis 2)

When considering the prediction of IAS scales by the PERM styles and affective states, the results showed that the accounted variances (adjusted R^2s) ranged from .05 to .20 in controls, .07 to .25 in BD I, and .26 in BD II. In controls, the Dependent style predicted Patho-thanatophobia and Symptom Effect, and Schizoid predicted Hypochondriacal Belief. In BD I, Histrionic predicted Patho-thanatophobia, HCL-32 predicted Symptom Effect, Narcissistic, Histrionic, HCL-32 and PVP together predicted Hypochondriacal Belief. In BD II, PVP and MDQ together predicted Symptom Effect, and PVP predicted Hypochondriacal Belief (Table 3).

Discussion

The current study was designed to look for the differences of hypochondriasis and their associations with affective states and personality variables in two types of bipolar disorder, and our results might help to explain the treatment-difficulty of the disorder. Compared to healthy controls, BD I and BD II scored significantly higher on MDQ, HCL-32, and PVP scales, on almost all PERM styles, and on IAS Symptom Effect and Treatment Seeking; and their score differences on PVP and IAS were relatively weak as indicated by the effect sizes (η^2: .08). Specifically, BD II scored higher on Patho-thanatophobia and Hypochondriacal Belief than healthy controls, and also scored higher on Patho-thanatophobia

Table 2 Scales scores (mean ± S.D.) of personality and affective states in healthy volunteers (controls, $n = 129$), and patients with bipolar I (BD I, $n = 86$) and II (BD II, $n = 92$) disorders

	Controls	BD I	95% Confidence Interval	BD II	95% Confidence Interval
Parker Personality Measure					
Paranoid	19.07 ± 6.65	24.51 ± 5.70a	3.11~7.76 vs. controls	26.27 ± 8.27a	4.86~9.43 vs. controls
Schizoid	18.67 ± 3.78	19.68 ± 4.00	−.27~2.28 vs. controls	21.15 ± 3.76a	1.12 ~ 3.64 vs. controls
Schizotypal	8.49 ± 3.13	10.07 ± 3.13a	1.02~3.41 vs. controls	12.36 ± 4.3a,b	2.69~5.03 vs. controls .36 ~ 2.93 vs. BD I
Antisocial	17.40 ± 5.62	21.05 ± 4.99a	1.78~5.52 vs. controls	22.92 ± 6.17a	3.44~7.12 vs. controls
Borderline	18.09 ± 5.68	23.09 ± 6.60a	2.67~7.33 vs. controls	26.56 ± 8.65a,b	6.26~10.84 vs. controls 1.04 ~ 6.06 vs. BD I
Histrionic	11.47 ± 3.62	14.44 ± 3.31a	1.71~4.23 vs. controls	15.31 ± 4.40a	2.52~5.00 vs. controls
Narcissistic	14.55 ± 5.00	18.44 ± 5.11a	2.11~5.66 vs. controls	19.91 ± 5.93a	3.42~6.91 vs. controls
Avoidant	23.40 ± 7.13	27.56 ± 6.36a	1.75~6.57 vs. controls	29.41 ± 8.04a	3.74~8.48 vs. controls
Dependent	20.38 ± 5.97	24.06 ± 5.07a	1.60~5.75 vs. controls	26.34 ± 7.45a,b	4.00~8.08 vs. controls .13 ~ 4.60 vs. BD I
Obsessive-compulsive	16.34 ± 4.22	18.39 ± 3.89a	.62~3.48 vs. controls	18.00 ± 4.70a	.34~3.15 vs. controls
Passive-aggressive	18.64 ± 5.36	22.10 ± 4.95a	1.62~5.31 vs. controls	23.97 ± 6.24a	3.35~6.98 vs. controls
Plutchik-van Praag	14.84 ± 12.30	14.94 ± 11.76a	1.44 ~ 8.99 vs. controls	21.92 ± 13.58 a,b	8.51 ~ 15.88 vs. controls
Depression Inventory					2.92 ~ 11.05 vs. BD I
Mood Disorder	2.30 ± 2.56	8.33 ± 3.08a	5.11 ~ 6.94 vs. controls	5.34 ± 2.60a,b	2.14 ~ 3.93 vs. controls
Questionnaire					-3.97~-2.01 vs. BD I
Hypomanic Checklist-32	11.62 ± 5.04	19.16 ± 6.32a	5.76 ~ 9.33 vs. controls	17.66 ± 4.67a	4.29 ~ 7.79 vs. controls

Note: a, $p < .05$ vs. controls; b, $p < .05$ vs. BD I

Table 3 The stepwise multiple linear regression analysis for the relationships between the IAS, PERM, PVP, MDQ, and HCL-32 scales in healthy volunteers (controls, $n = 129$), and patients with bipolar I (BD I, $n = 87$) and II (BD II, $n = 92$) disorders

	a-R^2	Controls beta (B, SE), predictor	a-R^2	BD I beta (B, SE), predictor	a-R^2	BD II beta (B, SE), predictor
Patho-thanatophobia	.20	.45 (.52,.09), Dependent	.07	.28 (.59,.22), Histrionic		
Symptom effect	.06	.26 (.13,.54), Dependent	.09	.30 (.19,.06), HCL-32	.26	.42 (.12,.02), PVP .26 (.41,.14), MDQ
Hypochondriacal Belief	.05	.24 (.18,.06), Schizoid	.25	−.42 (−.29,.08), Narcissistic .34 (.37,.13), Histrionic .30 (.17,.05), HCL-32 .26 (.07,.02), PVP	.26	.29 (.09,.30), PVP

Note: all predictors are significant ones at $p < .01$; a-R^2, adjusted R^2; B, beta; SE, Standardized error

than BD I. The results confirm previous reports that hypochondriac features are prominent in bipolar disorders [20], and confirmed our first hypothesis. Regarding associations with IAS scales, affective states were involved in both BD I and BD II, but some disordered personality symptoms or traits were in addition involved in BD I, which confirmed our second hypothesis. Our results therefore demonstrate that the belief regarding health is associated with personality symptoms, and that it mutually influenced the affective states, which supported the view that the implicit theories play a role in the etiopathology of bipolar disorder.

The higher scores of MDQ, HCL-32 and PVP in BD I and BD II were consistent with previous studies [24, 25]. Moreover, both BD I and BD II exhibited more comorbid personality disorders as they scored higher on most PERM scales, consistent with the previous reports [24, 35, 36]. BD II also scored higher on Borderline, Schizotypal and Dependent scales than BD I did in our study. Considering that patients with these personality disorders display more distressed emotions [23], our results are consistent with the description that BD II is associated with a high level of neuroticism [37] and explain its treatment difficulty due to the involvement of the pathological personality styles.

Previous results show that in manic or hypomanic states, hypochondriasis can be a manifestation of delusions or distorted beliefs in bipolar disorder [19]. The documentation in general explains the higher IAS scale scores in our BD I and BD II. The higher IAS scale scores in BD I and BD II were also consistent with a previous report that both patients with hypochondriasis and bipolar disorder showed cognitive dysfunctions [38]. For example, in bipolar disorder patients, individuals' defenses tend to indicate an increase in hypochondriasis when manic episodes begin to abate [21], while in depressive patients, individuals reported difficulties in describing feelings that specifically predict the degree of health anxiety and illness-related behaviors [39]. All these help to explain the higher score of IAS in bipolar disorder.

Patho-thanatophobia is the core characteristic of hypochondriasis, which covers the fears of death and dying [40] and is closely associated with anxiety [41]. BD II patients exhibit more lifetime phobia and other anxiety disorders [4, 42], which might account for the higher Patho-thanatophobia in BD II than that in BD I. Moreover, BD II scored higher on Dependent, Schizotypal and Borderline styles than BD I did, which supports the higher suspiciousness [43] and anxiety [8, 23] in BD II, and helps to explain the higher Patho-thanatophobia and Hypochondriacal Belief in BD II. Therefore, both our study and the literature show that the influences between illness attitudes and the affective states in bipolar disorder are reciprocal, which fits into the implicit theories.

In controls, the Dependent style predicted Patho-thanatophobia and Symptom Effect, which is consistent with the prevalence of dependent personality disorder in hypochondriac patients [23]. Other studies have shown that patients with dependent personality disorder are anxious [44], report more clinical symptoms, and rely more on doctors or medication in life or in the hospital [45], and thus are more apt to seek treatment, and use health services than patients without personality disorders [46]. There are also some related studies supporting that the Schizoid style predicts Hypochondriac Belief. Both schizoid and avoidant factors resided in the schizophrenia spectrum disorders [47], which have overlapping clinical features with each other [9], and avoidant personality disorder is often found in hypochondriasis [22, 23]. These observations indirectly point to the association between Schizoid and Hypochondriacal Belief.

In BD I, Narcissistic was negatively associated with Hypochondriacal Belief which was consistent with the clinical manifestations of narcissistic personality disorder. For instance, narcissistic patients are characterized by attention seeking or self-esteem demanding, in order to reduce their psychosocial distress, and then to reduce clinical hypochondriasis [23, 48, 49]. The mania helps these patients to elevate the self-esteem, thus present less distress and less hypochondriasis. On the other hand, the association between Histrionic and Patho-thanatophobia and Hypochondriacal Belief was consistent with the clinical features of histrionic personality patients, for instance the high rate of somatic disorders, conversion disorder, major depressive disorder [9], and increased anxiety disorder comorbidity [50], all of which are closely related to hypochondriasis. Previous results also pointed to the greater hypochondriac concerns in histrionic personality disorder [51]. Our results suggest that the pathological personality styles, such as Narcissistic and Histrionic which held different cognitions or beliefs, display different associations with the health-related anxiety or hypochondriasis in BD I.

In BD II, affective states have great effect on hypochondriasis. Regarding the association between PVP and Symptom Effect and Hypochondriacal Belief, previous studies showed that depression in BD II is more severe than that in BD I, especially somatic symptoms [5], which were linked to Symptom Effect, with BD II associated with increased retardation, guilt delusions, and suicidal ideations [3] which are linked with increased hypochondriacal belief. Generally, bipolar disorder patients mobilize their ego defense through mania to decrease their health-related symptoms, but they are still symptomatic and hypochondriac [21]. This paradox might be responsible for the association between MDQ and Symptom Effect found in our BD II.

There are four limitations of the present study. Firstly, our participants were between 17 and 49 years of age and so the current results might not be generalizable for elderly individuals, since hypochondriasis is ubiquitous in this population [52]. Secondly, our study lacked other disease controls such as unipolar depression, schizophrenia, personality disorder, or health-related anxiety disorder. Thirdly, we used self-report questionnaires, which might result in measurement profile-floating. Fourthly, our study was a cross-sectional design, which lacks a longitudinal perspective and precludes a conclusion about the causal-effective nature between these measures in a given group. Further comparisons with more clinical controls or conducting a cohort design would clear up our current associations.

Conclusions

Our study indicates the presence of more hypochondriac symptoms in bipolar disorder, especially BD II, and that the increased hypochondriasis has contributions from disordered personality symptoms. Specifically, mania in BD I and depression in BD II are predictive of some hypochondriac aspects, and personality symptoms contribute to the association between mood and hypochondriasis in BD I and more so in healthy controls. Our results thus offer more explanations for the treatment-recalcitrant features of bipolar disorder, especially of BD II.

Abbreviations

BD I: Bipolar I disorder; BD II: Bipolar II disorder; CT: Computed tomography; MRI: Magnetic resonance imaging; IAS: The Illness Attitude Scale; PERM: The Parker Personality Measure; MDQ: The Mood Disorder Questionnaire; HCL-32: The Hypomania Checklist-32; PVP: The Plutchik - van praag Depression Inventory

Acknowledgments

The authors thank other members of the Department of Psychiatry in the Second Affiliated Hospital for their support in the date collection.

Funding

Dr. *B. pan* was sponsored by a grant from the Zhejiang Provincial Health Science and Technology Project (2016KYA101), and Dr. W. Wang was sponsored by grants from the Natural Science Foundation of China (Nos. 81571336 and 81771475).

Authors' contribution

Study concept and design: WW. Acquisition of data: BP, QZ, HT. Analysis and interpretation of data: BP, BZ, and WW. Draft written of the manuscript: BP and WW. The authors have read the manuscript and approved for its publication.

Consent for publication

Not applicable.

Competing interests

The authors declare that they have no competing interests. Author Wei Wang is currently acting as a Section Editor for BMC Psychiatry.

Author details

[1]Department of Psychiatry, Second Affiliated Hospital, Zhejiang University College of Medicine, Hangzhou, China. [2]Department of Clinical Psychology and Psychiatry/ School of Public Health, Zhejiang University College of Medicine, Zhejiang 310058, Hangzhou, China.

References

1. Martinowich K, Schloesser RJ, Manji HK. Bipolar disorder: from genes to behavior pathways. J Clin Invest. 2009;119(4):726–36.
2. Belmaker RH. Bipolar disorder. N Engl J Med. 2004;351(5):476–86.
3. Baek JH, Park DY, Choi J, Kim JS, Choi JS, Ha K, Kwon JS, Lee D, Hong KS. Differences between bipolar I and bipolar II disorders in clinical features, comorbidity, and family history. J Affect Disord. 2011;131:59–67.
4. Judd LL, Akiskal HS, Schettler PJ, Coryell W, Maser J, Rice JA, Solomon DA, Keller MB. The comparative clinical phenotype and long term longitudinal episode course of bipolar I and II: a clinical spectrum or distinct disorders? J Affect Disord. 2003;73:19–32.
5. Mantere O, Melartin TK, Suominen K, Rytsälä HJ, Valtonen HM, Arvilommi P, Leppämäki S, Isometsä ET. Differences in Axis I and II comorbidity between bipolar I and II disorders and major depressive disorder. J Clin Psychiatry. 2006;67:584–93.
6. García S, Martínez-Cengotitabengoa M, López-Zurbano S, Zorrilla I, López P, Vieta E, González-Pinto A. Adherence to antipsychotic medication in bipolar disorder and schizophrenic patients: a systematic review. J Clin Psychopharmacol. 2016;36(4):355–71.
7. Simon GE, Gureje O, Fullerton C. Course of hypochondriasis in an international primary care study. Gen Hosp Psychiatry. 2001;23:51–5.
8. Abramowitz JS, Olatunji BO, Deacon BJ. Health anxiety, hypochondriasis, and the anxiety disorders. Behav Ther. 2007;38:86–94.

9. American Psychiatric Association. Diagnostic and statistical manual of mental disorders. 5th ed. Washington, DC: American Psychiatric Association; 2013.
10. Speckens AE, Van Hemert AM, Spinhoven P, Bolk JH. The diagnostic and prognostic significance of the whitely index, the illness attitude scales and the somatosensory amplification scale. Psychol Med. 1996;26:1085–90.
11. Sirri L, Grandi S. Illness behavior. Adv Psychosom Med. 2012;32:160–81.
12. Luo D, Zhang Y, Yu E, Tan Y, Tong Z, Zhou Y, Chen W, Chai H, Wang W. The development and validation of a Chinese version of the illness attitude scales: an investigation of university students. Int J Behav Med. 2014;21:638–45.
13. Dweck CS, Chiu C, Hong Y. Implicit theories and their role in judgments and reactions: a world from two perspectives. Psychol Inq. 1995;6:267–85.
14. Schroder HS, Dawood S, Yalch MM, Donnellan MB, Moser JS. The role of implicit theories in mental health symptoms, emotion regulation, and hypothetical treatment choices in college students. Cogn Ther Res. 2015;39: 120–39.
15. Rush AJ, Zimmerman M, Wisniewski SR, Fava M, Hollon SD, Warden D, Biggs MM, Shores-Wilson K, Shelton RC, Luther JF, Thomas B, Trivedi MH. Comorbid psychiatric disorders in depressed outpatients: demographic and clinical features. J Affect Disord. 2005;87:43–55.
16. Srivastava AS, Kumar R. Suicidal ideation and attempts in patients with major depression: sociodemographic and clinical variables. Indian J Psychiatry. 2005;47:225–8.
17. Neng JM, Weck F. Attribution of somatic symptoms in hypochondriasis. Clin Psychol Psychother. 2015;22:116–24.
18. Weck F, Nagel LC, Richtberg S, Neng JM. Personality disorders in hypochondriasis: a comparison to panic disorder and healthy controls. J Personal Disord. 2017;31(4):567–76.
19. Zaninotto L, Souery D, Calati R, Camardese G, Janiri L, Montgomery S, Kasper S, Zohar J, De Ronchi D, Mendlewicz J, Serretti A. Dimensions of delusions in major depression: socio-demographic and clinical correlates in an unipolar-bipolar sample. Clin Psychopharmacol Neurosci. 2015;13:48–52.
20. Bernstein EE, Rabideau DJ, Gigler ME, Nierenberg AA, Deckersbach T, Sylvia LG. Patient perceptions of physical health and bipolar symptoms: the intersection of mental and physical health. J Affect Disord. 2016;189:203–6.
21. Ablon SL, Carlson GA, Goodwin FK. Ego defense patterns in manic-depressive illness. Am J Psychiatry. 1974;131:803–7.
22. Sakai R, Nestoriuc Y, Nolido NV, Barsky AJ. The prevalence of personality disorders in hypochondriasis. J Clin Psychiatry. 2010;71:41–7.
23. Saulsman LM, Page AC. The five-factor model and personality disorder empirical literature: a meta analytic review. Clin Psychol Rev. 2004;23:1055–108.
24. Yao J, Xu Y, Qin Y, Liu J, Shen Y, Wang W, Chen W. Relationship between personality disorder functioning styles and the affective states in bipolar I and II disorders. PLoS One. 2015;10:e0117353.
25. Xu S, Gao Q, Ma L, Fan H, Mao H, Liu J, Wang W. The Zuckerman-Kuhlman personality questionnaire in bipolar I and II disorders: a preliminary report. Psychiatry Res. 2015;226:357–60.
26. Kellner R, Abbott P, Winslow WW, Pathak D. Fears, beliefs, and attitudes in DSM-III hypochondriasis. J Nerv Ment Dis. 1987;175:20–5.
27. Parker G, Hadzi-Pavlovic D. A question of style: refining the dimensions of personality disorders style. J Personal Disord. 2001;15:300–18.
28. Wang W, Hu L, Mu L, Chen D, Song Q, Zhou M, Zhang W, Hou J, Li Z, Wang J, Liu J, He C. Functioning styles of personality disorders and five-factor normal personality traits: a correlation study in Chinese students. BMC Psychiatry. 2003;3:11.
29. Hirschfeld RM, Williams JB, Spitzer RL, Calabrese JR, Flynn L, Keck PE Jr, Lewis L, McElroy SL, Post RM, Rapport DJ, Russell JM, Sachs GS, Zajecka J. Development and validation of a screening instrument for bipolar spectrum disorder: the mood disorder questionnaire. Am J Psychiatry. 2000;157:1873–5.
30. Yang HC, Yuan CM, Liu TB, Li LJ, Peng HJ, Rong H, Liao CP, Shen QJ, Fang YR. Validity of the Chinese version mood disorder questionnaire (MDQ) and the optimal cutoff screening bipolar disorders. Psychiatry Res. 2011;189:446–50.
31. Angst J, Adolfsson R, Benazzi F, Gamma A, Hantouche E, Meyer TD, Skeppar P, Vieta E, Scott J. The HCL-32: towards a self-assessment tool for hypomanic symptoms in outpatients. J Affect Disord. 2005;88(2):217–33.
32. Yang HC, Yuan CM, Liu TB, Li LJ, Peng HJ, Liao C, Rong H, Fang Y, Angst J. Validity of the 32-item hypomania checklist (HCL-32) in a clinical sample with mood disorders in China. BMC Psychiatry. 2011;11:84.
33. Plutchik R, van Praag HM. Interconvertability of five self-report measures of depression. Psychiatry Res. 1987;22:243–56.
34. Wang W, Cao M, Zhu S, Gu J, Liu J, Wang Y. Zuckerman-Kuhlman's personality questionnaire in patients with major depression. Soc Behav Pers. 2002;30:757–64.
35. Paris J, Gunderson J, Weinberg I. The interface between borderline personality disorder and bipolar spectrum disorders. Compr Psychiatry. 2007;48:145–54.
36. Zimmerman M, Morgan TA. The relationship between borderline personality disorder and bipolar disorder. Dialogues Clin Neurosci. 2013;15:155–69.
37. Kim B, Lim JH, Kim SY, Joo YH. Comparative study of personality traits in patients with bipolar I and II disorder from the five-factor model perspective. Psychiatry Investig. 2012;9:347–53.
38. Gomes BC, Rocca CC, Belizario GO, Lafer B. Cognitive-behavioral rehabilitation vs. treatment as usual for bipolar patients: study protocol for a randomized controlled trial. Trials. 2017;18:142.
39. Bailer J, Witthöft M, Erkic M, Mier D. Emotion dysregulation in hypochondriasis and depression. Clin Psychol Psychother. 2017;24(6):1254–62.
40. Sinoff G. Thanatophobia (death anxiety) in the elderly: the problem of the Child's inability to assess their own Parent's death anxiety state. Front Med (Lausanne). 2017;4:11.
41. Scarella TM, Laferton JA, Ahern DK, Fallon BA, Barsky A. The relationship of hypochondriasis to anxiety, depressive, and somatoform disorders. Psychosomatics. 2016;57:200–7.
42. Dell'Osso B, Holtzman JN, Goffin KC, Portillo N, Hooshmand F, Miller S, Dore J, Wang PW, Hill SJ, Ketter TA. American tertiary clinic-referred bipolar II disorder compared to bipolar I disorder: more severe in multiple ways, but less severe in a few other ways. J Affect Disord. 2015;188:257–62.
43. Fallon BA, Harper KM, Landa A, Pavlicova M, Schneier FR, Carson A, Harding K, Keegan K, Schwartz T, Liebowitz MR. Personality disorders in hypochondriasis: prevalence and comparison with two anxiety disorders. Psychosomatics. 2012;53:566–74.
44. Mroczkowski MM, Goes FS, Riddle MA, Grados MA, Bienvenu OJ, Greenberg BD, Fyer AJ, McCracken JT, Rauch SL, Murphy DL, Knowles JA, Piacentini J, Cullen B, Rasmussen SA, Pauls DL, Nestadt G, Samuels J. Dependent personality, separation anxiety disorder and other anxiety disorders in OCD. Personal Ment Health. 2016;10(1):22–8.
45. Bender DS. The therapeutic alliance in the treatment of personality disorders. J Psychiatr Pract. 2005;11(2):73–87.
46. Tyrer H, Tyrer P, Barrett B. Influence of dependent personality status on the outcome and health service costs of health anxiety. Int J Soc Psychiatry. 2013;59:274–80.
47. Bolinskey PK, Smith EA, Schuder KM, Cooper-Bolinskey D, Myers KR, Hudak DV, James AV, Hunter HK, Novi JH, Guidi JP, Gonzalez Y, McTiernan EF, Arnold KM, Iati CA, Gottesman II. Schizophrenia spectrum personality disorders in psychometrically identified schizotypes at two-year follow-up. Psychiatry Res. 2017;252:289–95.
48. Albarracin D. Narcissism and object relations in hypochondria. Psychoanal Rev. 2015;102(4):483–502.
49. Kacel EL, Ennis N, Pereira DB. Narcissistic personality disorder in clinical health psychology practice: case studies of comorbid psychological distress and life-limiting illness. Behav Med. 2017;43(3):156–64.
50. Grant BF, Hasin DS, Stinson FS, Dawson DA, Patricia Chou S, June Ruan W, Huang B. Co-occurrence of 12-month mood and anxiety disorders and personality disorders in the US: results from the national epidemiologic survey on alcohol and related conditions. J Psychiatr Res. 2005;39(1):1–9.
51. Demopulos C, Fava M, McLean NE, Alpert JE, Nierenberg AA, Rosenbaum JF. Hypochondriacal concerns in depressed outpatients. Psychosom Med. 1996; 58:314–20.
52. Thomas P, Hazif-Thomas C, Pareaud M. Hypochondriasis and somatisation in elderly. Rev Prat. 2008;58:1977–81.

16

Perception of inpatients following remission of a manic episode in bipolar I disorder on a group-based Psychoeducation program

Runsen Chen[1,2†], Yingjun Xi[1†], Xue Wang[1], Yaqiong Li[1], Yuyang He[1] and Jiong Luo[1*]

Abstract

Background: This forms the first study of a group-based psychoeducation program for inpatients following remission of a manic episode in patients suffering from bipolar I disorder in a Chinese population. The aim was to explore the patient's perspectives of the program and their suggestions regarding ways to improve the intervention in the future.

Methods: Semi-structured and in-depth interviews were conducted with 15 participants who had participated in 8 sessions of a group psychoeducation program over 2 weeks. The verbatim transcripts of those interviews were analysed using thematic analysis.

Results: Five themes emerged from the data, including the patients' perception of participating in the program, their perception of the setting, perception of participating in a group program, perception of the learning content and of the outcome of participating in the program.

Conclusions: The results presented here describe how the short-term group psychoeducation program was experienced by the patients. Recommendations are also offered to improve the setting, content, and delivery. Our findings provide evidence that the program is beneficial for manic patients with bipolar I disorder, and this intervention warrants further research especially in a Chinese population. If these benefits are confirmed in future studies, this program could be incorporated into routine psychiatric inpatient care in China.

Keywords: Bipolar disorder, Psychiatric inpatients, Group-psychoeducation, Qualitative, Cultural adaptations

Background

Bipolar disorder type I (BD-I) is the sixth leading cause of disability globally [1]. Manic episodes are a common feature of BD-I and the lifetime prevalence is about 1.5% in European countries [2]. The lifetime prevalence of BD-I in China is about 0.09% in the year of 2017 [3]. Acute manic episodes usually require emergency admission to a psychiatric hospital to facilitate rapid recovery [4]. A range of quantitative researches indicate that group-based psychoeducation interventions guide patients to greater awareness of relapse features [5], reduce time spent in bipolar episodes [6], raise treatment adherence levels and improve quality of life [7]. Poole, Smith and Simpson [8] conducted a qualitative study on the perspectives of bipolar outpatients' enrolled in a group-based psychoeducation program in the UK, and they found that psychoeducation had a positive impact on patients' medication adherence, social support, knowledge and acceptance of BD and access to the services. However, there are few psychoeducational studies have been conducted in psychiatric inpatient settings, inpatients are more severely impaired than outpatients [9] and most

* Correspondence: luojiong2004@163.com
†Equal contributors
[1]The National Clinical Research Center for Mental Disorders & Beijing key Laboratory of Mental Disorders, Beijing Anding Hospital, Capital Medical University, No. 5 Ankang Lane, Dewai Avenue, Xicheng District, Beijing 100088, China

patients suffering from manic episodes require hospital admission. It is unclear whether psychoeducational programs may benefit psychiatric routine care in severely manic patients in the literature. Dropout rates are very high in the outpatient settings, perhaps due to the long duration of psychoeducation programs [10], hence the present study adjusted the length of treatment to examine whether a short duration psychoeducational program could reduce drop-out rates whilst resulting in similar benefits.

Furthermore, research indicates a need to examine psychoeducation for BD as a tool to engage people from diverse ethnic backgrounds [8]. Chinese populations hold particularly stigmatized attitudes towards mental illness because of Confucian beliefs [11, 12]. The diagnosis and treatment of mental disorder leads to marginalization due to perceived humiliation within the community [13]. Thus, many discharged patients no longer feel the need to see a doctor regularly and go off medication use as a consequence. Psychoeducation may be an important way to address the stigma and other barriers to mental health treatment amongst those inpatients [14]. There is also evidence from a systematic review suggesting that mental health interventions targeted to a specific cultural group are four times more effective than interventions that do not target such cultural differences. The same is true for interventions conducted in the patients' native language (if other than English), being twice as effective than those using English [15]. It is unclear whether culturally adapted group-based psychoeducational programs are acceptable and feasible for Chinese patients.

As the present study is the first to conduct a group-based psychoeducation program for BD-I inpatients in China, a qualitative evaluation is the most appropriate way to understand unique cultural elements of engaging with the intervention [16]. Therefore, we aimed to explore the experiences of Chinese patients with bipolar disorder of being in a culturally adapted short group-based psychoeducation program and their perceptions of elements such as content, teaching, delivery methods, impact and suggestions for improvement of the program in China.

Method

Group-based intervention

The program was delivered by the Beijing Anding Hospital affiliated Capital Medical University research team. All BD-I patients admitted to the inpatient unit and who received standard hospitalized treatment between September 2015 and April 2016 were approached for participation. Participants were referred to the program when their clinical symptoms were alleviated [as defined by a Young Mania Rating Scale (YMRS) score of less than 8] and during their discharge period. The program delivered eight sessions of 40–60 min duration in two weeks. Three psychiatrists and two clinical psychologists directed these sessions and the facilitators were trained by an academic expert in psychoeducation. The psychoeducation handbook was culturally adapted from Colom and Vieta [17], and the group sessions included the following topics: Session 1: introduction of BD disease knowledge, such as biological etiology, epidemiology and concepts; Session 2: definition of mania and hypomania, depression mixed state and psychotic symptoms; Session 3: biological rhythm and manic/depressive episode; Session 4: the role of pharmacological treatment and different types of medication; Session 5: medication adherence and monitoring, electroconvulsive therapy and psychotherapy; Session 6: stress management, problem coping strategies and interpersonal relationships; Session 7: recurrent signal, early detection of episodes and how to seek help; Session 8: review and assessment, how to establish a management plan and how to monitor daily mood. *The psychoeducation materials in Chinese are available for request by email from the corresponding author.*

Sample

Purposive sampling was used to select 13 participants who successfully completed the program and 2 participants who did not complete the program. Participants who had been discharged from the hospital were invited to take part in this interview process through a letter/email, which was sent along with the informed consent form. If the participants were willing to take part in the study, they had two weeks to contact the author by telephone and arrange a suitable time for the interview in the hospital. Resident participants were recruited from the inpatients ward directly after they completed the program. Data saturation was achieved at the 12nd participant. Three more interviews were conducted to examine the saturation [18], giving a total sample of 15 participants (Table 1). Each individual interview lasted 40 to 60 min and was conducted by the authors. All interviews were audio-recorded.

Table 1 Socio-demographic characteristics of participants

Patients characteristics $N = 15$	
Gender	
Male	4
Female	11
Age	
Range	18–51
Mean	34
Education	
Middle school	3
High school	4
College and above	8
Times of Episode	
Mean	3.7

Data collection

This study aimed to understand underlying themes in patients' perspectives of the group-based psychoeducation program and any impact of the intervention. Hence, researchers used semi-structured interviews to obtain the data and used thematic analysis as this was the most appropriate method for qualitative analysis [19]. All interviews were conducted at the affective disorder inpatient unit. The interview questions were developed through literature review and discussion with qualitative experts. The expert panels include two experts in qualitative research and psychoeducation. The interview questions were revised after their review. Also, in order to compare the perception of Chinese patients with those of European patients, some of the questions were adapted from Poole, Smith and Simpson [8]. Some sample questions discussed in the interviews were as follows: How did you feel while participating in this program (initial question)? Would you recommend the program to others? How do you feel about the learning environment? How do you feel about the facilitators? What do you think of the learning content? How can this content be improved further? What is your experience of the group? What has been the benefit (s) of participating in the program?

Analysis

The transcripts were analyzed according to the thematic analysis method described by Braun and Clarke [19]. There are six phases of thematic analysis:

- familiarizing with data;
- generating the initial codes;
- searching themes from text;
- reviewing themes;
- defining and naming the themes;
- producing the report.

To ensure that conformability was established, two independent authors separately reviewed the coding and themes, one author with a background in clinical psychology, and a second author with a background in psychiatry [19]. Related words or sentences representing an underlying idea were identified and coded into a category for the analysis of emerging sub-themes [20]. Also, these two authors held several meetings to compare their notes on themes and sub-themes in order to achieve consensus upon an accurate interpretation of the data. The credibility of the data was established through a check by another staff member.

Ethics

This study was approved by the Human Research and Ethics Committee of Beijing Anding Hospital, Capital Medical University. Informed consent, including permission to record the interviews, was obtained from the participants. The participants were also informed that they could withdraw from the study at any time without reason or penalty.

Results

Five themes emerged from the thematic analysis: (1) perception of participating in the program; (2) perception of the setting; (3) perception of being in a group; (4) perception of learning content; and (5) perception of the outcome of participating in program.

Theme 1: Perception of participating in the program

Sub-theme 1: Engagement

For those participants who were willing to complete the program, the most common reason for doing so was their wish to understand more about their illness.

> "I have a better understanding of the illness, why not? It's cost-free" (Participant 10).

Sub-theme 2: Recommending the program to others

All participants would recommend the program to others. They commented that people would experience a range of benefits if they participated in this program.

> "I feel so lucky that I was selected to attend this program, I would definitely recommend the program to others I know suffering from a bipolar disorder." (Participant 6)

Sub-theme 3: Suggestions for the program

Some participants suggested that the research team should have made a comprehensive booklet for patients who wanted to learn further in their free time.

> "Can you print the handout for me before I am discharged from the hospital? I need it. I can review it when I am at home." (Participant 6)

Furthermore, participants expressed interest in any follow-up studies, where they hoped to learn suggestions for dealing with their illness.

> "I would like to have access to more up-to-date information about my illness and treatments from the doctor." (Participant 11)

Theme 2: Perceptions of the setting

Sub-theme 1: Learning environment

Most participants reported that the classroom was relaxed, and that the light background music created a pleasant environment.

"This ambiance with light music enhanced my mood and allowed me to focus on the class." (Participant 7)

"A big table can fit all of the people (group members) and I felt it's a teamwork and our heart tights junctions." (Participant 10)

Some participants suggested ways in which the setting could be improved, such as the need to create a quieter environment to avoid potential distractions and the need to improve lighting conditions to improve the readability of the powerpoint slides.

"um....the light was too dim, I felt sleepy and a bit depressed....it was hard to concentrate on the class. What I suggested is a change to a brighter light." (Participant 2)

"You know, I would wonder sometimes if I was hearing the noise from outside. I hope it's quiet." (Participant 3)

Also, some participates suggested that they required a short break, perhaps with a light refreshment, in order to increase their attention and participation.

"The session was long, and we should have had five minutes to rest in between." (Participant 1)

Sub-theme 2: Facilitators

Most of the participants reported that the facilitators performed at an expert level and their speech was clear and well structured. Participants observed that the facilitator were friendly, responsible, and were attentive and respectful listeners.

"The class was very organized; the devices, such as the laptop, projector and practice booklet, were well arranged by those doctors and every time they came to pick us up from the ward to the classroom, they were always on time; I appreciated that." (Participant 8)

However, the suggestions included a range of recommendations. The facilitator's slides should have included more interesting, flashy information and photos. Indeed, text-focused presentations may create the impression that the presentation is 'dry' or overly technical and boring.

"There are too many texts in some slides, I found the class quite boring." (Participant 9)

Furthermore, the facilitator should have allowed more time to answer questions from the class.

"I had many questions on the medication section; I wanted to ask more questions to the teacher but the time was ending." (Participant 9)

Also, it was suggested that the facilitators should improve their class-management skills, as participants reported discouragement or distress due to others' negative or irrelevant comments.

"Sometimes the class was in a little bit of chaos and I felt irritable towards the group members who were speaking loudly and dominating the group." (Participant 1)

Finally, it was suggested that facilitators could start each lesson with an offer to briefly review prior contents, as this could have enhanced understanding and retention.

"However, some contents are easy to forget, I wish the facilitator had repeated things again at the beginning of the class." (Participant 8)

Sub-theme 3: Time

Participants preferred to attend the class in the afternoon rather than in the morning, due to sleepiness.

"You know, we have to wake up at 6 am during the routine hospitalization. In the following 3 hours, I have to eat breakfast, read some books and play table tennis. Whenever the class started at 10 am, I felt tired and sleepy. So, I prefer to attend the 3pm class in the afternoon as I felt more energized then after my 2pm nap." (Participant 5)

Most participants agreed that each session should take about 40 min.

"Sometimes the class took longer than 40 minutes and I felt restless." (Participant 6)

Sessions had intervals of 2 to 3 days; because if the gap between the sessions is too long, some participants may lose interest and patience in the program.

Theme 3: Perception of participating in a group

Sub-theme 1: Group-versus individual-based intervention

Most of the participants commented that the group-based psychoeducation was favorable to the individual psychoeducation intervention. They reported that group--based programs can help participants realise that they are not alone in suffering from BD.

"I am not only the one who has bipolar disorder; many people around me have the same problems. Within the group, we can discuss bipolar disorder." (Participant 8)

They reported benefits of exposure to a wider range of perspectives on their situation when hearing from other members, such as how to communicate with friends and relatives regarding their illness.

"When I see what others are doing, I can push myself harder." (Participant 5)

Group therapy had a range of other benefits, such as participants being more likely to discuss and share the experiences on: medication use and side effects; treatment in the outpatient and inpatient unit; experience with family members and friends; and varying coping strategies that they found useful.

However, a few participants suggested that individual therapy sessions would have been better because they experienced difficulties talking in a group with 8–10 people. Some participants felt embarrassed after sharing their own experiences about the illness with others, because someone in the group was laughing.

"I was sharing my own experiences at the period of manic onset; I told everyone I earned salary of 10000 RMB in a month, my husband only earned 8000 RMB. I wanted to change my husband at that time....but then everyone in the group was laughing at me and I felt very embarrassed."

(Participant 13)

Two participates reported that they felt uncomfortable at first when discussing each other's problems in front of strangers.

"I didn't know what to expect from the course and I felt very anxious initially...many strangers were siting around me." (Participant 3)

Sub-theme 2: Class-taught versus discussion

Most of the participants preferred to be involved in the facilitator-directed class discussion compared with a teacher-directed class. Their reasons included difficulty maintaining attention when all they could hear was the teacher talking. An effective way to improve interest may be to require participants to think and connect with the content.

"If I only listened to the teaching talking, I would lose my interest in the class." (Participant 5)

A few participants reported that they preferred teacher-directed classes, because some participants from the group were likely to dominate the group discussion.

"She kept talking, talking and talking in the class, I felt restless and annoyed at her."

(Participant 2)

Sub-theme 3: Family involvement

Altogether, 80% of the participants mentioned that they would like to ask their family members to become involved in the program. Listening to the class would help some family members understand that they should not put too much pressure on BD sufferers, because some of the symptoms are due to biological or environment effects, rather than "stubbornness".

"If my mom could come to the class that would be helpful, she could listen more about bipolar disorder, the medication I am taking and this would help her understand more about me....maybe she will change her attitude towards me, that I am not lazy." (Participant4)

Some participants suggested that it was only necessary for their family to participate in some sessions, because some of the sessions are not relevant to them.

"Yes, especially in the psychological session, the doctor taught us how to identify, understand, express and manage our emotion; if my husband was here, it would definitely improve our relationship."

(Participant 13)

However, some participants did not show this interest; one participant expressed that their family members lived far from the hospital and would have trouble with transportation and taking time off work.

"That's too far, my dad is living in the Shandong province, I don't want him to come here everyday, you know traveling is difficult for him".

(Participate 14)

Two other participants reported that they had poor relationships with their mom/husband and would prefer not having them within the group.

"No, I don't. I don't want my mom to participate in the class because we argue very often at home". (Participant 2)

Sub-theme 4: Real stories sharing

Some participants suggested that the course could include one or more patients with bipolar disorder who had been cured or who are effectively managing their illness. Hearing from such individuals could inspire hope and confidence that recovery is possible for others.

> "It's better to listen to some real stories from real people who have been cured, such as how they recovered from the bipolar disorder, what they did during the treatment and recovery period... which medication they think is the best....this information could help me feel more authentic". (Participant 15)

Theme 4: Perception of learning content

Most of the participants commented that the content was professional, well structured and useful. The following results are specific to each session.

Sub-theme 1: Concept of BD

Participants said that the session on "bipolar disorder" increased their knowledge of BD, such as the symptoms of depression, manic behavior, and etiology.

> "No one has ever told me what is bipolar disorder, and now I know what has happened to me." (Participant 10)

Sub-theme 2: Treatment of BD

Most of the participants expressed that they were willing to take different medications for Bipolar disorder, and that they understood how important the medications were as an adjunct to other psychotherapeutic intervention.

> "I don't like to take medication, I always hide the medication under my pillow and then the nurse found out and forced me to take it. But now I understand why I should take the medication." (Participant 13)

Sub-theme 3: Psychological approach

Some patients participated in psychological exercises, such as imagery relaxation and group-based mindfulness practice. These were experienced as being useful and patients kept practicing them in their daily life. This session also included some basic cognitive therapy.

> "The imagery relaxation made me feel comfortable; I could imagine that I was in the ocean with my lover. I also practiced it before going to sleep every night and it enabled me to really calm down." (Participant 9)

Some participants expressed that they had learned how to replace some automatic negative thoughts and beliefs with new rational beliefs, which lead to their behavior becoming more reasonable. Particularly, two participants mentioned that they would continue to participate in cognitive behavioral therapies after their discharge from hospital.

> "In the past, I was always thinking that I was going to die, but I understand now this type of thought is called catastrophizing; catastrophizing means only expecting the worst outcome in everything, so actually I was not going to die." (Participant 7)

Sub-theme 4: Self-management

Some participants reported that they found the self-management session useful, such as learning how to list triggers and monitor mood. Participants' emotions have become more stable as a result of the self-management session; they know how to recognise, understand, express and self-manage their emotions.

> "I feel that I can actually recognize the dangerous triggers in the different environment settings as a result of an increased awareness of my mood." (Participant 5)

Sub-theme 5: Lifestyle management

All participants reported that maintaining a regular bio--clock rhythm, being physically active, and abstaining from alcohol, reinforce the importance of a healthy diet and lifestyle.

> "I always reversed my bio-clock, I used to work at night until 5 to 6 am and go to bed at daytime. I understand if I do not want to come back to hospital again, I should have a regular life." (Participant 7)

> "I will keep doing sports every day because my mood becomes more stable after playing badminton with my neighbor every time." (Participant 6)

Sub-theme 6: Relapse prevention

Some participants reported that the mood diary was the most helpful tool. They reported that monitoring their mood changes on a day-to-day basis would assist in making the most of their visit to see the doctors.

> "The mood diary was the most useful thing I have learned from the class, it can help me monitor my mood, if the score is higher than 4 or 4.5, I should

definitely see my doctor as soon as possible."(Participant 8)

Sub-theme 7: Suggestion for improving the learning content

Some participants suggested ways in which the content could be improved. Participants complained that they still had fears of modified electroconvulsive therapy (MECT), and therefore they thought the program should include more details on MECT, such as its mechanism of operation, side effects, and information on anesthesia.

> "I am still not very sure of electroconvulsive therapy, what's that for? Will I die after injecting something in my body by the doctor?" (Participant 8)

Participants also thought that the mood charting exercise should contain more examples of how to complete the diary.

> "The doctor gave me the sheet but I totally had no idea how to do that."(Participant 13)

Participants also suggested wanting to understand how to reduce or manage the side effects of their medication.

> "The side effects of the medication are common to everyone, not only me, but I still fear weight gain as result of taking long-term medication, I want to know how to reduce this side effect." (Participant 8)

> "I understand how important medication is to me, but the side effects....You know I am a girl and I am not married yet." (Participant 7)

Some female participants suggested that the content should include information about bipolar disorder and pregnancy.

> "I have bipolar disorder and want to get pregnant but I want to know the risks and benefits of medications and forms of birth control." (Participant 13)

Theme 5: Outcome of participating in program

Sub-theme 1: Self-acceptance

The majority of participants reported that the program reduced their feelings of embarrassment, shame and confusion regarding their illness. Hence, the program increased their acceptance of their illness.

> "I understand that my illness is not my fault." (Participant 11)

> "This is something I can't change by myself, but I should accept it." (Participant 15)

Sub-theme 2: Self-confidence

Some participants mentioned that they were struggling to speak up for themselves within their daily lives. However, whilst practicing skills introduced through group work, patients increased their confidence for confidently interacting with people outside the group.

> "I was struggling to speak up about my illness, but when someone was speaking up about their illness in the group discussions, that would give me the confidence to do the same." (Participant 8)

> "Since I started to share my own experiences in the group, I felt stronger within myself." (Participant 6)

Sub-theme 3: Self-awareness

Some participants reported that they had become more aware of warning signs of a bipolar episode, and this helped them address their mood when it was becoming excessively high or low.

> "Once I recognized the trigger and in the future I will know when my mood is becoming low or high." (Participate 15)

Sub-theme 4: Self-motivation

Some participants stated that they experienced increased motivation to participate in treatment and engage in lifestyle changes, and these feelings led to a sense of control.

> "My mom sent me to the hospital because I would always go on a shopping sprees... If I receive enough treatment, I won't waste the money again." (Participant 4)

> "I feel so sorry and regret towards my husband, I won't try to change my husband again despite my salary being higher than him, I will try my best to recover from the illness." (Participant 13)

Sub-theme 5: Social support

Some participants reported that they developed new friendships with group members and that they would continue to meet each other and offer social support at the end of the program.

"I am not only getting support from my family, but also from the group members." (Participant 8)

"She said I am her good friend, we did everything together during the hospitalization, we would wake up at the same time, go to the washroom, watch TV, sit together when eating breakfast and lunch." (Participant 6)

Sub-theme 6: Relationship with the doctor

Some participants mentioned that the program enhanced the relationship with their doctor and they also reported an increase in trusting their resident doctor at the end of program.

"I was reluctant to talk to my resident doctor before attending this program, because I thought he had lied to me about my condition and that he just wouldn't let me go home but I found out I was wrong....we did have a pleasant conversation yesterday in the ward and I believed him." (Participant 12)

Some participants said this change in trust may result in greater adherence to outpatient visits and check-up sessions.

"If I keep up taking the medication that my doctor prescribes me then everything will be okay for me." (Participant 5)

Discussion

Perception of participating in the program

Those patients who showed a higher understanding of their illness would encourage positive treatment outcomes, and this formed the main motivation to complete the program. The participants showed interest in recommending the program to others. These findings are in agreement with an earlier qualitative study in outpatient sample [8]. The patients recommended that the program should provide a comprehensive educational booklet. This may be due to some patients favouring written materials as they can then review them at any time [21]. Finally, participants expressed interest in further participating in follow-up studies after discharge from the hospital.

Perception of the setting

Most of the participants reported that the learning environment facilitated their attention and attendance, with the presence of light music enhancing their mood and focus while in class. The single-table seating led to feelings of equality and solidarity. Some participants suggested that the learning environment could improve, with suggestions including enhancing the ambient light and introducing breaks and refreshment, as well as ensuring a quiet and undisturbed environment.

Participants reported preferring afternoon sessions due to morning sleepiness and the disruption to preferred daily routines. Instead of attending classes in the mornings, participants would like to attend classes during the afternoon, perhaps after a nap. Most participants agreed that each session should take about 40 min to achieve a balance between the content covered and the toll on attentional and emotional resources. All participants in our sample were presently in a recovery period from acute BD symptoms and therefore they could experience disruptions to mood during longer sessions. The present study agreed that each session should have intervals separated by 2 to 3 days as participants may lose interest and patience to the program if the gap between sessions is excessive. Our program delivered eight sessions in a period of two weeks. This might explain why the drop out rate was low in our study.

Most of the facilitators were perceived as professional, friendly, respectful and responsible. There were suggestions for the facilitators to: (i) improve the powerpoint slides to include more interesting, flashy information, photos and videos, in order to enhance the class's learning atmosphere; (ii) expand even further upon main points offered in the lecture slides; (iii) allow more time to answer participants' questions; (iv) improve class-management skills to prevent dominant group-members offering disruptive or irrelevant content. Indeed, in a study by Poole, Smith and Simpson [8], it was found that participants dominating the group members was one of the reasons for dropping out the program. Lastly, participants suggested that the facilitators (v) should offer a revision of the previous session at the beginning of each new session, as participants reported difficulties remembering all the information.

Perception of the learning content

The content and the lecturer were both judged of being of expert quality, clear and well structured. Participants especially enjoyed the sessions that included: definition of bipolar disorder; a treatment approach; a psychosocial approach; self-management; and healthy lifestyle in order to prevent relapse. However, the lack of detailed knowledge about MECT caused some participants to feel anxious. Hence, participants suggested that the MECT session should cover the mechanisms of operation, side effects, anxious relaxation and some basic knowledge of anesthesia. More information about bipolar disorder and pregnancy and how to reduce the side effects from the medication were requested from female participants. Female patients appeared more prone to worry about their weight gain as result of taking medication. Excessive weight gain was the most common cause of non-adherence of treatment [22]. Crucially, further instruction and practice on mood charting is necessary as most of the participants reported that they did not know how to complete the exercise sheet at the end of program.

Perception of participating in a group

Most of the participants stated that the group-based psychoeducation was preferred over individual intervention. This result supports earlier findings, as learning that the patient is not alone in suffering the illness can alleviate feelings of shame and isolation [23]. Participants were able to learn how to communicate with their friends and relatives from interacting with the group. In the Chinese society, the role of "teacher" has long been respected. Chinese people think the teacher is the expert they can trust and rely to receive valuable suggestions [24]. Interestingly, there are psychotherapy studies, such as those including cognitive behavior therapy, suggesting that didactic teaching is the desirable approach during the treatment process, since it can improve the trust relationship between patients and psychotherapists [24–26]. Surprisingly, in our study, most of the participants preferred to be involved in a facilitator-directed class discussion rather than in didactic teaching. Some participants felt embarrassed after sharing their own experiences as some group members were laughing at them. In order to partially address these concerns, perhaps the facilitator should remind participants of the principle of information confidentiality. Also, the facilitator should emphasize the key points from the slides by asking questions to participants, hence refocusing any discussion that approaches an irrelevant topic. For those participants who feel uncomfortable during initial sessions, the facilitator should provide a more natural icebreaker exercise [8]. Many participants suggested that involving family members would be useful, as this would promote an understanding of the patient's illness and their current condition. However, whether the relatives should become involved in the program depends on the patients' personal and financial situation. Poole, Smith and Simpson [8] suggested that future programs could provide sessions specifically for family member to become involved in the therapeutic process. Lastly, some participants suggested that the program should invite patients who are effectively managing or have been cured of BD. Sharing their treatment and recovery experiences with the group may encourage hope and confidence within these group-members. This point also was raised in previous study [8].

Outcome of participating in the program

Poole, Smith and Simpson [8] demonstrated that a UK-based group pychoeducation intervention had positive impact on the patient's knowledge, acceptance, social support and attitude towards taking medication. Our results are comparable to findings from European patients, as participants reported that the program increased their personal acceptance of their illness, reducing their feeling of confusion and self-doubt. Patients became more confident to communicate with the people outside the group, which can reduce self-stigma and promote prosocial behaviours. A number of participants stated that they have a strong motivation to stay in treatment and experience lasting changes as a result. Some participants reported that they would continue to meet each other at the end of the program, therefore increasing their social support. Some participants increased their awareness as they became more capable to recognise personal triggers. Others reported that the program enhanced their "trust relationship" with their doctor. A more trusting relationship could increase compliance and help achieve better treatment outcomes [27].

Strengths and limitations

The aim of this study was to qualitatively explore experiences of group-based psychoeducation for BD-I via thematic analysis. The data analysed during the process evaluation helped the authors understand the strengths and weaknesses of the program. This addresses a gap within existing literature regarding the efficacy of group psychoeducation for individuals with BD. This study is the first to assess group-based psychoeducation programs for inpatients following remission of a manic episode in bipolar I disorder within a Chinese sample. The findings indicate that the program was helpful for patients with BD-I. Patients offered a range of recommendations that future research on group-based psychoeducation programs should explore. There are some limitations in this study: the methodological design did not include direct questions asking for participants' potential discomfort and non-beneficial aspect of the program; our sample had a large proportion of female patients, hence future studies may wish to explore differences in group dynamics across a range of gender ratios; family was not involved in this study, so future research needs to explore family-based intervention for BD in Chinese populations; finally, since this study was conducted on a single hospital ward, future research may consider implementing this intervention across multiple sites and include community based psychoeducation programs to explore its generalisability.

Clinical implications

Future programs should include further details about MECT and more information about BD and pregnancy for female patients. More support from facilitators is required when patients work on mood charting. Importantly, participants may benefit from less didactic teaching and more discussions during each session. Finally, it would be helpful for patients to have access to a comprehensive education booklet, which they can then review at any time, at their own pace.

As recommended by many participants, future psychoeducation education programs should involve family members, as this could help them better understand the patients' illness and current condition. Future programs may also consider to invite BD patients who have been successfully treated, as sharing their treatment and recovery experiences with the group may encourage hope and confidence.

Our study demonstrated that a culturally adapted group-based psychoeducation program for BD is feasible and acceptable in a Chinese population. Different social and cultural backgrounds could impact on the patient's perception of their symptoms and services engagement [28]. The role of Confucianism in the Chinese culture as well as its collectivistic tradition discourages open displays of emotions in order to maintain social and familial harmony or avoid exposing personal's weakness/perception. As a result, some Chinese patients are reluctant to share negative feelings due to fears of creating interpersonal conflicts (and hence damage their connections with others) and bring shame to their family ("lose face"), which could result in the avoidance of interactions in group interventions. For instance, Lin [25] indicated that Chinese American patients may experience difficulties with straightforward discussions about some problems between family members during cognitive behavior therapy. Thus, when working with Chinese patients, the notion of "saving face" is an important element that needs to be considered through the course of intervention [24]. In our study, we found that most of the participants were willing to discuss and share personal experiences with others in the group. Facilitators can therefore educate patients to recognize the importance of actively engaging in group discussions in the beginning and during the course of the sessions. Also, culturally adapted interventions are an effective way to facilitate group discussions and promote a good trusting relationship, such as using local folk stories, idioms, image and examples from religious [28].

Conclusion

This qualitative study provides positive evidence on the benefits of a group-based psychoeducation program in enhancing patient knowledge, confidence, acceptance, motivation, social support and a trusting relationship with the doctor. Based on the benefits of our program on patients, this intervention could potentially be incorporated into routine psychiatry inpatient care. Therefore, it is suggested that policy makers should consider placing more efforts on the provision of more accessible psychoeducation interventions to patients with bipolar disorder in China.

Abbreviations

BD: Bipolar disorder; BD-I: Bipolar disorder type I

Acknowledgements

The authors would also like to thank Dr. Liliana Capitao (Department of Psychiatry, Oxford University) and Dr. Lloyd C. Williams for proofreading the final version of the Manuscript and for useful suggestions.

Funding

This work was supported by the Capital Characteristic Clinical Application Research [grant numbers Z141107002514032]; the funding body had no role in the design of the study and collection, analysis, and interpretation of data and in writing the manuscript.

Authors' contributions

Study design: CR, XY, LJ, LY, WX, HY. Study Implementation: CR, XY, LY, HY. Data analysis: CR, XY, HY. Manuscript preparation: CR, XY, LJ, LY, WX, HY. All authors read and approved the final manuscript.

Consent for publication

The informed consent for publication obtained from the patient had been in writing.

Competing interests

The authors declare that there is no conflict of interests.

Author details

[1]The National Clinical Research Center for Mental Disorders & Beijing key Laboratory of Mental Disorders, Beijing Anding Hospital, Capital Medical University, No. 5 Ankang Lane, Dewai Avenue, Xicheng District, Beijing 100088, China. [2]Department of Psychiatry, University of Oxford, Oxford, UK.

References

1. Inder ML, Crowe MT, Luty SE, Carter JD, Moor S, Frampton CM, Joyce PR. Randomized, controlled trial of interpersonal and social rhythm therapy for young people with bipolar disorder. Bipolar Disord. 2015;17(2):128–38.
2. Pini S, de Queiroz V, Pagnin D, Pezawas L, Angst J, Cassano GB, Wittchen H-U. Prevalence and burden of bipolar disorders in European countries. Eur Neuropsychopharmacol. 2005;15(4):425–34.
3. Zhang L, Cao X-L, Wang S-B, Zheng W, Ungvari GS, Ng CH, Zhong B-L, Wang G, Xiang Y-T. The prevalence of bipolar disorder in China: a meta-analysis. J Affect Disord. 2017;207:413–21.
4. Karamustafalıoğlu O, Reif A, Atmaca M, Gonzalez D, Moreno-Manzanaro M, Gonzalez MA, Medina E, Bellomo A. Hospital stay in patients admitted for acute bipolar manic episodes prescribed quetiapine immediate or extended release: a retrospective non-interventional cohort study (HOME). BMC Psychiatry. 2014;14(1):246.

5. Colom F, Vieta E, Martínez-Arán A, Reinares M, Goikolea JM, Benabarre A, Torrent C, Comes M, Corbella B, Parramon G. A randomized trial on the efficacy of group psychoeducation in the prophylaxis of recurrences in bipolar patients whose disease is in remission. Arch Gen Psychiatry. 2003;60(4):402–7.
6. Bauer MS, McBride L, Williford WO, Glick H, Kinosian B, Altshuler L, Beresford T, Kilbourne AM, Sajatovic M. Collaborative care for bipolar disorder: part I. Intervention and implementation in a randomized effectiveness trial. Psychiatr Serv. 2006;57(7):927-36. doi:https://doi.org/10.1176/ps.2006.57.7.927.
7. Colom F, Vieta E, Sanchez-Moreno J, Palomino-Otiniano R, Reinares M, Goikolea J, Benabarre A, Martinez-Aran A. Group psychoeducation for stabilised bipolar disorders: 5-year outcome of a randomised clinical trial. Br J Psychiatry. 2009;194(3):260–5.
8. Poole R, Smith D, Simpson S. Patients' perspectives of the feasibility, acceptability and impact of a group-based psychoeducation programme for bipolar disorder: a qualitative analysis. BMC Psychiatry. 2015;15(1):184.
9. George LS, Sharma P, Nair S. Effect of psycho-education on quality of life and disability among persons. Indian J Health Wellbeing. 2015;6(5):461.
10. Gumus F, Buzlu S, Cakir S. Effectiveness of individual psychoeducation on recurrence in bipolar disorder; a controlled study. Arch Psychiatr Nurs. 2015; 29(3):174–9.
11. Mellor D, Carne L, Shen YC, McCabe M, Wang L. Stigma toward mental illness: a cross-cultural comparison of Taiwanese, Chinese immigrants to Australia and Anglo-Australians. J Cross-Cult Psychol. 2013;44(3):352-64.
12. Xi Y, Chen R, Yan F, Ma X, Rakofsky JJ, Tang L, Guo H, Wu X, Li X, Zhu H. Low post-traumatic stress disorder rate in Chinese in Beijing, China. Asian J Psychiatr. 2017;30:79–83.
13. Lin T-Y, Lin M-C. Love, denial and rejection: responses of Chinese families to mental illness. A Kleinman, T Lin. Reidel, Dordrecht. In: Normal and abnormal behavior in Chinese culture: Springer; 1981. p. 387–401.
14. Alvidrez J, Snowden LR, Rao SM, Boccellari A. Psychoeducation to address stigma in black adults referred for mental health treatment: a randomized pilot study. Community Ment Health J. 2009;45(2):127–36.
15. Griner D, Smith TB: Culturally adapted mental health intervention: a meta-analytic review. In.: Educational Publishing Foundation. Psychotherapy: Theory, Research, Practice, Training. 2006;43(4):531-48. https://doi.org/10.1037/0033-3204.43.4.531.
16. Breitmayer BJ, Ayres L, Knafl KA. Triangulation in qualitative research: evaluation of completeness and confirmation purposes. Image J Nurs Sch. 1993;25(3):237–43.
17. Colom F, Vieta E. Psychoeducation Manual for Bipolar Disorder. Cambridge: Cambridge University Press; 2006. Crossref https://www.cambridge.org/core/books/psychoeducation-manual-for-bipolardisorder/331739037E4D1C8E83D8A78E57B52C1D.
18. Francis JJ, Johnston M, Robertson C, Glidewell L, Entwistle V, Eccles MP, Grimshaw JM. What is an adequate sample size? Operationalising data saturation for theory-based interview studies. Psychol Health. 2010;25(10):1229–45.
19. Braun V, Clarke V. Using thematic analysis in psychology. Qual Res Psychol. 2006;3(2):77–101.
20. Shorey S, Chan SW, Chong YS, He HG. Perceptions of primiparas on a postnatal psychoeducation programme: the process evaluation. Midwifery. 2015;31(1):155–63.
21. Renkert S, Nutbeam D. Opportunities to improve maternal health literacy through antenatal education: an exploratory study. Health Promot Int. 2001;16(4):381–8.
22. Berken GH, Weinstein DO, Stern WC. Weight gain: a side-effect of tricyclic antidepressants. J Affect Disord. 1984;7(2):133–8.
23. Yalom ID, Leszcz M: Theory and practice of group psychotherapy: basic books; 2005.
24. Chen SW, Davenport DS: Cognitive-behavioral therapy with Chinese American clients: cautions and modifications. Psychother Theory Res Pract Train 2005, 42(1):101.
25. Lin Y-N. The application of cognitive-behavioral therapy to counseling Chinese. Am J Psychother. 2002;56(1):46.
26. Chen CP. Counseling applications of RET in a Chinese cultural context. J Rational-emotive Cogn Behav Ther. 1995;13(2):117–29.
27. O'Connor C, Gordon O, Graham M, Kelly F, O'Grady-Walshe A. Service user perspectives of a psychoeducation group for individuals with a diagnosis of bipolar disorder: a qualitative study. J Nerv Ment Dis. 2008;196(7):568–71.
28. Husain MI, Chaudhry IB, Rahman RR, Hamirani MM, Mehmood N, Haddad PM, Hodsoll J, Young AH, Naeem F, Husain N. Pilot study of a culturally adapted psychoeducation (CaPE) intervention for bipolar disorder in Pakistan. Int J Bipolar Disord. 2017;5(1):3.

Reasons for lithium discontinuation in men and women with bipolar disorder

Louise Öhlund[1], Michael Ott[2], Sofia Oja[3], Malin Bergqvist[4], Robert Lundqvist[5], Mikael Sandlund[6], Ellinor Salander Renberg[6] and Ursula Werneke[1,7*]

Abstract

Background: Lithium remains first choice as maintenance treatment for bipolar affective disorder. Yet, about half of all individuals may stop their treatment at some point, despite lithium's proven benefits concerning the prevention of severe affective episodes and suicide.

Methods: Retrospective cohort study in the Swedish region of Norrbotten into the causes of lithium discontinuation. The study was set up to (1) test whether patients with bipolar affective disorder or schizoaffective disorder, treated with lithium maintenance therapy, were more likely to discontinue lithium because of adverse effects than lack of therapeutic effectiveness, (2) explore gender differences, (3) understand the role of diagnosis and (4) identify who, patient or doctor, took the initiative to stop lithium. Review of medical records for all episodes of lithium discontinuation that had occurred between 1997 and 2013 with the intent to stop lithium for good.

Results: Of 873 patients treated with lithium, 54% discontinued lithium, corresponding to 561 episodes of lithium discontinuation. In 62% of episodes, lithium was discontinued due to adverse effects, in 44% due to psychiatric reasons, and in 12% due to physical reasons interfering with lithium treatment. The five single most common adverse effects leading to lithium discontinuation were diarrhoea (13%), tremor (11%), polyuria/polydipsia/diabetes insipidus (9%), creatinine increase (9%) and weight gain (7%). Women were as likely as men to take the initiative to stop lithium, but twice as likely to consult a doctor before taking action ($p < 0.01$). Patients with type 1 BPAD or SZD were more likely to discontinue lithium than patients with type 2 or unspecified BPAD ($p < 0.01$). Patients with type 1 BPAD or SZD were more likely to refuse medication ($p < 0.01$). Conversely, patients with type 2 or unspecified BPAD were three times as likely to discontinue lithium for lack or perceived lack of effectiveness ($p < 0.001$).

Conclusions: Stopping lithium treatment is common and occurs mostly due to adverse effects. It is important to discuss potential adverse effects with patients before initiation and continuously during lithium treatment, to reduce the frequency of potentially unnecessary discontinuations.

Keywords: Lithium, Bipolar disorder, Physical health, Compliance, Side effects

* Correspondence: uwerneke@gmail.com
[1]Sunderby Research Unit, Department of Clinical Sciences, Division of Psychiatry, Umeå University, Umeå, Sweden
[7]Sunderby Hospital – Psychiatry, 97180 Luleå, Sweden
Full list of author information is available at the end of the article

Background

Ever since publication of the BALANCE trial in 2010 [1], lithium has experienced a renaissance as maintenance treatment for bipolar affective disorder (BPAD) in Europe. In 2014, the UK National Institute for Clinical Excellence (NICE) endorsed lithium as a first-line, long-term pharmacological treatment for bipolar disorder [2]. Two recent large observational register studies have demonstrated lithium's therapeutic superiority regarding prevention of suicide and recurrence of acute affective episodes [3, 4].

Yet, despite its therapeutic superiority, patients may find it difficult to take lithium long-term. Non-adherence is common in the treatment of serious mental disorders, irrespective of the substance in question [5]. For lithium, non-adherence rates vary from 14% to 61% [6, 7]. Both doctors and patients may discontinue lithium, albeit for different reasons [8]. But as lithium may remain the treatment of choice for most patients requiring maintenance treatment even in the face of adverse renal effects [9, 10], it is important to understand the reasons for discontinuing lithium. Equally important is it to understand the factors that influence the initiative to stop.

Aim

We conducted a retrospective historical cohort study to (1) test whether patients with BPAD or schizoaffective disorder (SZD), treated with lithium maintenance therapy, were more likely to discontinue lithium because of adverse effects than lack of therapeutic effectiveness, (2) explore gender differences, (3) understand the role of diagnosis and (4) identify who, patient or doctor, took the initiative to stop lithium.

Method

Study design

We designed a retrospective (historical) cohort study (LISIE) into effects and side effects of lithium treatment as compared to other mood stabilizers for the maintenance treatment of BPAD. The Regional Ethics Review Board at Umeå University, Sweden, had approved this study (DNR 2010-227-31 M, DNR 2011-228-32 M, DNR 2014-10-32 M).

The participants were informed about the nature of the study in writing and provided verbal informed consent. The consent was documented in our research files, dated and signed by the research worker who obtained the consent. In accordance with the ethics approval granted, for deceased patients, no consent was obtained. The ethics committee approved these consent procedures prior to commencement of this study.

Participants

For LISIE, we identified all patients in the Swedish region of Norrbotten, who had been either diagnosed with BPAD (F31) or SZD (F25), or who had been prescribed lithium and were at least 18 years of age. We screened the medical records of all patients who had either given informed consent to participate, or who we were approved to include because they had deceased.

For this study, we retrospectively examined routine clinical data recorded until 31 December 2015. The extraction, validation and analysis were performed in 2016 and 2017. We defined as "exposed", patients who had received a diagnosis of BPAD or SZD on at least two occasions at least six months apart any time between 1997 and 2013, and for whom at least two positive lithium serum levels were available. We determined when lithium had been started and validated the diagnoses in the medical records at this point.

Patients were potentially eligible for inclusion into this study, when we found a lithium prescription that had been discontinued in the electronic prescription database. We included all episodes for which the medical records then indicated that lithium was indeed discontinued with the intention to stop for good. At this point, we also checked the records for the exact point of time lithium was discontinued, since this may have preceded discontinuation of the prescription.

Chart review, variable definitions and outcomes

For each patient, we systematically abstracted the case records to obtain information regarding (1) baseline characteristics including diagnosis, (2) date of and reason for lithium discontinuation and (3) communication about the initiative to stop lithium. All episodes of lithium discontinuation were registered in the time frame studied. We used this information to quantify overall reasons for lithium discontinuation. We also explored for how long a patient had coped with a side effect or a doctor had accepted an adverse effect before discontinuing lithium.

We stratified diagnosis in two groups, BPAD type 1 or SZD on the one hand and BPAD type 2 or unspecified on the other. We divided reasons for lithium discontinuation into three main categories. The first category concerned psychiatric reasons, related to the mental disorder itself or associated circumstances, such as not being able to pay for medication. The second category related to physical health reasons that could interfere with lithium. The third category covered adverse effects. We allocated intentional overdoses to the first category of psychiatric reasons. We allocated unintentional overdoses and unintended increases in lithium serum concentration to the second category of physical health reasons, such as chronic kidney disease, dehydration or co-medications interfering with lithium pharmacokinetics. For the psychiatric reason category, we created a variable called "non-adherence". Under this variable, we summed up discontinuation of lithium due to fear of adverse effects, being in disagreement with the diagnosis, refusing medication, feeling subjectively well and not adhering to monitoring.

We determined who initiated lithium discontinuation, patient or doctor. This, we called “agent who took the initiative to discontinue lithium”. For the decision process, we explored whether patients had consulted their doctor before. Some patients had discontinued lithium only once in the time frame of our study. But others had discontinued and then reinstated lithium on at least one occasion. Thus, we divided episodes of discontinuation into first and subsequent episodes.

We conducted a sub-analysis, to assess how long a patient had coped with or a doctor had accepted an adverse effect before discontinuing lithium. To avoid overestimation of the length of time a problem had persisted before it led to discontinuation of lithium (lead time), we only considered *proven* first but not subsequent episodes of lithium discontinuation. For this sub-analysis, we traced back medical records until 1965 to make sure that we had not missed any previous episodes of lithium discontinuation, which might have occurred prior to 1997. Here, we excluded patients for whom such prior episodes of lithium discontinuation were found or where information was missing.

Control for bias

Of all patients approached, 75% consented to inclusion into the LISIE study. In accordance with the ethical approval granted, we controlled for selection bias in the whole LISIE study, comparing age, sex, maximum recorded lithium and creatinine level as key parameters, available in anonymized form. We did not find any significant difference between participating and non-participating patients. To minimize observer and recording bias, all reasons for discontinuation were assessed by two separate reviewers. Patients, who were excluded from the final sample since the reasons for stopping lithium had not been recorded, had the same age and sex distribution as patients who were included.

Sub-analysis lead time

In a sub-analysis, we explored the lead time from start of lithium treatment until the first episode of discontinuation. We included only patients for whom we could unequivocally define the first episode of lithium discontinuation. Age and sex were not significantly different in patients included and excluded from this sub-analysis.

Statistical analysis

We conducted a descriptive analysis, establishing the frequency of all variables in our database. We divided the sample according to category of reason, and stratified then further according to gender, diagnosis and agent, patient or doctor, who took the initiative to discontinue lithium. To assess potential group differences, we used chi square test for categorical variables and t-test and ANOVA for continuous variables. Statistical significance level was set at $p \leq 0.05$. We conducted the statistical analysis with IBM SPSS Statistics (Version 23). We checked our whole method against the Strobe checklist (Appendix 1).

Results

Baseline characteristics

The total cohort comprised of 1566 patients. Of these, 873 had received lithium at some point during the study period. 468 (54%) patients discontinued lithium at least on one occasion with intention to stop for good. Of these, 81% of patients had stopped lithium on one occasion and 19% on more than one occasion after at least one futile attempt at lithium reinstatement. In total, there were 589 episodes of lithium discontinuation. For 561 (95%) episodes, the reasons of lithium discontinuation were known (Fig. 1). For these episodes, 922 individual reasons were recorded (Table 1).

Reasons for lithium discontinuation

Adverse effects dominated reasons for lithium discontinuation with 62% of the 561 episodes. Psychiatric reasons were given in 44% and physical health reasons in 12% of all episodes ($p < 0.001$) (Table 2). In 37% of episodes, there were more than one reason for lithium discontinuation reported. As there were more reasons than episodes, the percentages did not add up to 100.

Concerning psychiatric reasons, non-adherence was reported in 22% of episodes and perceived or actual lack of effectiveness in 21% of episodes. Of all patients who had discontinued lithium due to perceived or actual lack of effectiveness, 26% reinstated lithium subsequently. The five single most common adverse effects leading to lithium discontinuation included diarrhoea (13%), tremor (11%), polyuria/polydipsia/diabetes insipidus (9%), creatinine increase (9%) and weight gain (7%). Hyperparathyroidism, hypernatraemia and sexual dysfunction were only rarely given as reasons for discontinuation and accounted for less than five episodes each. Intentional overdoses were rarely a cause for discontinuing lithium for good. Unintentional overdoses and risk of increasing lithium concentration accounted for 7% of all discontinuation episodes.

Gender differences

Men with BPAD or SZD were more often treated with lithium (59%) than women (54%, $p < 0.05$). There was no significant difference in proportion of women and men who had continued lithium compared to those who had discontinued lithium. But women had

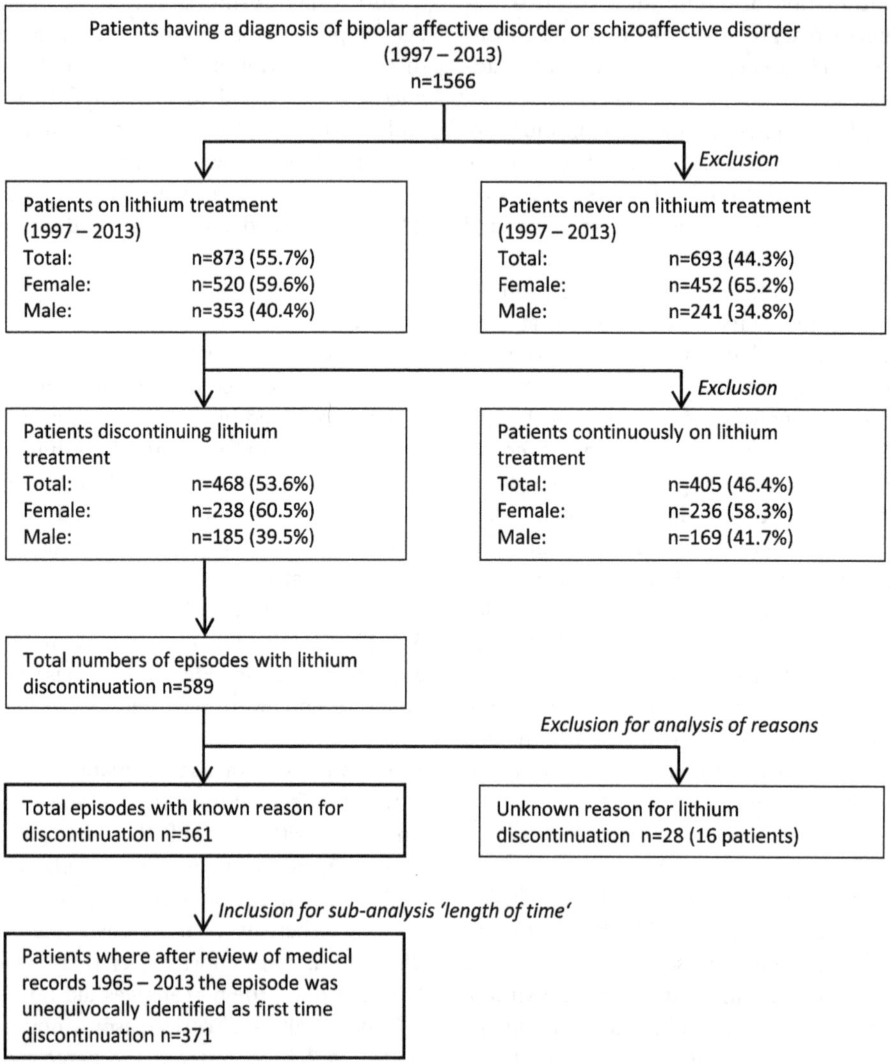

Fig. 1 Selection of study sample

three times more often discontinued lithium because of weight gain ($p < 0.01$) and five times as often because of oedema ($p < 0.01$). In 4 % of episodes, women discontinued lithium due to pregnancy. Conversely, men had three times more often stopped lithium for feeling well ($p < 0.01$). Men had twice as often discontinued lithium without consulting a doctor ($p < 0.01$).

Type of disorder

Patients with type 1 BPAD or SZD were more likely to discontinue lithium than patients with type 2 or -unspecified BPAD ($p < 0.01$). Patients with type 1 BPAD or SZD were more likely to refuse medication ($p < 0.01$). Conversely, patients with type 2 or unspecified BPAD were three times as likely to discontinue lithium for lack or perceived lack of effectiveness ($p < 0.001$). Creatinine increases accounted for three times as many episodes of lithium discontinuation in patients with type 1 BPAD or SZD ($p < 0.001$). Unintentional increase of lithium concentration accounted for twice as many episodes of lithium discontinuation in patients with type 1 BPAD or SZD ($p < 0.05$) (Table 2).

Agent who took the initiative to discontinue lithium

Patients were more likely to take the initiative to stop lithium than doctors ($p < 0.001$). Of all discontinuation episodes, 28% were attributable to lack of adherence on the part of the patient ($p < 0.001$). Concerning adverse effects, patients discontinued lithium more often than doctors because of emotional blunting ($p < 0.001$), diarrhoea ($p < 0.05$) and stomach ache ($p < 0.01$). Doctors discontinued prescribing lithium if patients had not stuck to the required follow-up ($p < 0.01$). Doctors also stopped prescribing lithium for fear of intoxications, irrespective of whether such were intentional or not ($p < 0.01$). Finally,

Table 1 Baseline characteristics of the sample of patients having discontinued lithium treatment at least once between the years of 1997-2013

Gender, n (%)	
Female	238 (60.5)
Male	185 (39.5)
Type of disorder, n (%)	
BPAD 1/SZD	199 (42.5)
BPAD 2/Other	269 (57.5)
Total number of episodes with lithium discontinuation, n (%)	589
Patients with one episode only	378 (80.8)
Patients with more than one episode	90 (19.2)
Total number of episodes with known reason for discontinuation, n (%)	561
Episodes with one reason only	355 (63.3)
Episodes with more than one reason	206 (35.7)
Total number of reasons for lithium discontinuation, n (%)	922
Patients where first episode of discontinuation where identified, n (%)	371 (79.3)
Lead-time to first lithium discontinuation, years	
Mean (SD)	3.6 (6.1)
Median (min-max)	1.1 (0.02-39.9)

n number, *BPAD* bipolar affective disorder, *SZD* schizoaffective disorder, *Other* unspecified bipolar affective disorder or subgroup specified otherwise; *SD* standard deviation

doctors stopped lithium more commonly due to creatinine increases and chronic kidney disease ($p < 0.001$).

Top 10 reasons for lithium discontinuation in relation to duration of treatment

This sub-analysis was based on the first episode of lithium discontinuation in those 371 patients for whom we could be sure that this was unequivocally their first episode of lithium discontinuation. In this subgroup, patients had taken lithium for a mean of 3.6 years (SD 6.1) before stopping treatment. 50% of patients discontinued within 1.1 years (min 6 days, max 39.9 years). Judged on the duration of lithium treatment before discontinuation, patients with type 1 BPAD or SZD coped with adverse effects for significantly longer periods of times than patients with type 2 or unspecified BPAD ($p < 0.01$). Nausea and diarrhoea tended to lead to early discontinuation of lithium. Nausea accounted for discontinuation of lithium in 21 episodes and diarrhoea in 49 episodes (Table 3). Nausea was tolerated for half a year on average. The longest time nausea was tolerated for was one year and seven months. Diarrhoea was tolerated for one year and seven months on average. Yet, a substantial number of patients tried to cope with diarrhoea for a much longer time. There were thirteen patients who took lithium for at least two years before finally stopping due to diarrhoea. Renal factors tended to lead to lithium discontinuations later. Polyuria, polydipsia and diabetes insipidus led to lithium discontinuation usually within five years. Lithium discontinuation due to rising creatinine level occurred on average after 17 years. Four patients discontinued lithium after 30 years due to increased creatinine.

Discussion

In our study, 54% of patients treated with lithium discontinued their medication on at least one occasion with the intention to stop for good. This is well in the range of estimates reported (6). This is the first study that systematically identifies reasons for discontinuation of lithium in a large sample of patients, over a sufficiently long follow-up period to take into account adverse effects occurring late during the course of the illness. We found four more studies exploring reasons for lithium discontinuation. These stem from the 1980s and 90s, with sample sizes ranging from 20 to 64 patients and follow-up times from 6 months to 7 years (11-14).

Usual suspects?

Adverse effects were the most common cause for lithium discontinuation. Among the adverse effects, diarrhoea, tremor, creatinine increase, polyuria/polydipsia/diabetes insipidus and weight gain were the top five reasons for discontinuing lithium. This is in line with findings of three of the previous studies, which also found that adverse event was the most common reason for lithium discontinuation [11–13]. However, Schumann et al. found that lithium discontinuation occurred more commonly due to "internal resistance to treatment" than adverse effects [14]. Yet, due to the relative short follow-up times, neither of the previous studies were designed to capture concerns about impairment of glomerular function. This kind of problem tends to appear only after decades of treatment [15, 16]. Only very few patients had their lithium stopped because of hypercalcaemia/hyperparathyroidism, an adverse effect classically associated with lithium [17].

Psychiatric reasons were given in 44% of all episodes. This calls for further developing of strategies to improve adherence. One fourth of patients who had discontinued lithium due to actual or perceived lack of effectiveness had to reinstate lithium subsequently. Better identification of subgroups of patients who have the most to gain from lithium treatment may help to reduce the amount of lithium discontinuation leading to recurrence of affective episodes.

Gender differences

Men and women were equally likely to discontinue lithium. However, men and women discontinued for different

Table 2 Reasons for lithium discontinuation

	Total, n (%)	Type of disorder, n (%)		Agent, n[a] (%)	
		BPAD 1/SZD	BPAD2/ Other	Doctor	Patient
Episodes, n	561	253	308	225	334
Psychiatric reasons					
Total	249 (44.4)	97 (38.3)	152 (49.4)**	81 (36.0)	167 (50.0)**
Non-adherence	121 (21.6)	65 (25.7)	56 (18.2)*	26 (11.6)	95 (28.4)***
Fear for adverse effects	17 (3.0)	6 (2.4)	11 (3.6)	2 (0.9)	15 (4.5)*
Not agreeing with diagnosis	6 (1.1)	5 (2.0)	1 (0.3)	0 (0)	6 (1.8)*
Refusing medication	34 (6.1)	23 (9.1)	11 (3.6)**	0 (0)	34 (10.2)***
Feeling subjectively well	26 (4.6)	12 (4.7)	14 (4.5)	0 (0)	26 (7.8)***
Not adhering to monitoring	38 (6.8)	19 (7.5)	19 (6.2)	24 (10.7)	14 (4.2)**
Perceived or actual lack of effectiveness	116 (20.7)	25 (9.9)	91 (29.5)***	46 (20.4)	69 (20.7)
Intentional Li intoxication	5 (0.9)	0 (0)	5 (1.6)*	5 (2.2)	0 (0)**
Other reasons[b]	22 (3.9)	13 (5.1)	9 (2.9)	11 (4.9)	11 (3.3)
Physical health reasons					
Total	68 (12.1)	36 (14.2)	31 (10.1)	53 (23.6)	17 (4.2)***
Unintentional Li intoxication	11 (2.0)	6 (2.4)	5 (1.6)	10 (4.4)	1 (0.3)**
Increase of Li concentration	30 (5.3)	19 (7.5)	11 (3.6)*	28 (12.4)	2 (0.6)***
Pregnancy or planned pregnancy	15 (2.7)	5 (2.0)	10 (3.2)	5 (2.2)	10 (3.0)
Physical health problem[c]	12 (2.1)	6 (2.4)	6 (1.9)	11 (4.9)	1 (0.3)***
Adverse effects					
Total	350 (62.4)	164 (64.8)	186 (60.4)	142 (63.1)	207 (62.0)
Kidneys and urinary tract					
Creatinine increase, Li-nephropathy	51 (9.1)	37 (14.6)	14 (4.5)***	44 (19.6)	7 (2.1)***
Nephrogenic DI, polyuria, polydipsia	52 (9.3)	27 (10.7)	25 (8.1)	25 (11.1)	27 (8.1)
Endocrine system					
TSH increase, hypothyroidism	11 (2.0)	4 (1.6)	7 (2.3)	6 (2.7)	5 (1.5)
CNS					
Tremor	61 (10.9)	32 (12.6)	29 (9.4)	27 (12.0)	34 (10.2)
Dizziness	12 (2.1)	4 (1.6)	8 (2.6)	6 (2.7)	6 (1.8)
Headache	8 (1.4)	1 (0.4)	7 (2.3)	2 (0.9)	6 (1.8)
Restless legs	5 (0.9)	2 (0.8)	3 (1.0)	2 (0.9)	3 (0.9)
Psychological adverse effects					
Emotional blunting	31 (5.5)	9 (3.6)	22 (7.1)	2 (0.9)	29 (8.7)***
Irritability/anxiety	12 (2.1)	2 (0.8)	10 (3.2)*	4 (1.8)	8 (2.4)
Other, not specified	20 (3.6)	7 (2.8)	13 (4.2)	5 (2.2)	15 (4.5)
Cognitive adverse effects					
Fatigue	30 (5.3)	11 (4.3)	19 (6.2)	13 (5.8)	17 (5.1)
Imoaired concentration	17 (3.0)	3 (1.2)	14 (4.5)*	11 (4.9)	6 (1.8)*
Impaired memory	8 (1.4)	1 (0.4)	7 (2.3)	6 (2.7)	2 (0.6)*
Gastrointestinal tract					
Diarrhoea	71 (12.7)	33 (13.0)	38 (12.3)	21 (9.3)	50 (15.0)*
Nausea	24 (4.3)	6 (2.4)	18 (5.8)*	7 (3.1)	17 (5.1)
Stomach ache	10 (1.8)	4 (1.6)	6 (1.9)	0 (0)	10 (3.0)**
Other, not specified	7 (1.2)	2 (0.8)	5 (1.6)	2 (0.8)	5 (1.6)

Table 2 Reasons for lithium discontinuation *(Continued)*

	Total, n (%)	Type of disorder, n (%)		Agent, n[a] (%)	
		BPAD 1/SZD	BPAD2/ Other	Doctor	Patient
Skin					
Psoriasis	10 (1.8)	6 (2.4)	4 (1.3)	6 (2.7)	4 (1.2)
Acne	8 (1.4)	4 (1.6)	4 (1.3)	3 (1.3)	5 (1.5)
Other					
Weight gain	41 (7.3)	19 (7.5)	22 (7.1)	12 (5.3)	29 (8.7)
Edema	19 (3.4)	10 (4.0)	9 (2.9)	8 (3.6)	10 (3.0)
Muscle weakness	13 (2.3)	6 (2.4)	7 (2.3)	7 (3.1)	6 (1.8)
Xerostomia	5 (0.9)	2 (0.8)	3 (1.0)	1 (0.4)	4 (1.2)
Other adverse effects[b]	64 (11.4)	29 (11.5)	35 (11.4)	27 (12.0)	37 (11.1)

n number, *BPAD* bipolar affective disorder, *SZD* schizoaffective disorder, *Other* unspecified or otherwise specified bipolar affective disorder, *DI* diabetes insipidus
[a]$n = 559$, data missing in 2 (0.4%) episodes; [b]frequency less than five episodes; [c]i.e. comorbidities as dementia, chronic heart failure, cancer, non-lithium related chronic kidney disease, $^{*}p < 0.05$, $^{**}p < 0.01$, $^{***}p < 0.001$

reasons. More men stopped because they felt well. Also, they were less likely to speak to a doctor before ceasing medication. This suggests that clinicians need to engage more actively with men. Subjective well-being, although being desirable, may increase the risk of treatment discontinuation. Strategies, such as shared decision-making (SDM) [18, 19], motivational interviewing, psychoeducation and involvement of relatives [7, 20], dedicated mood disorder clinics [7], taking account of executive function in older patients [21], or offering financial incentives for patients with psychotic disorders [22], may improve adherence. However, we do not know how well such strategies work specifically in the context of lithium treatment. Neither do we know how far such strategies can help patients to cope with adverse effects of their treatment.

Women were more likely to stop lithium for fear of weight gain. Women may be more susceptible to changes in body image and pressures of social norms that can make lithium mediated weight gain unacceptable [23, 24]. This finding is in line with a study by Kriegshauser et al. 2010 [25]. In that study, men and women had the same risk of weight gain. Yet, women were twice as likely to regard weight gain as the worst of all adverse effects. Interventions could target the underlying aetiology. For instance, lithium associated weight gain could be secondary to hypothyroidism. This underlines the importance of regular thyroid function tests. Polyuria, leading to polydipsia, leading to an increased intake of high caloric sugary drinks is another potential cause. When thinking diet, patients and doctors alike may focus on foods rather than drinks. Yet, sugar-sweetened drinks, such as soft drinks *and* juices, are a major contributor to obesity world-wide [26]. Finally, lithium may also have direct weight increasing properties. As demonstrated in animal experiments, lithium can increase the expression of melanin concentrating hormone (MCH), a powerful orexic peptide [27]. Women were also more likely to discontinue lithium because of oedema. Such may occur due to higher oestrogen

Table 3 Top 10 reasons for lithium discontinuation in relation to duration to lithium treatment ($n = 371$)[a]

		n (%)	Lead time to lithium discontinuation	
			Years, mean (SD)	Years, median (min-max)
1.	Perceived or actual lack of effectiveness	90 (24.6)	2.3 (4.9)	1.1 (0.04-39.9)
2.	Non-adherence	85 (22.4)	2.9 (3.6)	1.2 (0.1-15.0)
3.	Diarrhoea	49 (13.2)	1.6 (2.2)	0.7 (0.02-10.5)
4.	Tremor	45 (12.1)	3.7 (5.4)	1.6 (0.02-23.3)
5.	Weight gain	35 (9.4)	2.6 (3.3)	1.3 (0.1-12.9)
6.	Nephrogenic diabetes insipidus, polyuria, polydipsia	32 (8.6)	4.8 (5.5)	2.7 (0.1-20.6)
7.	Emotional blunting	24 (6.5)	2.2 (1.9)	1.8 (0.1-6.4)
8.	Fatigue	22 (5.9)	2.6 (4.8)	0.4 (0.02-17.3)
9.	Nausea	21 (5.7)	0.5 (0.5)	0.3 (0.02-1.6)
10.	Creatinine increase, Li-nephropathy	20 (5.4)	17.2 (11.2)	17.0 (0.1-38.8)

n number, *SD* standard deviation
[a]Sub-analysis of 371 patients

levels in women, which could promote water retention in body tissues [28].

Type of disorder

Patients with type 1 BPAD or SZD were more likely not to accept lithium treatment in the first place, whereas patients with type 2 or unspecified BPAD discontinued lithium treatment due to lack of perceived effectiveness. This calls for a further evaluation of the role of lithium maintenance treatment for type 2 BPAD. Concerns about renal function and creatinine increases led more frequently to lithium discontinuation in patients with type 1 BPAD or SZD. Patients with type 2 or unspecified BPAD may be more likely to discontinue earlier because they seem to have less therapeutic benefit. Thus, they may be less likely to accrue sufficiently long lithium exposure for clinically significant glomerular impairment to develop.

Agent who took the initiative to discontinue lithium

Unsurprisingly, patients were more likely to discontinue lithium when lacking insight or not wanting to take medication. Significantly more patients with type 1 BPAD or SZD discontinued lithium. This may reflect a greater loss of function leading to lower adherence. Equally, doctors may be more likely to prescribe lithium to patients with type 1 BPAD or SZD. In this patient group, doctors may be particularly concerned about the risk of recurrence and suicide and hence more likely to disregard patients' concerns about adverse effects. They may also be less likely to inform these patients about potential adverse effects due to fear that this may decrease adherence.

Regarding adverse effects, emotional blunting and diarrhoea were greater concerns for patients. Doctors were more likely to discontinue lithium for fear of intoxications. Yet, lithium intoxications are relatively rare events, which can be safely managed in most cases [29]. Doctors were also more likely to stop lithium due to decreases in glomerular function. But even in many patients with a decrease in glomerular function, lithium can be continued, since the risk of suicide and recurrence of an acute manic or depressive episode tends to outweigh the risk of end-stage renal disease [1, 9, 10, 30, 31]. In any case, it has been suggested that renal function declines irrespective of lithium discontinuation – albeit slowly and after decades of treatment [16]. If this suggestion was confirmed, lithium discontinuation would be of no benefit at all.

Length of time adverse effects are coped with

Our results suggest that some patients tried to cope with diarrhoea and polyuria over long periods of time, before they discontinued. As such adverse effects are perceived as stigmatising, patients may not bring them up. The same applies for side effects concerning sexual dysfunction, which in our study, only very few patients reported. Doctors may underestimate the personal significance of such adverse effects. The impact of adverse effects on quality of life of patients treated with lithium has not been studied [8]. Particularly polyuria and diabetes insipidus can become disabling, making patients virtually house-bound in extreme cases. Schou et al. considered nausea an early adverse event that became less common after long-term lithium use [32]. But our findings suggest that waiting for nausea to pass is not an option for most patients. Tremor is another adverse effect thought to improve over time [8]. However, our study does not confirm this assumption. Patients stayed on lithium for an average of four years before they discontinued lithium due to tremor.

Strengths

Register studies have access to large sample sizes with little detailed clinical information. Conversely, clinical studies have access to detailed clinical information, but samples sizes tend to be small. In our study, we combined the best of both worlds, a large sample size and detailed clinical information. Thus, we established lithium treatment status, not only by prescription but also by lithium serum levels and information recorded in the medical notes. We were also able to validate diagnoses from the case records and distinguish between the various types of BPAD. All reasons for lithium were assessed by two separate reviewers to minimize observer bias. Our long follow-up time allowed to take account both, adverse effects occurring early and late during lithium treatment. A further strength was the high rate of consent for participation into the study. As age and sex distribution of consenting or not consenting patients was similar, the likelihood of selection bias was low.

Limitations

Our study was retrospective and observational in nature. Hence, the quality of our data depended on the quality of the information recorded in the medical notes. Doctors may record selectively problems they find most relevant. This could lead to an underestimation of patients' concerns. Besides, most patients have contact with more than one health professional, each of whom may focus on different issues.

Compared to retrospective observational studies, prospective studies run a higher risk that the very act of observation modifies the outcome under study. As described above, we took extensive measures to ensure that the data abstracted from the clinical notes was correct. Lithium discontinuation can be difficult to define in terms of time frames. Some patients may discontinue lithium nearly immediately after initiation. Others may have longer periods of lithium interruption due to physical illness, but finally resume treatment. Therefore, we considered lithium to be truly discontinued, when there was a stated intention to discontinue for good. Some patients had episodes of lithium treatment before our observation period began. Thus, it was possible to misclassify adverse effects as occurring early, when in fact they occurred late. For avoiding such misclassification, we needed to avoid missing such prior episodes of lithium discontinuation. For this analysis, we only included a subset of patients. For this subset, we could establish that patients had not had any episodes of lithium treatment that could potentially have gone unnoticed.

Conclusions

With the mortality gap between individuals with bipolar affective disorder and the general population widening [33], we need to understand why patients and doctors discontinue lithium. It is important that patients who may benefit from lithium can continue to take it, striking the right balance between benefits and risks [9, 10]. Particularly men may require proactive follow-up since they may be more likely not to consult with their doctor before discontinuing treatment. Understanding the reasons why patients and doctors discontinue lithium can assist us to develop strategies to improve adherence. In this context, management of adverse effects plays a major role. Our results show that regular monitoring of laboratory parameters is necessary but not sufficient to manage adverse effects. Regular blood tests are no substitute for regular personal follow-up. Adverse effects such as diarrhoea and polyuria substantially impair quality of life, which must not be ignored. Unnecessary termination of treatment could possibly be avoided if patient received comprehensive information about their pharmacological treatment at an appropriate time. Being responsive to patients' concerns and needs may substantially improve treatment adherence [34] Shared decision making (SDM), which has already been tested in primary care and psychiatric settings, may be a way forward [18, 19]. Finally, close collaboration between psychiatric and internal medicine/nephrology service is imperative to minimize discontinuation of lithium in patients who have capacity to benefit.

Abbreviations

ANOVA: Analysis of variance; BALANCE trial: Bipolar Affective Disorder: Lithium/ Anticonvulsant Evaluation trial; BPAD: Bipolar affective disorder; i.e: id est; Li: Lithium; LISIE study: Lithium Effects and Side Effects study; MCH: Melanin concentrating hormone; n: Number; Nephrogenic DI: Nephrogenic diabetes insipidus; NICE: the UK National Institute for Clinical Excellence; SD: Standard deviation; SDM: Shared decision-making; SZD: Schizoaffective disorder

Acknowledgements

We wish to thank Amanda Keinström Sihvonen, Sofia Månsson and Nazanin Shayeghi for their help with the validation of the clinical information, and Annika Essner, Anna Granberg, Annika Johansson, Ulrika Lundmark, Anna Nyberg, Eva Lång Rhyn for their help with assistance in conduct of the study.

Funding

This work was supported by a grant of the Research & Development Fund of Norrbotten Region, Research and Innovation Unit, Sweden.

Authors' contributions

UW, MO and LÖ conceptualized the initial study design and developed the initial draft of the manuscript. UW, MO, LÖ, RL, MS and ESR provided constructive feedback on the initial study design. LÖ, SO, MB, MO, and UW extracted the clinical data. LÖ, MO, RL and UW analysed the data. All authors interpreted the data, provided constructive feedback during manuscript development, and read and approved the final manuscript.

Consent for publication

Not applicable.

Competing interests

Ursula Werneke has received funding for educational activities on behalf of Norrbotten Region (Masterclass Psychiatry Programme, EAPM 2016 Luleå, Sweden): Astra Zeneca, Janssen, Eli Lilly, Novartis, Otsuka/Lundbeck, Servier, Sunivion and Shire.
Louise Öhlund, Michael Ott, Sofia Oja, Malin Bergqvist, Robert Lundqvist, Mikael Sandlund and Ellinor Salander Renberg declare that there is no conflict of interest.

Author details

[1]Sunderby Research Unit, Department of Clinical Sciences, Division of Psychiatry, Umeå University, Umeå, Sweden. [2]Department of Public Health and Clinical Medicine, Division of Medicine, Umeå University, Umeå, Sweden. [3]Department of Psychiatry, Sunderby Hospital, Luleå, Sweden. [4]Department of Psychiatry, Piteå Älvdals Hospital, Piteå, Sweden. [5]Research and Innovation Unit, Luleå, Norrbotten Region, Sweden. [6]Department of Clinical Science, Division of Psychiatry, Umeå University, Umeå, Sweden. [7]Sunderby Hospital – Psychiatry, 97180 Luleå, Sweden.

References

1. BALANCE investigators. Lithium plus valproate combination therapy versus monotherapy for relapse prevention in bipolar I disorder (BALANCE): a randomised open-label trial. Lancet. 2010;375:385–95.
2. NICE (2014). 2016. Bipolar disorder: assessment and management. Clinical guideline 185. London, UK: National Institute for Health and Care Excellence. Available at: https://www.nice.org.uk/guidance/cg185 (Accessed 6 Oct 2017).
3. Hayes JF, Pitman A, Marston L, Walters K, Geddes JR, King M, et al. Self-harm, unintentional injury, and suicide in bipolar disorder during maintenance mood stabilizer treatment: a UK population-based electronic health records study. JAMA Psychiat. 2016;73:630–7.
4. Joas E, Karanti A, Song J, Goodwin GM, Lichtenstein P, Landén M. Pharmacological treatment and risk of psychiatric hospital admission in bipolar disorder. Br J Psychiatry. 2017;210:197–202.
5. Baldessarini RJ, Tondo L, Viguera AC. Discontinuing lithium maintenance treatment in bipolar disorders: risks and implications. Bipolar Disord. 1999;1:17–24.
6. Perlick D, Rosenheck R, Kaczynski R, Kozma L. Medication non-adherence in bipolar disorder: a patient-centered review of research findings. Clin Approach Bipolar Disord. 2004;3:56–64.
7. Rosa AR, Marco M, Fachel JM, Kapczinski F, Stein AT, Barros HM. Correlation between drug treatment adherence and lithium treatment attitudes and knowledge by bipolar patients. Prog Neuropsychopharmacol Biol Psychiatry. 2007;31:217–24.

8. Gitlin M. Lithium Side effects and toxicity: prevalence and management strategies. Int J Bipolar Disord. 2016;4:27.
9. Werneke U, Ott M, Renberg ES, Taylor D, Stegmayr B. A decision analysis of long-term lithium treatment and the risk of renal failure. Acta Psychiatr Scand. 2012;126:186–97.
10. Kessing L, Feldt-Rasmussen B, Andersen P, Gerds T, Licht R. Continuation of lithium after a diagnosis of chronic kidney disease. Acta Psychiatr Scand. 2017;136:615–22.
11. McCreadie RG, McCormick M, Morrison DP. The impact of lithium in South-West Scotland. III. The discontinuation of lithium. Br J Psychiatry. 1985;146:77–80.
12. Maarbjerg K, Aagaard J, Vestergaard P. Adherence to lithium prophylaxis: I. Clinical predictors and patient's reasons for nonadherence. Pharmacopsychiatry. 1988;21:121–5.
13. Nilsson A, Axelsson R. Factors associated with discontinuation of long-term lithium treatment. Acta Psychiatr Scand. 1989;80:221–30.
14. Schumann C, Lenz G, Berghöfer A, Müller-Oerlinghausen B. Non-adherence with long-term prophylaxis: a 6-year naturalistic follow-up study of affectively ill patients. Psychiatry Res. 1999;89:247–57.
15. Bendz H, Schön S, Attman P, Aurell M. Renal failure occurs in chronic lithium treatment but is uncommon. Kidney Int. 2010;77:219–24.
16. Bocchetta A, Ardau R, Fanni T, Sardu C, Piras D, Pani A, et al. Renal function during long-term lithium treatment: a cross-sectional and longitudinal study. BMC Med. 2015;13:12.
17. McKnight RF, Adida M, Budge K, Stockton S, Goodwin GM, Geddes JR. Lithium toxicity profile: a systematic review and meta-analysis. Lancet. 2012; 379:721–8.
18. Hamann J, Leucht S, Kissling W. Shared decision making in psychiatry. Acta Psychiatr Scand. 2003;107:403–9.
19. Elwyn G, Frosch D, Thomson R, Joseph-Williams N, Lloyd A, Kinnersley P, et al. Shared decision making: a model for clinical practice. J Gen Intern Med. 2012;27:1361–7.
20. Pakpour AH, Modabbernia A, Lin C, Saffari M, Asl MA, Webb T. Promoting medication adherence among patients with bipolar disorder: a multicenter randomized controlled trial of a multifaceted intervention. Psychol Med. 2017;47:2528–39.
21. Corréard N, Consoloni J, Raust A, Etain B, Guillot R, Job S, et al. Neuropsychological functioning, age, and medication adherence in bipolar disorder. PLoS One. 2017;12:e0184313.
22. Priebe S, Yeeles K, Bremner S, Lauber C, Eldridge S, Ashby D, et al. Effectiveness of financial incentives to improve adherence to maintenance treatment with antipsychotics: cluster randomised controlled trial. BMJ. 2013;347:f5847.
23. Owens TE, Allen MD, Spangler DL. An fMRI study of self-reflection about body image: sex differences. Personal Individ Differ. 2010;48:849–54.
24. Helfert S, Warschburger P. The face of appearance-related social pressure: gender, age and body mass variations in peer and parental pressure during adolescence. Child Adolesc Psychiatr Ment Health. 2013;7:16.
25. Kriegshauser K, Sajatovic M, Jenkins JH, Cassidy KA, Muzina D, Fattal O, et al. Gender differences in subjective experience and treatment of bipolar disorder. J Nerv Ment Dis. 2010;198:370–2.
26. Werneke U, Taylor D, Sanders TA. Behavioral interventions for antipsychotic induced appetite changes. Curr Psychiatry Rep. 2013;15:347.
27. Presse F, Cardona B, Borsu L, Nahon J. Lithium increases melanin-concentrating hormone mRNA stability and inhibits tyrosine hydroxylase gene expression in PC12 cells. Mol Brain Res. 1997;52:270–83.
28. Stachenfeld NS, Taylor HS, Leone CA, Keefe DL. Oestrogen effects on urine concentrating response in young women. J Physiol (Lond). 2003;552:869–80.
29. Ott M, Stegmayr B, Salander Renberg E, Werneke U. Lithium intoxication: incidence, clinical course and renal function–a population-based retrospective cohort study. J Psychopharmacol. 2016;30:1008–19.
30. Kessing LV, Gerds TA, Feldt-Rasmussen B, Andersen PK, Licht RW. Use of lithium and anticonvulsants and the rate of chronic kidney disease: a nationwide population-based study. JAMA Psychiat. 2015;72:1182–91.
31. Song J, Sjölander A, Joas E, Bergen SE, Runeson B, Larsson H, et al. Suicidal behavior during lithium and Valproate treatment: a within-individual 8-year prospective study of 50,000 patients with bipolar disorder. Am J Psychiatry. 2017;174:795–802.
32. Schou M, Baastrup PC, Grof P, Weis P, Angst J. Pharmacological and clinical problems of lithium prophylaxis. Br J Psychiatry. 1970;116:615–9.
33. Hayes JF, Marston L, Walters K, King MB, Osborn DPJ. Mortality gap for people with bipolar disorder and schizophrenia: UK-based cohort study 2000-2014. Br J Psychiatry. 2017;211:175–81.
34. Kraemer S, Minarzyk A, Eppendorfer S, Henneges C, Hundemer H, Wilhelm S, et al. Comparably high retention and low relapse rates in different subpopulations of bipolar patients in a German non-interventional study. BMC Psychiatry. 2013;13:193.

18

Understanding the emotions of patients with inadequate response to antidepressant treatments: results of an international online survey in patients with major depressive disorder

Rajnish Mago[1*], Andrea Fagiolini[2], Emmanuelle Weiller[3] and Catherine Weiss[4]

Abstract

Background: Evidence suggests that nearly half of patients with major depressive disorder (MDD) do not achieve an adequate response to antidepressant treatments (ADTs), which impacts patients' functioning, quality of life (QoL), and well-being. This patient survey aimed to better understand patient perspectives on the emotional impact of experiencing an inadequate response to ADTs.

Methods: An online survey was conducted in 6 countries with respondents diagnosed with MDD and experiencing an inadequate response to ADTs. The survey was designed to explore how patients felt about their medications and health care provider (HCP). Those indicating they were 'frustrated' with their medications and/or HCP were asked to provide reasons for their frustration and its impact on their relationship with their HCP and decisions about their treatment.

Results: Overall, 2096 respondents with MDD and inadequate response to ADT completed the survey. The most frequent emotion reported by patients regarding their medication was frustration (29.8% of respondents) followed by hopeless (27.4%) and apprehensive/anxious/scared (27.4%). Regarding their HCP, patients reported feeling understood (31.6%) and trusting/confident (28.8%) most often; however, 19.2% reported feelings of frustration. Main reasons for frustration with medication were poor symptom control/lack of efficacy (59.3%) and tolerability issues (19.7%), and the main reasons for frustration with their HCP were not feeling heard (22.4%), ineffective treatment (13.5%) and feeling rushed/lack of quality visit (12.5%). The longer the current episode duration and the greater the disruption to daily living, the more likely the respondents experienced feelings of frustration with medication. Feelings of frustration lead to adherence issues, with 33.3 and 27.3% of respondents indicating their frustration with their medication and HCP, respectively, made them want to quit their medication. Approximately one in six patients frustrated with either their medication and/or HCP indicated their frustration had resulted in them not taking their medication regularly. Frustration with their HCP also impacted patient's confidence in HCPs abilities (34.7%), sharing less information with their HCP (28.9%) as well as missing appointments (17.4%) and medications (14.5%).

Conclusions: Feelings of frustration are frequent in patients with inadequate response to ADT and this frustration may impact treatment adherence and the patient-HCP relationship.

Keywords: Major depressive disorder, Inadequate response to ADTs, Frustration, Patient survey

* Correspondence: mago@simpleandpractical.com
[1]Simple and Practical Mental Health, Philadelphia, PA, USA
Full list of author information is available at the end of the article

Background

The treatment of major depressive disorder (MDD) has progressed over the past several decades with greater awareness and understanding of the disease, better diagnosis, and medications with improved tolerability. However, despite the treatment advances and availability of multiple antidepressant classes/medications, approximately 50% of patients with MDD do not achieve an adequate response to antidepressant treatment (ADT) [1–3], as defined by a failure to achieve a response (50% or greater reduction in the severity of the depression) after treatment with an antidepressant at an adequate dose and duration (i.e., at least 6–8 weeks) [4]. From the patient perspective, people with MDD want their treatment to help them return to their usual level of functioning, return to their 'usual self' and to regain optimism and self-confidence [5].

Patients with inadequate response to ADT experience significant impairments in social functioning and often fail to regain a normal quality of life [6]. Work productivity loss of those employed and higher unemployment, along with higher emergency room utilization and hospitalization are also associated with an inadequate response to ADT [7]. Timely and effective treatment is important to prevent the long-term consequences of prolonged inadequately-treated MDD [2].

While the personal burden of an inadequate response can be significant and wide-ranging [8], little is known on the emotional impact of inadequate response to ADT. This survey set out to better understand the patient perspective on the emotional impact of experiencing an inadequate response to ADTs.

Specifically, the survey was designed to assess how frequently different emotions were reported in people with MDD experiencing an inadequate response to ADT, including the frequency of feelings of frustration with medication and their HCP. For those respondents who reported feeling frustrated with their medication and/or HCP, we sought to understand the reasons for their frustration and the impact this frustration had on their behavior.

Methods

Survey design and respondent criteria

This survey was conducted in the United States, Canada, UK, Germany, France, and Spain between 15 March and 16 June, 2016. Respondents were recruited using consumer panels where all panelists have provided consent to participate in research. An online questionnaire was used to screen respondents and collect quantitative data. Access to the survey was secure, ensuring the anonymity of respondents.

All respondents were eligible for the survey if they met the following criteria: age 18 to 65 years, diagnosed with depression by a healthcare professional; no comorbid diagnoses of bipolar disorder, schizoaffective disorder, or schizophrenia; experiencing symptoms of depression most of the time over the past week; their depression has a moderate to extreme impact on overall functioning as measured by the Sheehan Disability Scale (SDS) [9]; has a psychiatrist or primary care physician (or, in the US, a nurse practitioner or physician assistant) who is primarily responsible for their treatment; currently on an ADT for at least 6 weeks at an adequate dose (see Appendix); they felt that their depression has not improved or only a little since the onset of the current episode (as measured by the Patient Global Impression of Improvement (PGI-I), and, finally, not working for a biasing employer (advertising agency or marketing research company or a company that manufactures, distributes or sells pharmaceuticals or health care products). Finally, per pharmacovigilance compliance regulations, all eligible respondents were required to provide consent for disclosure of any adverse-events reported within their responses.

Defining an "inadequate response" to ADT

Eligible survey participants all suffered from MDD with a current episode having moderate to extreme impact on overall functioning as measured by SDS, and to be on at least one ADT at an adequate dose for at least 6 weeks. Participants were considered as having an inadequate response to their current ADT if they indicated that their current symptoms had little to no improvement (based on the 7-item PGI-C, ranging from very much worse to very much improved).

Assessments

The survey was conducted as an online 20-min questionnaire. All data collected was self-reported by participants and included both close-ended and open questions on the following topics: history of depression (onset of first episode, number of lifetime episodes, length of current episode), treatment history (hospitalizations, psychotherapy, treatment received for current episode, reason for discontinuation); change on current treatment (patients' global impression of change, PGI-C), current symptoms of depression, other current symptoms, impact of depression on functioning (SDS), treatment goals, emotional feelings about their experience with medication, healthcare providers and overall healthcare system, including feelings of frustration, intensity of frustration and reasons for feeling frustrated. Here we present the results pertaining to their feeling towards medication and HCP.

Current symptoms of depression were assessed using a modified version of the Patient Health Questionnaire (PHQ-9) [10], excluding the question about suicidal ideation. The scale was the standard PHQ-9 where 0 = Not at all, 1 = Several days, 2 = More than half of the days and 3 = Nearly every day. Other (non-PHQ-9) current symptoms were elicited from a check list of clinical symptoms associated with depression (see list in Fig. 1). The lists of emotional feelings regarding their treatment and HCP, included in the survey were created using direct patient input from qualitative interviews conducted during the survey development (not shown). Reasons for frustration were asked using a voluntary open-end format and responses were manually coded. Coded responses were validated by a second coder and quality checked by a research analyst. A list of consequences of frustration was also included in the survey based on patient and physician input during pre-survey qualitative interviews. To gauge the patient's perception on the overall level of impairment caused by their depression, the survey included the additional PHQ item 10 "*How difficult have these problems made it for you to do your work, take care of things at home, or get along with other people?*", where the scale included was 1 = Not difficult at all, 2 = Somewhat difficult 3 = Very difficult and 4 = Extremely difficult.

Statistical analyses

Descriptive statistics included means and frequency of responses (%). A driver analyses was conducted using random forest analysis [11]. A random forest is a method where many decision trees (500 in our analysis) are constructed. The analysis selects a random sample of cases as the training set for each tree, and at each potential branching of the tree, a random subset of variables is evaluated as potential splits. The output of a random forest analysis provides ratio-level data of the influence that each characteristic has on the presence of dependent variable. Higher scores mean that, on average, the nodes created when the tree splits on this variable are more homogenous than nodes created by splitting on variables with lower scores – in other words they are considered more important. Patient characteristics entered as independent variables into the analysis included time since first episode, past hospitalization, past psychotherapy, number of episodes experienced, length of current episode, number of ADT failures, current treatment of monotherapy vs. combination therapy, change on current treatment (PGI-C), level of impairment (PHQ item 10) and disruption of daily living (SDS mean score). The dependent variable was the presence of moderate-to-severe frustration with their treatment. The random forest analysis was performed using the "randomForest" statistical package in R. Validity testing was done using a logistic regression to determine the explanatory power of the entered predictors.

Results

Respondent characteristics

A total of 18,083 adult (age 18–65) respondents diagnosed with MDD by a health care professional with no comorbid diagnoses of Bipolar Disorder, Schizoaffective or Schizophrenia were identified through our screening process using consumer panels (Fig. 1). Of the respondents with MDD, 11,466 were currently suffering from symptoms of depression and 93.5% of these (10,715) had at least a moderate impact on functioning. Approximately 56.3% (n = 6037)

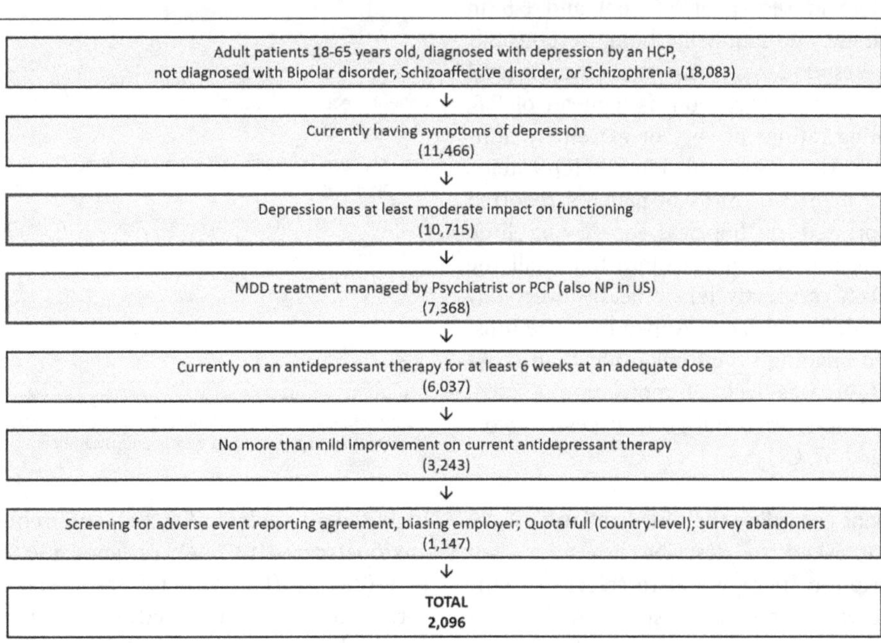

Fig. 1 Screening disposition for participation in online patient survey

were being treated with an adequate dose of ADT for at least six weeks under the supervision of a psychiatrist, primary care physician (or nurse practitioner in the US). Of those adequately treated, 54% (3243) were experiencing an inadequate response to ADT. Finally, with drop-outs and quota caps at a country level, a total of 2096 respondents with inadequate response to ADT, completed the survey from six countries. These included the US (597, 28.5%), Canada (301, 14.4%), UK (300, 14.4%), Germany (299, 14.3%), France (299, 14.3%) and Spain (300, 14.4%).

The mean age of our survey respondents was 42.1 years and 56.7% were female (Table 1). While more than half of the respondents were working, 10% were on sick-leave or disability due to depression. The mean duration since onset of first episode was 10.5 years. Most respondents (91.1%) had suffered recurrent episodes and 39.6% had experienced over 10 episodes of depression. A third (34%) had been hospitalized for depression and 79% had received psychotherapy at some point.

Per the screening requirements, all respondents were suffering from a current episode of depression. Just over half (51.7%) had been experiencing their current episode of depression for a year or less. Just over a third (38.1%) were taking combination ADT (at least two classes), and 16.4% were taking an adjunctive antipsychotic (AP).

Despite ongoing AD treatment, nearly a quarter of patients (23.7%) indicated their depression had gotten worse since the onset of their current episode, while another 20.4% indicated no change, 48.7% indicated minimal improvement, and only 7.2% indicated moderate-great improvement (PGI-C). The SDS mean score was 6.9, with mean domain scores of 7.5, 6.9 and 6.5 in work/school, social life, and family life/home responsibilities, respectively. Respondents' rated their overall level of impairment caused by depression as a mean of 2.8, with 60.6% indicating ratings of very or extremely difficult (PHQ item 10). Analysis of individual PHQ-9 items revealed that more than two-thirds of patients reported feeling down, depressed or hopeless, or having little interest or pleasure in doing things more than half the days (33.3 and 30.6%, respectively) or nearly every day (36.5 and 38.0%) (Additional file 1: Appendix). The most frequently reported ongoing symptoms other than those measured by PHQ-9, was lack of motivation (77.2%) followed by anxiousness, irritability and excessive worries, (67.1%, 58.1 and 57.4%).

Table 1 Demographic and clinical characteristics of respondents ($n = 2096$)

CHARACTERISTIC	$N = 2096$
Age; mean (years)	42.1
Gender; n (%) female	1188 (56.7)
Employment status; n (%)	
Working full/part time	923 (44.0)
Working, but currently on a sick leave/disability due to depression	219 (10.4)
Working, but currently on a sick leave/disability for another reason	80 (3.8)
Unemployed	308 (14.7)
Retired	184 (8.8)
Student	80 (3.8)
Homemaker	170 (8.1)
Other	132 (6.3)
Time since first episode; mean (years)	10.5
Number of total episodes; n (%) of respondents	
1	186 (8.9)
2–5	564 (26.9)
6–10	328 (15.6)
> 10	829 (39.6)
Don't know	189 (9.0)
Recurrent episodes; n (%) of respondents	1721 (91.1)
Ever hospitalized for their depression; n (%) of respondents	713 (34.0)
Ever had psychotherapy; n (%) of respondents	1655 (79.0)
Duration of current episode; n (%) of respondents	
0–6 months	766 (36.5)
7–12 months	319 (15.2)
2–5 years*	457 (21.8)
> 5 years*	554 (26.4)
Patients receiving two or more classes of ADT; n (%) of respondents	799 (38.1)
Patients receiving adjunctive antipsychotic**; n (%) of respondents	345 (16.4)
Number of ADT failures in current episode; n (%) of respondents	
1	361 (17.2)
2	722 (34.4)
3+	1013 (48.3)

*Patients may have difficulties remembering symptom-free periods in between 2 episodes, leading to report of long lasting single episodes
**includes both atypical and typical antipsychotics

Respondent emotions regarding their medication

Respondents were asked to describe how they felt about their prescription therapy and to select as many feelings that were relevant to their situation. Frustration was the emotion selected most often (29.8%) by respondents. Other emotions most often cited included, hopeless (27.4%), apprehensive/ nervous/ anxious/scared (27.4%), resigned (26.9%), and dissatisfied (25.4%) (Fig. 2a). Of the respondents that indicated they were frustrated with their treatment, 85.9% rated their frustration as being moderate-to-severe (Fig. 2b). In addition, these respondents reported high

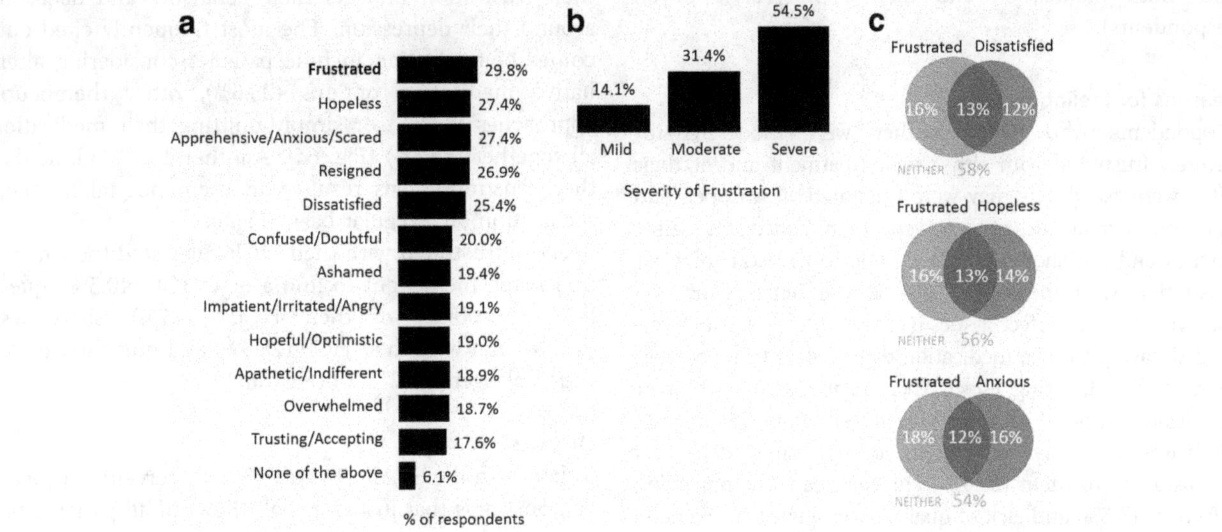

Fig. 2 Respondent emotions regarding their medication (**a**) survey population ($n = 2096$), (**b**) severity of frustration when reported ($n = 536$), (**c**) overlap of frustration with hopelessness, anxiousness and dissatisfaction

levels of concomitant hopelessness (44.8% of those frustrated), anxiousness (48.2%) and dissatisfaction (44.8%) (Fig. 2c).

Respondent emotions regarding their HCP

Patients with an inadequate response to their ADT were also asked how they felt about their HCP by selecting as many feelings that were relevant to their situation. The two most frequently chosen emotions were 'feeling understood' (31.6%) and 'trusting/confident' (28.8%). However, 19.2% of respondents reported frustration (Fig. 3a). Of those indicating they were frustrated with their HCP, 78% rated their frustration as being moderate-to-severe (Fig. 3b). Finally, of the 38.0% of patients who reported being frustrated with medication and/or their HCP, nearly a third reported frustration

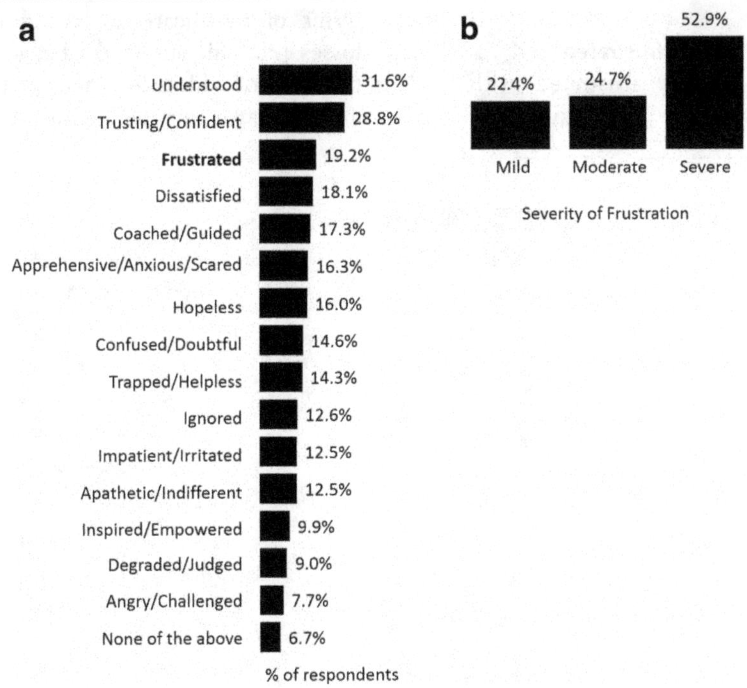

Fig. 3 Respondent emotions regarding their HCP (**a**) survey population ($n = 2096$), (**b**) severity of frustration when reported ($n = 311$)

with both medication and their HCP (10.9% of all respondents).

Reasons for feeling frustrated

Respondents who indicated they were moderately-to-severely frustrated with either their treatment and/or their HCP were asked why they were frustrated via an open-end question format. Responses were then coded for select themes and are shown in Fig. 4. The top reason for their frustration with medication was lack of efficacy (59.3%) followed by side-effect issues (19.7%). Other reasons included having to take medication daily, failing to meet their expectations, tapering effect, their relationship with their physician and onset of action (Fig. 4). Frustration with their HCP was driven by respondents feeling dismissed/HCP is not listening to them (22.4%), current treatment not being effective (13.5%) and lack of quality time spent with patient/too rushed (12.5%) among other reasons shown in Fig. 4b.

Clinical characteristics associated with higher frequency of frustration

Random forest analyses indicated that for both frustration with medication and frustration with HCP the three largest drivers of frustration, of those entered in the model, were length of current episode, time since first episode and impact on function (SDS). Further, these three were twice as important as PGI-C and number of treatment failures (Fig. 5). The validity results however yielded a very small effect (Nagelkerke R-square = 0.074 for medication and 0.087 for HCP).

Consequences/impact of feeling frustrated

Patients moderately-to-severely frustrated with their treatment for depression were asked to identify how their frustration impacts their behaviors and decisions around their depression. The most frequently cited outcomes of frustration include patients considering alternative medication options (35.5%), other therapeutic approaches (33.8%) or simply quitting their medication all together (33.3%) (Fig. 6a). Another 14.7% admit that their frustration has resulted in them not taking their medication on a regular basis (Fig. 6a).

Those frustrated with their HCP suggested the frustration made them want to find a new HCP (40.5%), question the ability of their HCP (34.7%), share less information with their HCP (28.9%) and quit their medication altogether (27.3%) (Fig. 6b).

Discussion

In line with the STAR*D study [3], our screening process demonstrates that just over half (54%) of all patients being treated for an ongoing episode of depression experience an inadequate response, and that this is associated with significant impairment in functioning (mean SDS score of 6.9). Beyond the presence of unresolved symptoms and impaired functioning, the results of this patient survey further suggest that an inadequate response to antidepressants may have other consequences that are important to consider as a healthcare provider.

It has been suggested that protracted depressive illness and treatment failure can lead to the erosion of critical social support, along with increased interpersonal, vocational and economic stress [12]. Studies have shown that having an inadequate response increases the duration of MDD and imposes a significant burden to society in terms of healthcare costs and workplace productivity losses [7]. This survey further supports the critical importance of addressing inadequate response in a timely and effective manner. Our results suggest that an

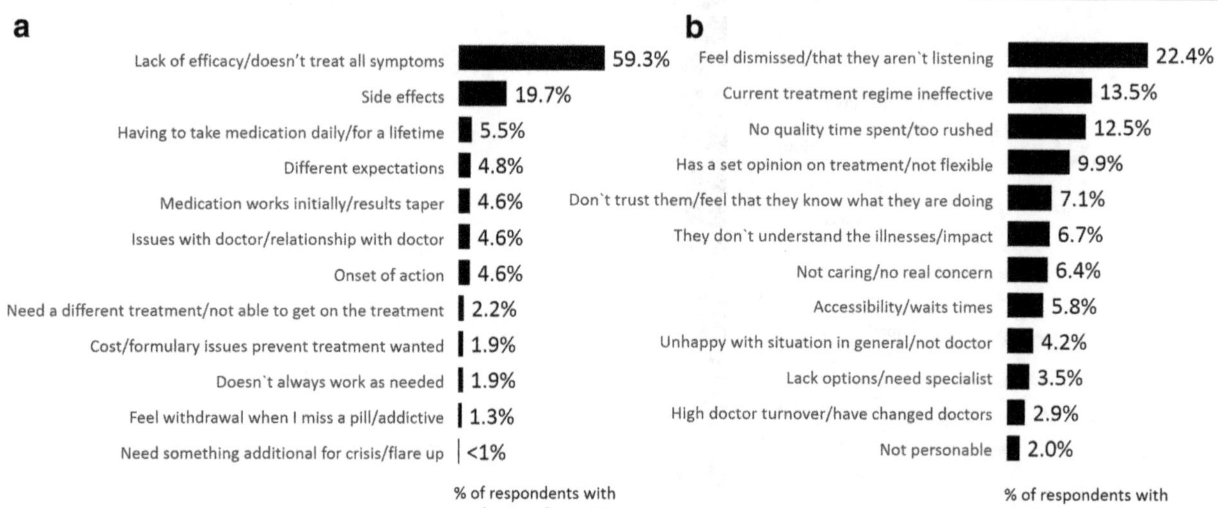

Fig. 4 Reasons for frustration with (**a**) medication ($n = 536$) and (**b**) HCP ($n = 311$)

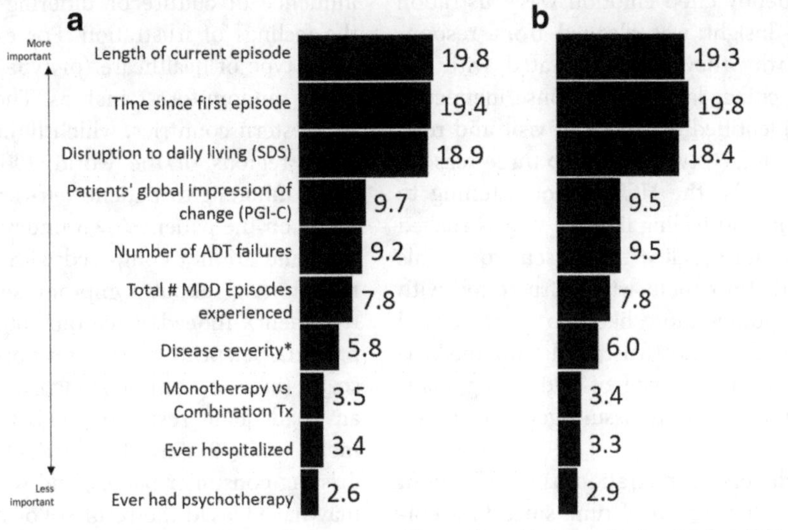

Fig. 5 Relative contribution of respondent characteristics on the presence of frustration with (**a**) medication (**b**) their HCP

inadequate response to antidepressants is often associated with negative emotions towards medication and HCP, including feelings of frustration, hopelessness and dissatisfaction. Frustration was the most frequently cited emotion regarding medication, with two in five patients indicating their frustration. The primary reasons for frustration with medication were directly related to the unresolved symptoms and side-effects of ADTs. A major finding of STAR*D was that likelihood of responding to a third or fourth step treatment after failing the initial two steps was < 20% [3]. Thus, the high levels of frustration with medication may reflect the fact that current treatment approaches/medications have not been effective, and that there is still an unmet need for treatments with an improved efficacy-tolerability profile.

In regards to HCPs, the most frequent emotions reported by respondents included two positive feelings of being understood, (31.6%) and confidence (28.8%), but

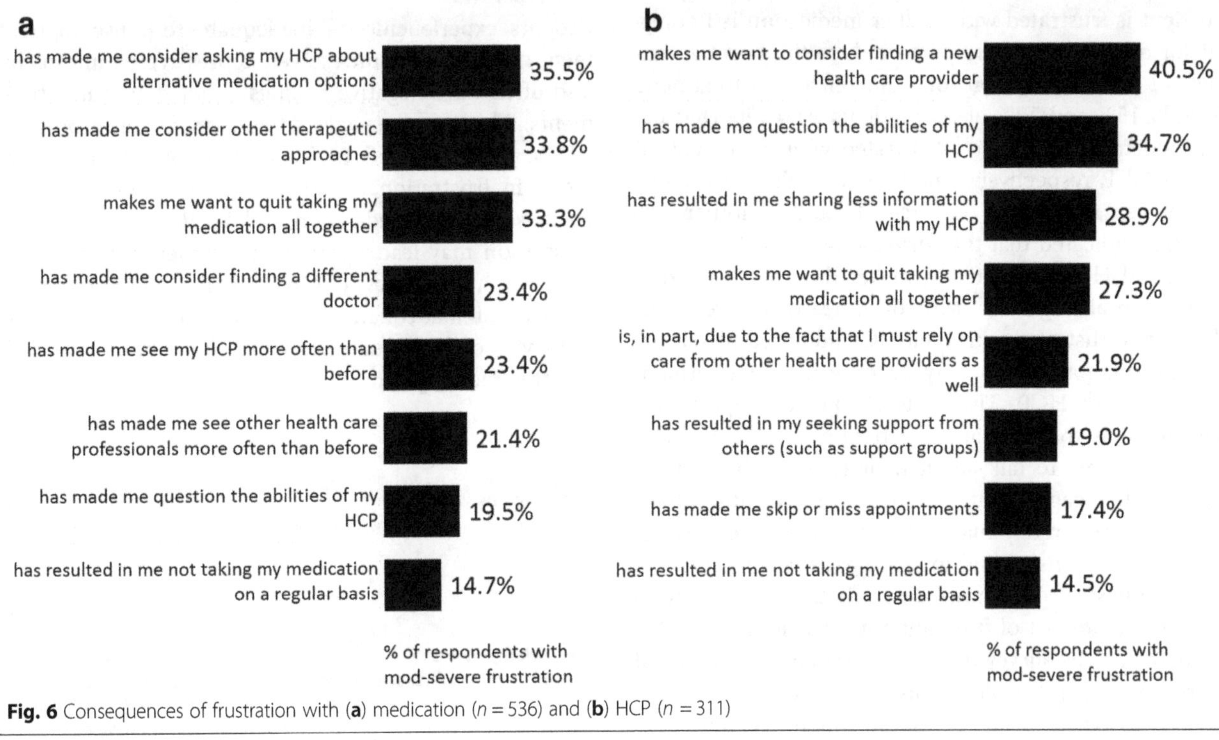

Fig. 6 Consequences of frustration with (**a**) medication ($n = 536$) and (**b**) HCP ($n = 311$)

the third most frequently cited emotion was frustration (19.2%). Interesting insight was gleaned from respondents when asked why they were frustrated with the HCP. Along with citing lack of response/ineffective treatment, patients identified dynamics of visit and relationship with HCPs. In fact, two of the top three reasons cited included feeling like the HCP is not listening to them/dismissing them and feeling like the visit is rushed and does not allow for quality time/discussion. This study also suggests that a patient who is frustrated with their medication is 4 times more likely to be frustrated with their HCP than those not frustrated with medication, underscoring the importance of addressing inadequate response to medication to assure good relations/collaboration.

Evaluation of the drivers of frustration using a random forest model showed that length of time since first episode, length of current episode and impact on functioning were the three highest predictors/drivers of frustration, both with medication and with HCP. However, it is important to remember that our explanation power, or lift in this case, is low suggesting there are many things influencing feelings of frustration that are not included in the model. For example, we observed that patients in France were less likely to report frustration with medication or HCPs than patients in the US, UK and Canada (data not shown). This may be due to cultural differences or differences in the healthcare system, but we were unable to explore this interesting observation within the limits of the survey design.

The results of this survey suggest that recognizing that a patient is frustrated with his/her medication is important for a timely intervention to reduce the negative impact of this frustration on adherence to treatment. Overall, 15% and 17% of respondents who reported being moderately-to-severely frustrated with their medication or HCP, respectively, said they have already stopped taking their medication on a regular basis. Another 33% and 27% indicated that their frustration with their medication and HCP, respectively, makes them want to "quit medication all together". Moreover, nearly a third (29%) of patients frustrated with their HCP admitted to sharing less information, which may be critical to a treatment approach with HCP. Thus, frustration may represent a warning sign that a change in treatment is warranted. Asking patients to talk about their feelings about treatment and engaging patients on communicating their frustration concretely may help strengthen the patient/physician relationship and improve patient outcomes.

To the best of our knowledge, it is the first survey to evaluate the impact of frustration in patients with MDD. Strengths of this survey include its size and international approach. While this allowed us to note some interesting differences between countries, we did not explore the influence of culture or differing healthcare systems on the feelings of frustration. For example, we did not include type of healthcare (or type of healthcare provider) in the random forest analysis. The survey was conducted in Western countries, which limits its generalizability to other regions of the world. Other limitations include those inherent to patient self-report surveys, which are based on the patient's own understanding of their condition, and are not compared with objective clinical information (e.g. about symptom severity, or response to treatment). Indeed, since our intent was to examine the patient perspective, we purposefully used subjective scales (instead of more standard clinical scales) to define an 'inadequate response' (PGI-C) and level of impairment (PHQ-9 item 10). Patients were recruited from existing consumer panels, and we do not know how this may have biased the results. For example, it may be that patients who are frustrated with their healthcare are more likely to respond to health surveys. Conversely, they could be less motivated to reply to the invitation.

In summary, this survey findings suggest that patients with prolonged disease (total or current episode), multiple treatment failures and impact on daily living may lead to feelings of frustration. In turn this frustration can lead to destructive behaviors such as non-compliance, mistrust of the HCP and patient's withholding information that may be relevant to treatment decisions.

Conclusions

Patients experiencing an inadequate response to treatment not only have unresolved depressive symptoms but also often have negative feelings about their failed treatments. This survey suggests that inadequate response to ADTs and continued trial-and-error of treatments can result in frustration, dissatisfaction, and other negative feelings towards medication and HCP. Since feelings of frustration may lead to adherence issues it is important that health care providers realize the emotional consequences of inadequate treatment and strive to reduce the levels of inadequate responses by exploring alternative treatment options.

Abbreviations

ADT: Antidepressant therapy; HCP: Healthcare professional; MDD: Major depressive disorder

Acknowledgements

The authors wish to thank all the respondents who kindly participated in the survey. In addition, we thank Alexandra Bonello and Katy Palmer of Market Strategies International (funded by H.Lundbeck A/S and Otsuka) for supporting the online survey and data collection. RM is Editor-in-Chief of Simple and Practical Mental Health and is a Clinical Assistant Professor of Psychiatry at the Perelman School of Medicine, University of Pennsylvania, Philadelphia, PA.

Funding

Medical writing support was provided by Katy Palmer, PhD of Market Strategies International and Anita Chadha-Patel, PhD of ACP Clinical Communications (funded by H.Lundbeck A/S and Otsuka). H.Lundbeck A/S and Otsuka supported the survey design, data collection and analysis and preparation of this report. The companies employed two of the authors (Emmanuelle Weiller and Catherine Weiss) who participated in interpretation of data and in writing the manuscript.

Authors' contributions

All authors conceptualized the survey and contributed to the interpretation of results and to the final version of the article. EW and CW wrote the first draft of the paper with direction from RM and AF. All authors read and approved the final manuscript.

Consent for publication

Not applicable.

Competing interests

RM reports that in the previous 12 months, he received research grants from Alkermes, Allergan, Genomind, Takeda. He has been a consultant for GuidePoint Global, Lundbeck, Neurocrine, and Otsuka. He has developed and delivered educational activities for PsychU, funded by Otsuka Pharmaceuticals. He receives book royalties from On Demand Publishing and Kindle Direct Publishing. AF reports that he is /has been a consultant and/or a speaker and/or has received research grants from Allergen, Angelini, Astra Zeneca, Bristol-Myers Squibb, Boehringer Ingelheim, Pfizer, Eli Lilly, Ferrer, Janssen, Lundbeck, Novartis, Otsuka, and Roche. EW was employed by H.Lundbeck A/S at the time of the study and CW is employed by Otsuka.

Author details

Simple and Practical Mental Health, Philadelphia, PA, USA. [2]University of Siena Medical Center, Siena, Italy. [3]H. Lundbeck A/S, Valby, Denmark. [4]Otsuka Pharmaceutical Development & Commercialization, Inc., Princeton, NJ, USA.

References

1. Han C, Wang SM, Kato M, Lee SJ, Patkar AA, Masand PS, Pae CU. Second-generation antipsychotics in the treatment of major depressive disorder: current evidence. Expert Rev Neurother. 2013;13(7):851–70.
2. Papakostas GI. Managing partial response or nonresponse: switching, augmentation, and combination strategies for major depressive disorder. J Clin Psychiatry. 2009;70(Suppl 6):16–25.
3. Rush AJ, Trivedi MH, Wisniewski SR, Nierenberg AA, Stewart JW, Warden D, Niederehe G, Thase ME, Lavori PW, Lebowitz BD, et al. Acute and longer-term outcomes in depressed outpatients requiring one or several treatment steps: a STAR*D report. Am J Psychiatry. 2006;163(11):1905–17.
4. Dold M, Kasper S. Evidence-based pharmacotherapy of treatment-resistant unipolar depression. Int J Psychiatry Clin Pract. 2017;21(1):13–23.
5. Zimmerman M, McGlinchey JB, Posternak MA, Friedman M, Attiullah N, Boerescu D. How should remission from depression be defined? The depressed patient's perspective. Am J Psychiatry. 2006 Jan;163(1):148–50.
6. IsHak WW, Mirocha J, James D, Tobia G, Vilhauer J, Fakhry H, Pi S, Hanson E, Nashawati R, Peselow ED, et al. Quality of life in major depressive disorder before/after multiple steps of treatment and one-year follow-up. Acta Psychiatr Scand. 2015;131(1):51–60.
7. Knoth RL, Bolge SC, Kim E, Tran QV. Effect of inadequate response to treatment in patients with depression. Am J Manag Care. 2010;16(8):e188–96.
8. Kessler RC. The costs of depression. Psychiatr Clin North Am. 2012;35(1):1–14.
9. Sheehan DV, Harnett-Sheehan K, Raj BA. The measurement of disability. Int Clin Psychopharmacol. 1996;11(Suppl 3):89–95.
10. Gilbody S, Richards D, Brealey S, Hewitt C. Screening for depression in medical settings with the patient health questionnaire (PHQ): a diagnostic meta-analysis. J Gen Intern Med. 2007;22(11):1596–602.
11. Breiman L, Forests R. Mach Learn. 2001;45(1):5–32.
12. Thase ME, Rush AJ. When at first you don't succeed: sequential strategies for antidepressant nonresponders. J Clin Psychiatry. 1997;58(Suppl 13):23–9.

19

The effect of CBT and its modifications for relapse prevention in major depressive disorder

Zuojie Zhang[1,2,3], Lingli Zhang[1,2,5,6*], Guorong Zhang[3], Jianing Jin[3] and Zhenyang Zheng[4]

Abstract

Background: The risk of relapse in major depressive disorder (MDD) is associated with high worldwide disease burden. Cognitive behavioral therapy (CBT) and its modifications might be effective in relapse prevention. The aim of this review was to evaluate the efficacy of these treatments for reducing relapse of MDD.

Methods: The retrieval was performed in the databases of MEDLINE via Pubmed, EMBASE and PsycINFO via OVID, The Cochrane Library and four Chinese databases. Clinical trials registry platforms and references of relevant articles were retrieved as well. Hazard ratio (HR) and corresponding 95% confidence interval (CI) were used to pool evidences.

Results: A total of 16 eligible trials involving 1945 participants were included. In the first 12 months, CBT was more efficacious than control in reducing the risk of developing a new episode of depression for MDD patients in remission (HR:0.50, 95%CI:0.35–0.72, $I^2 = 11\%$). Mindfulness-based cognitive therapy (MBCT) was more efficacious than control only among patients with 3 or more previous depressive episodes (HR:0.46, 95%CI:0.31–0.70, $I^2 = 38\%$). Besides, compared with maintenance antidepressant medication (m-ADM), MBCT was a more effective intervention (HR:0.76, 95%CI:0.58–0.98, $I^2 = 0\%$). These positive effects might be only maintained at two and nearly 6 years follow up for CBT.

Conclusion: The use of CBT for MDD patients in remission might reduce risk of relapse. Besides, the effect of MBCT was moderated by number of prior episodes and MBCT might only be effective for MDD patients with 3 or more previous episodes. Further exploration for the influence of previous psychological intervention is required.

Keywords: major depressive disorder, remission, relapse, cognitive behavioural therapy

Background

Major depressive disorder (MDD) is one of the most common and prevalent mental disorders, which is characterized by low vigor, low mood, low self-confidence, and aversion to activity without a specific reason [1, 2]. It is one of the leading causes of worldwide disability and is associated with approximate 16% lifetime prevalence rate [3, 4]. Besides, it is related with continuous high risk of recurrence which represents an increased disease burden [5, 6]. Following each new episode, the condition of depression becomes worse and risk of next relapse increases [7, 8]. Researchers found that risk of relapse after experiencing one episode of major depression was 50%, after two was 80% and after three might be up to 90% [9, 10].These relapses are associated with considerable high cost to individual, family, and society [6, 11]. Therefore, in view of the nature of depression-related impairments and future implication of recurrent depression, attempting to prevent the relapse of depression is an important clinical therapeutic goal for long-term management of MDD.

The most commonly used treatment for reducing depression relapse rate after successful pharmacotherapy

* Correspondence: zhlingli@sina.com
[1]Department of Pharmacy, Evidence-based Pharmacy Center, West China second hospital, Sichuan University, Chengdu, China
[2]Key Laboratory of Birth Defects and Related Diseases of Women and Children (Sichuan University), Ministry of Education, Chengdu, China

might be sequential pharmacotherapy [12]. But long-term use is associated with enormous side effects such as drug interaction [13, 14]. In addition, even if the discontinuation reaction is gradual [15], patients who reluctant to continue pharmacotherapy are possible to relapse when discontinue the medicine [16]. In clinical practice, sequential pharmacotherapy is associated with high risk of noncompliance [17, 18] and psychotherapy is chosen with intense patient preference [19]. A research found that preference was a powerful influence for the effect of intervention [20]. Compared to unfavorable intervention, favorable intervention brings more positive results to patient [21].In addition, different from pharmacotherapy which might be invalid in the phase of discontinuation, psychotherapy brings with potential long-term benefit [22]. The lasting effect may be attributed to the fact that these patients could either improve the cause of recurrent risk or understand many useful techniques to hold back the risk of relapse [23]. As a result, looking for alternative suitable psychotherapy is a public health priority.

Cognitive behavioral therapy (CBT) is one of the most frequently used psychosocial treatment for mental disorders, which targets at changing tactic of patients to cope problems in cognitions (such as belief and thought) and behaviors [24, 25]. Different kinds of modifications of CBT were found to be effective as well, such as mindfulnessbased cognitive therapy (MBCT) [26–28]. MBCT uses conventional methods of CBT which combined with mindfulness meditation. It is a class-based skills training program and developed for increasing the ability of patients to prevent the recurrence of depression in the long term [29]. MBCT could not only help patients to be more aware of negative thoughts in the period of potential relapse but also allow them to get rid of rumination after depression [30]. Through MBCT, therapists could empower participants to process their experiences via mindfulness and meditation skills, and thus participants could improve their undesirable feelings [31].

However, many investigators found that MBCT might not reduce the risk of developing a new relapse of depression in patients with 2 previous episodes [28, 32]. Investigators offered two hypotheses. The first one was that depressive thoughts were derived from repeated connections between the depressed condition and negative thinking modes. The enhancement of these connections with higher numbers of episodes was thought to result in increasing the risk of relapse after each episode. The increased risk of relapse for patients with 3 or more previous episodes was assumed to be attributable to autonomous relapse processes involving reactivation of depressogenic thinking patterns by dysphoria. For patients with higher numbers of episodes, less environmental stress is needed to motivate relapse [33]). The preventative effect of MBCT was assumed to attribute to disrupt these processes at times of potential relapse by decreasing the extent of depressive thought reactivated by negative feelings [28, 34]. The second was that there might be different categories of depression. One category might be associated with reaction to life events, namely among patients with fewer numbers of previous episodes. Another category of depression might be associated with heightened rumination, namely among patients with a higher number of previous episodes [28].

Previous researches paid attention to the role of psychotherapy on the prevention of relapse. Jacob Piet and Esben Hougaard reported their researches in 2011 which investigated the effect of MBCT for preventing relapse or recurrence among patients with MDD in remission, but some comparisons included few evidences [35]. Currently, the incremental number of clinical trials make it a necessary to conduct an update metaanalysis. Katherine Clarke and colleagues identified the efficacy of all nonpharmacological interventions for preventing further episode, but they did not evaluate the influence of number of previous episodes and they defined control arms as any intervention, which might bring clinical heterogeneous [28, 32, 36]. The study by van der Velden et al. only investigated mechanism of MBCT in the treatment of recurrent MDD [37]. In light of the above evidences and the unclear comprehensive effectiveness of CBT and its modifications for reducing relapse rate in subjects with MDD in remission (a specific period of MDD), we conducted this review and meta-analysis to extend prior studies. The purpose of this review was to describe relevant research in this topic, and then to evaluate the short and long term efficacy of CBT and its modifications. In addition, in order to evaluate the influence of number of previous episodes, we separately analyzed the efficacy of trials which only included patients with 3 or more than 3 previous episodes.

Methods

Overall, our review was performed in line with the PRISMA statement [38, 39].

Inclusion and exclusion criteria.

The selection criteria was formulated as follows:

1. Patient: Aged ≥18 years old with MDD in full or partial remission based on a strict diagnostic definition, such as Diagnostic and Statistical Manual of Mental Disorders (DSM) or International Classification of Diseases 10th revision (ICD- 10). Full remission is defined as a relative brief period during which the individual is asymptomatic. Asymptomatic is not defined as a complete absence of symptoms but instead is defined as no more than minimal symptoms. Asymptomatic is operationalized as a score of < 8 on

the 17-item Hamilton Depression Rating Scale (HDRS). Partial remission is defined as persons whose depression do not meet the full remission criterion but who have clinical meaningful reductions in baseline, which refers to a HDRS-17 score<12 [40, 41].

2. Intervention: All CBT and its modifications (such as CBT, cognitive therapy(CT), behavioral therapy(BT), Cognitive Behavioral Analysis System of Psychotherapy (CBASP), and MBCT) will be selected regardless of their different modalities(face-to-face, Internet, or other), formats (group or individual), number of sessions, duration of each session, and frequency.
3. Comparison: Any comparator intervention, including control (treatment-as-usual (TAU), (psychological or pill) placebo (PLA), wait-list (WL), and psychoeducation) and maintenance antidepressant medication (m-ADM).
4. Study design: Randomized controlled trials (RCT).

Furthermore, the eligible articles were limited to report in English or Chinese.

Discontinuation researches were excluded.

Search strategy and study selection

The retrieval of eligible studies was performed from 1976 to September 1, 2016 in the following databases: MEDLINE via Pubmed, EMBASE and PsycINFO via OVID, The Cochrane Library, Chinese Biomedical Literature Database (CBM), China Knowledge Resource Integrated Database (CNKI), VIP Database and Wanfang Database. References of relevant articles were retrieved manually. In addition, unpublished trials were retrieved with the help of International Clinical Trials Registry Platform (ICTRP) (http://www.who.int/ictrp/search/en/) and clinical trial registries platform (http://clinicaltrials.gov/). The search used all relevant terms of 'depression', 'relapse', and 'cognitive behavioural therapy', with a limit to 'randomized controlled trial'. Additional file 1 showed a detailed systematic search strategy.

After removing duplicate articles, two investigators reviewed the remaining articles independently according to the selection criteria and decided whether the full-text reports should be reviewed. And then, after reviewing the eligible full-text reports, studies which met the selection standard were included in our review.

Disagreements were discussed and resolved by joining a third investigator.

Data extraction and quality assessment

Two investigators independently extracted the following data through a pre-designed Excel table: basic information (surname of the first investigator, year of publication, baseline relapse status of depression, the criteria used to measure relapse, inclusion and exclusion criteria, pharmacological interventions used before enrolment), characteristics of participations (sample size at randomization and dropout, age, sex, proportion of ADM used at baseline, mean age of first onset), interventions and comparisons (explicit definition, form of intervention, number of sessions, duration of each session, frequency, length of follow-up). Two investigators independently assessed risk of bias of individual studies according to the methods in Cochrane Handbook [42].

Any missing data were requested from some authors through e-mail to replenish our analysis. A third investigator checked the consistency of extractions and coordinated any discrepant data.

Statistics analysis

In our meta-analysis, we defined outcome measure as hazard ratio (HR) and corresponding 95% confidence interval (CI) of developing a new episode of depression. If study reported HR with 95%CI, these data would be recorded preferentially. If not and only Kaplan-Meier curve or observed event data could be reached, HR with 95%CI would be calculated through survival plots or observed event data according to the method provided by Tierney et al. [43]. For outcome at the specific time (such as the results at 12 months or 24 months in the follow up), we preferred to get the designated HR from Kaplan-Meier curves as we could.

Statistical heterogeneity of pooled HRs was examined by Q test and I^2 statistics. $P < 0.1$ or $I^2 > 50\%$ demonstrated that there was substantial heterogeneity. If that, we would identify potential factors which generated heterogeneity (clinic, methodology, and statistics). The random-effect model was chosen to pool HRs. Separate meta-analyses were conducted among: 1) different follow-up durations (12 months, 24 months, and longer than 24 months); 2) different kinds of comparison (control arm and maintenance antidepressant medication (m-ADM)); 3) different numbers of prior episodes (subjects with < or ≥3 previous episodes). Pre-designed subgroup analyses of different kinds of CBT were carried out. Because CBT and CT were essentially the same treatment but with some minor differences, we did not distinguish them and treated CT as CBT. In our meta-analysis, control arm was defined as treatment-as-usual condition. Studies with other kinds of comparator were only included in narrative analysis and excluded from statistics meta-analysis.

Funnel plots were chosen to test publication bias if any of the separate outcome included 10 or more trials as recommended by Cochrane Handbook [42], because the study number less than 10 was thought to be lack of statistical power to receive a reliable result. All the above statistical analyses were performed with the help of Review Manager 5.

Results

Studies included

Our search initially reached 53 articles which potentially met the inclusion and exclusion criteria. Finally, a total of 20 eligible articles (16 trials with 1945 participants, sample sizes ranged from 40 to 424) were included in our narrative review [26–28, 32, 44–59], of which 18 articles were included in our meta-analysis. Two were failed to be included because of either inappropriate control arm or lacking sufficient relapse data [56, 57]. One trial was conducted by Stangier et al., which was a multicenter prospective randomized observer-blinded study. Patients ($n = 180$) with three or more previous MDD were assigned to maintenance CBT or manualized psychoeducation. Analysis found that maintenance CBT was only significantly more efficacious than manualized psychoeducation in subjects with five or more previous episodes. Because the control arm was manualized psychoeducation, which did not meet our criterion of statistics analysis for meta-analysis. We excluded this trial from meta-analysis. Another trial was by Teismann et al., in which participants ($N = 60$) were randomly assigned to either CBT or wait-list control condition. Although the aim of this study was to investigate whether CBT group treatment was effective in reducing residual depression by targeting depressive rumination, authors reported outcome of relapse as secondary outcome. Authors found that CBT was effective for depressive rumination. For the relapse prevention, they only reported that one person (3.2%) suffered from a relapse in the first 6 months and eight persons (25.8%) suffered a relapse within the first year. We failed to calculate HR from these data, so we excluded this study from our meta-analysis as well.

PRISMA flow chart was depicted in Fig. 1.

The characteristics of included 16 trials were depicted in Table 1. The mean age was 46.8 (range: 24–75). For the outcome measure, apart from one trial by Teismann et al., all these trials used relapse as primary outcome measure. For all the modifications of CBT, our retrieval found that only MBCT has been investigated for reducing relapse rate in subjects with MDD in remission.

CBT

There were many differences in CBT manuals of included CBT trials, including mediums (face-to-face, Internet, or other), formats (group or individual), number of sessions, duration of each session, and frequency. In addition, the inclusion criteria of eligible patients, such as previous interventions of these patients, in these trials were different as well.

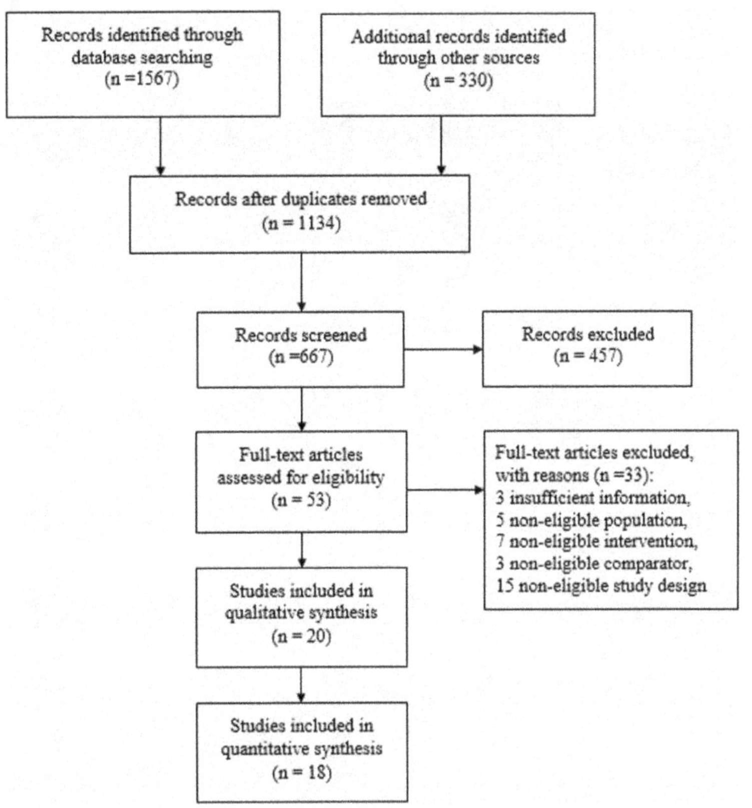

Fig. 1 Flow chart of meta-analysis

Table 1 Characteristics of included trials

Study ID		Pre randomization /eligibility				Patients						Interventions			
Author	Year	Condition	Previous episodes	Criteria used to measure relapse	Previous pharmacology interventions	N	Age[a]	Male (N/%)	Previous episodes[a]	% on ADM at baseline	Mean age of first onset[a]	Groups (n/dropouts)	Form of intervention	N(Number of sessions, frequency, Mean duration + boost sessions)	Length of Follow-Up(months)
Bockting	2005	recurrent MDD, in remission for 10 weeks - 2 years	2 + recent episodes in the previous 5 years	SCID-I	NR	187	44.7/9.5	46/27	3.5/3.8	51	28.4/12.5	CBT:97/16	group	8,weekly,2 h	24
												Control(TAU):90/6			
Bondolfi	2010	recurrent MDD, in remission for 3 + months	3 + episodes (2 in the past 5 years and at least one in the past 2 years)	SCID	a history antidepressants treatment but off medication for 3 + months before enrolment.	60	47.5 (24–66)	17/28	4(3–14)	30	24.5 (8–55)	MBCT:31/4	group	8,weekly,2 h + 4 sessions each 3 months	14
												Control(TAU):29/1			
Fava	1994	primary MDD, in full remission	NR	RDC-defined MDE	successfully response to antidepressant drugs according to a standardized protocol	40	43.7/2.3	16/40	NR	100	NR	CBT:20/0	individual	10,every other week,40 min	24
												Control(PLA):20/0			
Fava	1998	MDD, in full remission for 10 week +	3 or 3 + episodes	RDC-defined MDE	successfully response to antidepressant drugs according to a standardized protocol.	40	46.1/3.7	13/32.5	3.6/0.8	100	NR	CBT:20/0	individual	10,every other week,30 min	24
												Control(PLA):20/0			
Godfrin	2010	MDD, in remission for 8 + weeks	3 or 3 + episodes	DSM-IV diagnosis of MDE	No special	106	45.7/10.5	20/19	NR	76.4	29.8/10.2	MBCT:52/18	group	8,weekly, 2.75 h + homework exercises (meditation practices) for 45 + min/d	14
												Control (TAU):54/12			
Hollandare	2013	MDD, in partial remission	1 + episodes in the previous 5 years	SCID	No special	84	45.3/12.8	13/15	5.96/9.1	50	NR	CBT:42/10	individual	16 internet modules + general e-mails for 10 weeks	24
												Control(PLA)::42/7			
Kuyken	2008	recurrent MDD, in full or partial remission	3 or 3 + episodes	SCID	on a continuing dose of m-ADM for 6 + months	123	49.2/11.2	29/24	6.4/3.0	100	26.2/12.1	MBCT-TS:61/9	group	8,weekly,2 h + 4 sessions	15
												m-ADM:62/10			
kuyken	2015	recurrent MDD, in full or partial remission	3 or 3 + episodes	SCID	on a continuing dose of m-ADM for 6 + months	424	49.5/12.5	99/23	46% 6 +	100	24.9/12.4	MBCT-TS: 212/23	group	8,weekly, 2.25 h + 4 refresher sessions/ 3 months	24
												m-ADM: 212/18			
	2004					75	44.5/9.0	18/24	3/2.0	100	30.6/12.4	MBCT:37/6	group		13

Table 1 Characteristics of included trials *(Continued)*

Study ID		Pre randomization /eligibility				Patients						Interventions			
Author	Year	Condition	Previous episodes	Criteria used to measure relapse	Previous pharmacology interventions	N	Age[a]	Male (N/%)	Previous episodes[a]	% on ADM at baseline	Mean age of first onset[a]	Groups (n/dropouts)	Form of intervention	N(Number of sessions, frequency, Mean duration + boost sessions)	Length of Follow-Up(months)
Ma and Teasdale		MDD, in remission for 12 + weeks	2 or 2 + episodes in the previous 5 years	modeled on the SCID	a history antidepressants treatment but off medication for 3 + months before enrolment.									8,weekly, 2.75 h + homework exercises	
												Control(TAU):38/1			
Paykel	1999	MDD, in remission for 2–18 months	residual symptoms	DSM-III-R criteria for MDD for at least 1 month AND Minimum symptom score	all on a history antidepressants treatment	158	43.4/10.5	80/51	37% 3 +	100	NR		CBT:80/19	individual	16 sessions over 20 weeks + 2 sessions 6 and 14 weeks later
		Control(PLA): 78/12										15.8			
Segal	2010	MDD, in remission for 7+ months	3 + episodes	16 + on the HRSD-17 assessed twice then criteria for MDD measured with SCID	all on a history antidepressants treatment	54	44.1/11	31/37	4.7/2.3	55	31/11.6	MBCT:26/5	group	8,weekly,2 h + option 1 h/month mindfulness mediation class	18
												m-ADM:28/7			
Stangier	2013	MDD, in full remission	3 or 3 + episodes	DSM-IV diagnosis of MDE (LIFE)	NR	180	48.6/11.6	50/27.8	7.4/8.3	74.8	30.9/12.4	Maintenance CBT: 90/15	individual	16,NR,50 min	12
												Manualized psychoeducation: 90/31	individual	16,NR,20 min	
Teasdale	2000	MDD, in remission (0-24 months)	3 + episodes (2 in the past 5 years and at least one in the past 2 years)	SCID	a history antidepressants treatment but off medication for 3 + months before enrolment.	145	43.3/10.3	35/24	3.3/3.0	100	26.8/10.2	MBCT:76/13	group	8,weekly, 2 h + 4 more sessions over trial duration	12
												Control(TAU):69/0			
Teismann	2014	MDD, in partial remission	NR	SCID	No special	60	47.1/11.8	17/28	22.45% 5 +	40	NR	CBT:31/2	group	11,weekly,90 min	12
												WL:29/5			
Wilkinson	2009	MDD, in remission for 2 + months	NR	MADRS score of 10 + at 6/12 months	Received antidepressant medication	45	74.0/7.3	17/38	3.0/1.9	100	NR	CBT:22/4	group	8,NR,90 min	12
												Control(PLA):23/5			

Table 1 Characteristics of included trials *(Continued)*

Study ID		Pre randomization /eligibility				Patients						Interventions			
Author	Year	Condition	Previous episodes	Criteria used to measure relapse	Previous pharmacology interventions	N	Age[a]	Male (N/%)	Previous episodes[a]	% on ADM at baseline	Mean age of first onset[a]	Groups (n/dropouts)	Form of intervention	N(Number of sessions, frequency, Mean duration + boost sessions)	Length of Follow-Up(months)
Williams	2014	MDD, in remission for 8 + weeks	3 or 3 + episodes	SCID	NR	164	43.4/12	76/28	77% 5 +	44	21.3/10.7	MBCT:108/9	group	individual pre class interview + 8,weekly, 2 h + follow-up classes taking place 6 weeks and 6 months in the follow-up	12
												Control(TAU): 56/3			

Note:
[a] Mean/SD, Median(range)
CBT cognitive behavioral therapy, *CPE* cognitive psychological education, *MBCT* mindfulness-based cognitive therapy, *MBCT-TS* MBCT with support to taper or discontinue antidepressant treatment, *TAU* treatment as usual, *m-ADM* Maintenance antidepressant medication, *WL* wait-list, *PLA* (psychological or pill) placebo
Criteria used to measure relapse:
DSM Diagnostic Statistical Manual, *LIFE* Longitudinal Interval Follow-up Evaluation, *MDD* MDD Disorder, *MDE* MDD Episode, *RDC* Research Diagnostic Criteria, *SCID* Structured Clinical Interview for DSM Disorders, *MADRS* Montgomery–Asberg Depression Rating Scale, *HRSD* Hampton Roads Sanitation District

Two trials by Fava et al. [46, 49] implemented the intervention of CBT as described by Beck et al. [60], while others respectively used their own manuals which were modified from that by Beck et al. [60]. All the authors delivered CBT in face-to-face modality other than Holländare et al. [52], who delivered it in the modules of internet communication and encrypted e-mails which largely decreased time of therapist. Apart from three trials which delivered CBT in the format of group [26, 57, 58], others delivered in the format of individual. The explanation to group format was that it was more cost-effective and patients included were current free of psychopathology [26]. Sessions ranged from 8 to 16 and durations ranged from 30 to 90 min.

MBCT

In general, in contrast to CBT, the therapeutic manual, mediums, number of sessions, and duration of each sessions of MBCT in included MBCT trials were mainly consistent, namely eight weekly 2-h group training sessions in line with the manual published by Segal, Williams, & Teasdale [31], while the adjunction sessions had several unconformities among trials as displayed in Table 1. In order to eliminate the influence of previous other psychological interventions, all MBCT trials excluded patients with concurrent psychotherapy or more than one psychiatric consultation per month, four of which unequivocally excluded patients undergoing more than four sessions of CBT ever or positive response to CBT [28, 32, 45, 59].

Meta-analytic results

12 months

CBT and its modifications VS control This separate meta-analysis included 9 trials. Compared with control, risk of depression relapse was reduced by 37% for CBT and its modifications (HR: 0.63, 95%CI:0.44–0.90) (Fig. 2).

CBT VS control

This subgroup included 4 trials. Compared with control, risk of depression relapse was reduced by 50% for CBT (HR:0.50, 95%CI:0.35–0.72, $I^2 = 11\%$).

One trial by Bockting et al. [26]. randomized 187 recurrent depressive patients in remission for 10 weeks to 2 years to either brief CBT plus control ($N = 97$) or control($N = 90$), with continuing use of medication in both groups. Patients who recently received CBT or other psychotherapies were excluded. One was a medium trial by Hollandare et al. [52], which compared the efficacy of Internet-based CBT (16 CBT-based modules via a secure internet communication platform plus encrypted e-mail communication with a personal therapist, $N = 42$) to control group (only the e-mail communication, $N = 42$) for reducing the risk of relapse in partially remitted depressive patients. Medication was allowed to receive. In the trial conducted by Paykel et al. [54], 158 major depressive subjects who partially remitted from receiving antidepressant for at least previous 8 weeks were randomized to either 16 sessions of CBT for 20 weeks or control. Antidepressants were continued and maintained in all subjects. The last trial was conducted by Wilkinson et al. [58], they randomized 45 patients with MDDs in remission for at least 2 months to brief group CBT (CBT-G)($N = 22$) or control($N = 23$).

MBCT VS control

There were 5 trials among this subgroup. Compared with control, overall HR did not show a significant preventive effect for MBCT(HR:0.78, 95%CI:0.50–1.22, $I^2 = 69\%$) with high heterogeneity (Fig. 2).

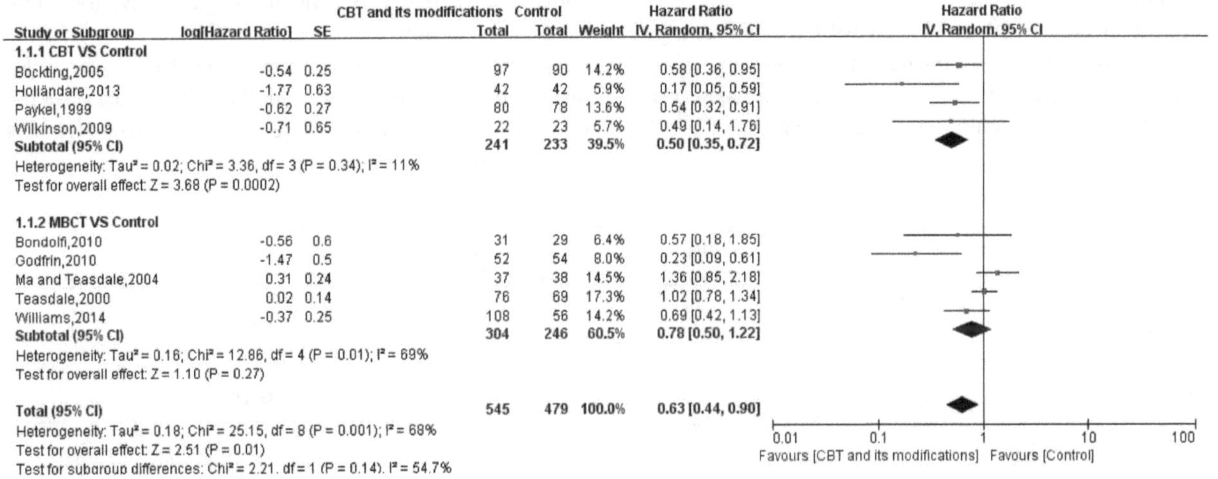

Fig. 2 Relapses in 12 months in CBT and its modifications vs Control

Of these trials, three, respectively conducted by Bondolfi et al. [45], Ma and Teasdale [32], and Teasdale et al. [28], were largely identical in inclusion/exclusion criteria and treatment framework. For the administration of medication, in the section of enrolment, subjects were required to receive antidepressants previously but discontinue them for at least 3 months before inclusion, and in the section of experiment, some of the antidepressants were reinstated.

For the study by Godfrin et al. [51], it randomized 106 MDD patients in remission for at least 8 weeks to MBCT or control. As to medication such as antidepressants, subjects were permitted to receive.

Williams and colleagues [59] conducted a three arm trial (MBCT, cognitive psychological education and control). As to the use of medication in experimental stage, subjects were encouraged to continue their administrations at enrolment.

CBT and its modifications VS m-ADM MBCT VS m-ADM

Pooled HR from three trials showed that MBCT was associated with a lower risk of relapse rate than m-ADM at 1 year follow-up (HR:0.76, 95% CI:0.58–0.98, I^2 = 0%) (Fig. 3). Two trials were reported by Kuyken and colleagues in 2008 (pilot trial) and 2015, respectively. They evaluated whether MBCT plus taper or discontinue antidepressant treatment (MBCT-TS) outperformed m-ADM in preventing depressive relapse or recurrence. Before the enrolment, all the subjects received a maintain antidepressant dose according to the British National Formulary (BNF) and NICE guidance. The last trial was by Segal et al. [55], in which MBCT (n = 26) and m-ADM (n = 28) were randomized to remitted depressive patients with at least 3 past episodes.

24 months

CBT and its modifications VS control CBT VS Control

There were 3 trials among this subgroup. Compared with control, risk of depression relapse was reduced by 76% for CBT (HR:0.24, 95%CI:0.12–0.46, I^2 = 0%)(Fig. 4).

One trial by Hollandare et al. [52] was described above. The remaining two trials (number of subjects both were 40) were all conducted by Fava and colleagues. The first one (1994) aimed at evaluating the efficacy of CBT for treating residual symptoms of primary major depressive and the other one (1998) was conducted in patients with recurrent depression (at least 3 episodes of depression). All the subjects were in full remission after successfully receiving standardized antidepressant. And then they were randomly assigned to either CBT or control (both with discontinuing ADM).

CBT and its modifications VS m-ADM MBCT VS m-ADM

For this comparison, only one trial conducted for 24 months [27]. Compared to m-ADM, MBCT did not show a significant relapse prevention effect (HR:0.89, 95%CI:0.67–1.17).

Longer than 24 Month

Three trials reported efficacy of CBT for preventing relapse at more than 24 months follow-up.

Bockting et al. [44] followed up their trial for 5.5 years and reported the results, which showed that there was a significant relapse preventive effect of CBT for MDD patients(HR:0.71, 95%CI:0.52–0.97) and the effect reinforced with the number of previous episodes. More narrowly, compared to control, patients with 4 or more previous episodes showed a more significant effect for CBT(HR:0.46, 95%CI:0.28–0.75), and patients with less than 4 previous episodes showed a non-significant effect (HR:0.86, 95%CI:0.51–1.45).

The other two trials by Fava et al. [48, 50] were followed-up for 6 years, which found that compared to control, CBT had a significant relapse prevention effect at 6-years follow-up (HR:0.36, 95%CI:0.18–0.72). Of note, one of these two trials reported the 4-year follow-up result [47], which showed that CBT was associated with a lower relapse rate than control (HR:0.45, 95%CI:0.16–0.97) as well.

Study or Subgroup	log[Hazard Ratio]	SE	MBCT Total	m-ADM Total	Weight	Hazard Ratio IV, Random, 95% CI
Kuyken,2008	-0.46	0.25	61	62	28.3%	0.63 [0.39, 1.03]
Kuyken,2015	-0.22	0.18	212	212	54.5%	0.80 [0.56, 1.14]
Segal,2010	-0.17	0.32	26	28	17.2%	0.84 [0.45, 1.58]
Total (95% CI)			**299**	**302**	**100.0%**	**0.76 [0.58, 0.98]**

Heterogeneity: Tau² = 0.00; Chi² = 0.75, df = 2 (P = 0.69); I² = 0%
Test for overall effect: Z = 2.10 (P = 0.04)

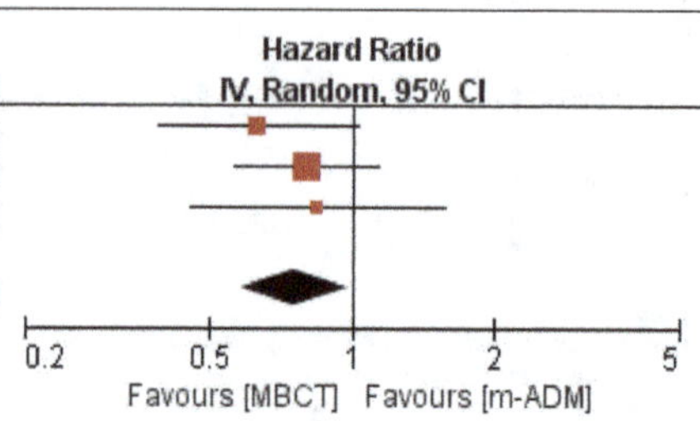

Fig. 3 Relapses in 12 months in MBCT vs m-ADM

Study or Subgroup	log[Hazard Ratio]	SE	CBT Total	Control Total	Weight	Hazard Ratio IV, Random, 95% CI
Fava,1994	-1.86	0.5	20	20	48.0%	0.16 [0.06, 0.41]
Fava,1998	-1.17	0.58	20	20	35.7%	0.31 [0.10, 0.97]
Holländare,2013	-0.84	0.86	42	42	16.2%	0.43 [0.08, 2.33]
Total (95% CI)			**82**	**82**	**100.0%**	**0.24 [0.12, 0.46]**

Heterogeneity: Tau² = 0.00; Chi² = 1.41, df = 2 (P = 0.49); I² = 0%
Test for overall effect: Z = 4.18 (P < 0.0001)

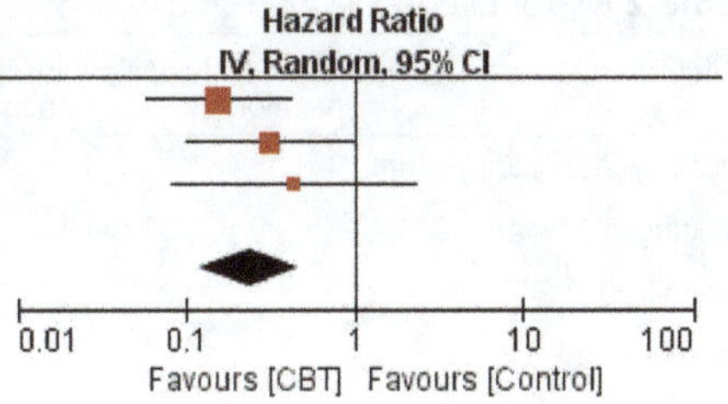

Fig. 4 Relapses in 24 months in CBT vs Control

Number of prior episodes

CBT VS Control

Only one trial by Fava et al. (1998) [49] reported subjects with 3 or more previous MDD episodes. They found that compared to control, CBT had a preventive effect (HR:0.31, 95%CI:0.10–0.97).

MBCT VS Control

Apart from two trials by Ma and Teasdale [32] and Teasdale et al. [28], all trials of MBCT only included MDD patients with 3 or more previous episodes. These two also included subjects with 2 previous episodes and separately evaluated relapse rates in the subgroup of patients with < or ≥3 previous episodes. Pooling data of patients with 3 or more previous episodes together, we found that compared to control arm, MBCT reduced the risk of developing a new depressive episode by 54% (HR:0.46, 95%CI:0.31–0.70, $I^2 = 38\%$) (Fig. 5).

Quality assessment Risk bias of the included 20 studies were displayed in Table 2. The majority of studies reported methodology of random sequence generation ($N = 15$) and allocation concealment ($N = 13$), while others provided insufficient information, leading to "unclear risk". Owning to the characteristic of psychotherapy, all the studies had a high risk of bias in the blinding of participants and personnel. 15 studies (75%) were judged to be prone to a low risk of bias in blinding of outcome assessment. 60% studies had a low risk of incomplete outcome data, while others had unclear or high risk due to either insufficient information or high scale of dropout. ITT analyses were available for 11 studies, while others only reported results of completer analyses. 6 studies (30%) were judged to be high risk of selective reporting.

Publication bias As the explanation showed in Cochrane Handbook, visual examination analysis of funnel plots have limited power to detect bias if the number of studies is small [42]. Because any one of the separate meta-analyses did not cover 10 or more than 10 trials, we did not identify publication bias through visual inspection of funnel plots.

Discussions

For short-term follow-up (12 months), our meta-analyses demonstrated that CBT was more efficacious in reducing the risk of developing a new relapse of depression than control, while compared to control, MBCT only showed a significant effect in patients with 3 or more previous depressive episodes. Besides, compared with m-ADM, MBCT was an effective intervention for relapse prevention. For long-term follow-up (24 or more than months), the preventive effect of CBT were maintained for 2 to 6 years in recurrent prevention. For MBCT, the only one trial found that MBCT and m-ADM were not significantly different from each other after 2 years in terms of relapse/recurrence.

For heterogeneity among comparisons, we thought it was associated with substantial differences in either the regimens of administration or the inclusion criterion regarding the use of psychotherapy or pharmacotherapy in MDD patients before enrolment.

Study or Subgroup	log[Hazard Ratio]	SE	MCBT Total	Control Total	Weight	Hazard Ratio IV, Random, 95% CI
Bondolfi,2010	-0.56	0.6	31	29	10.0%	0.57 [0.18, 1.85]
Godfrin,2010	-1.47	0.5	52	54	13.4%	0.23 [0.09, 0.61]
Ma and Teasdale,2004	-1.27	0.39	37	38	19.0%	0.28 [0.13, 0.60]
Teasdale,2000	-0.6	0.29	76	69	26.8%	0.55 [0.31, 0.97]
Williams,2014	-0.37	0.25	108	56	30.8%	0.69 [0.42, 1.13]
Total (95% CI)			**304**	**246**	**100.0%**	**0.46 [0.31, 0.70]**

Heterogeneity: Tau² = 0.08; Chi² = 6.42, df = 4 (P = 0.17); I² = 38%
Test for overall effect: Z = 3.66 (P = 0.0003)

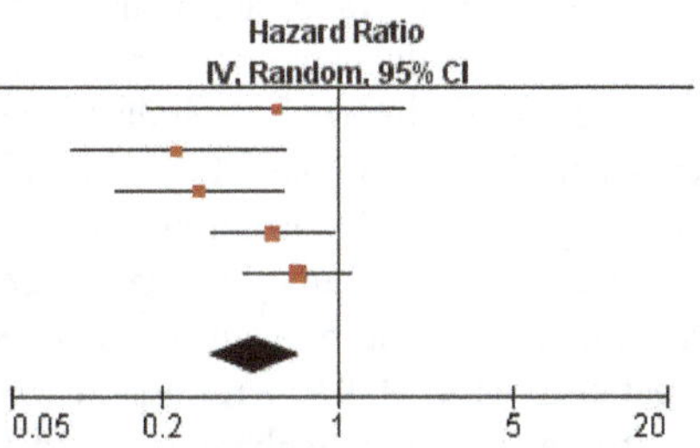

Fig. 5 Relapses in MBCT vs Control for participants with three or more previous episodes of major depression

Table 2 Risk of bias in included studies

Study ID	Random sequence generation	Allocation concealment	Blinding of participants and personnel	Blinding of outcome assessment	Incomplete outcome data	Selective reporting	Other sources of bias
Bockting, 2005 [26]	L	L	H	L	U	H	L
Bockting,2009 [44]	L	L	H	L	U	H	L
Bondolfi,2010 [45]	L	L	H	L	L	L	L
Fava,1994 [46]	U	U	H	L	L	L	L
Fava,1996 [47]	U	U	H	L	L	L	L
Fava,1998 a [48]	U	U	H	L	L	L	L
Fava,1998 b [49]	U	U	H	L	H	L	L
Fava,2004 [50]	U	U	H	L	L	L	L
Godfrin,2010 [51]	L	L	H	H	U	L	L
Hollandare,2013 [52]	L	U	H	U	L	L	L
Kuyken,2008 [53]	L	L	H	L	L	L	L
Kuyken,2015 [27]	L	L	H	L	L	L	L
Ma and Teasdale,2004 [32]	L	L	H	L	L	H	L
Paykel,1999 [54]	L	L	H	L	U	H	L
Segal,2010 [55]	L	L	H	L	U	H	L
Stangier,2013 [56]	L	U	H	H	H	H	L
Teasdale,2000 [28]	L	L	H	L	L	L	L
Teismann,2014 [57]	L	L	H	H	L	L	L
Wilkinson,2009 [58]	L	L	H	L	U	L	L
Williams,2014 [59]	L	L	H	H	L	L	L

Note: *H* high risk, *L* low risk, *U* unclear

Overall, our findings largely agreed with previous studies. Compared with the reviews by Beshai et al. and Bockting et al. [61, 62], our findings was from qualification of "best evidence" by using quantitative meta-analysis approach, which could illustrate the reliability and size of preventive effect of intervention on reducing relapse rate. Meta-analysis could also illustrate whether significant effect found in some studies are systematic or random. Our meta-analysis focused on evaluating the effect of CBT and its modifications for reducing relapse rate in subjects with MDD in remission (a specific period of MDD). This clinical question were more specific than the above two reviews. Therefore, the findings was more targeted. In addition, we used a different outcome measure of HR to summarize results. This measure has the advantage of applying more available information of the trial, including the number of patients who fail to complete the trial and time of patients occurring event in the duration of follow-up [63].

So far, two meta-analyses have been performed to evaluate the relapse prevention effect of psychotherapy in patients with MDD in remission [35, 36]. Compared with these two meta-analyses, we also found CBT to be effective in the prevention of a new depressive episode. The article conducted by Piet et al. [35] found that MBCT significantly reduced the risk of relapse compared to control and did not significantly reduce the risk of relapse compared to m-ADM. We reached different results. We found that compared to control, MBCT only significantly reduced the risk of relapse in patients with 3 or more previous episodes, not in all patients. It is to say that the effect was moderated by number of prior episodes. Compared to m-ADM, MBCT might have a preventive effect, but our effect size was at the edge(HR: 0.76, 95%CI:0.58–0.98). This inconsistency might because we included two more studies than this meta-analysis and used a different outcome measure. However, the evidences we included were insufficient to ascertain and relevant trials needed repetition to confirm or overturn our findings. Compared to another article by Clarke et al. [36] which did not evaluate the effect of MBCT at 2 years follow-up, we found that MBCT might not show a significant preventive effect at 2 years follow-up owning to our update retrieval. Although our analyses were somewhat similar to theirs which aimed to respectively display the effect of psychological interventions at 1 and 2 years follow up, the outcome measure we used could reach to these two particular time points which were thought to be more precise. The time points of outcome of the meta-analysis by Clarke et al. might be nearly 1 or 2 years and were vague. On the other hand, in their analyses, they mixed all control arms into meta-analysis without separate analyses, but we thought this brought clinical heterogeneity into results because these control arms were different from each other in clinic. Therefore, we evaluated them in separate analyses. In addition to these above differences, compared to these two meta-analyses, we also investigated the longer-term (more than 24 months) effect of CBT and MBCT, which haven't be investigated in other previous meta-analyses.

There are some other strengths we want to display in our meta-analysis. To make sure the comprising of all relevant trials regardless of whether the results have been published and reduce the possibility of publication bias, we performed a comprehensive retrieval, especially including clinical trial registry platforms. To reduce random error which might generate from literature selection, data extraction, or quality assessment, two investigators took part in the preliminary stage and then a third investigator joined to check and coordinate the disagreements.

However, limitations were also required to be considered when interpreting our results. The main limitation was that the number of trials and sample sizes for some comparisons, especially MBCT versus m-ADM, were too small to address firm conclusion. Besides, our conclusion could not be popularized to patients in other status of depression because the inclusion criteria of our participants was MDD in full or partial remission. We excluded other patients to ensure the homogeneity as needed by meta-analysis. Finally, no formal protocol was set up at the start of this meta-analysis, although this research was conducted with specific pre-designed purpose and rigorous methods.

Some significance aspects were needed to be focused on in future studies. Firstly, we only displayed some information about previous interventions, including pharmacotherapy and psychotherapy, but failed to evaluate the influence of these interventions on result. Further studies are suggested to pay more attention to the influence of previous interventions, especially sequential psychotherapy interventions. Trials which reported efficacy result at long-term follow-up were still insufficient, and future researches are suggested to provide more data about this. Since preferences of patient and patient-specific clinical variations (such as preferences for particular psychotherapy in previous treatment and severity of every episode of depression) might moderate the effect of psychological interventions [20, 64], future researchers should notice that more flexible and available interventions are important and focus on how to choose better intervention for a particular individual. If these factors are considered, the potential effect of psychological strategies might enlarge. There is also need for trials with head-to-head comparisons of these different psychotherapies.

Conclusion

There were evidences that for MDD patients in remission, CBT was an effective intervention for relapse prevention at either short or long term follow-up. Compared to control, MBCT demonstrated benefit in relapse prevention but only among subjects with 3 or more previous episodes, which meant that the effect of MBCT might be moderated by number of prior episodes. Further studies are suggested to pay more attention to evaluate the influence of previous interventions, especially sequential psychological interventions. There are also need for trials with psychological head-to-head comparisons.

Abbreviations

ADM: Antidepressant medication; BNF: British National Formulary; BT: Behavioral therapy; CBASP: Cognitive Behavioral Analysis System of Psychotherapy; CBT: Cognitive behavioral therapy; CI: Confidence interval; CT: Cognitive therapy; HDRS: Hamilton Depression Rating Scale; HR: Hazard ratio; m-ADM: Maintenance antidepressant medication; MBCT: Mindfulness-based cognitive therapy; MBCT-TS: Mindfulness-based cognitive therapy plus taper or discontinue antidepressant treatment; MDD: Major depressive disorder; PLA: (Psychological or pill) placebo; RCT: Randomized controlled trials

Acknowledgements

We thank Group of People with Highest Risk of Drug Exposure of International Network for the Rational Use of Drugs, China for providing support to coordinate circulation of the manuscript to all co-authors and collect comments from all co-authors.

Funding

This study was funded by Natural Science Foundation of China:Evidence based establishment of evaluation index system for pediatric rational drug use in China (No. 81373381). The sponsor had no role in the study design, writing of the manuscript, or decision to submit this or future manuscripts for publication.

Authors' contributions

ZZ was responsible for Draft the protocol,Develop and run the search strategy,Select which studies to include and exclude, Carry out the analysis and Draft the final review; LZ was responsible for Draft the protocol, Interpret the analysis and Draft the final review; GZ was responsible for Carry out the analysis, Develop and run the search strategy, Data Extraction and Quality Assessment, Interpret the analysis; JJ was responsible for, Select which studies to include and exclude, Data Extraction and Quality Assessment, Interpret the analysis, Draft the final review; ZZ was responsible for Draft the protocol, Select which studies to include and exclude, Data Extraction and Quality Assessment, Interpret the analysis. All authors read and approved the final manuscript.

Consent for publication
Not applicable

Competing interests
The authors declare that they have no competing interests.

Author details
[1]Department of Pharmacy, Evidence-based Pharmacy Center, West China second hospital, Sichuan University, Chengdu, China. [2]Key Laboratory of Birth Defects and Related Diseases of Women and Children (Sichuan University), Ministry of Education, Chengdu, China. [3]West China School of Pharmacy, Sichuan University, Chengdu, China. [4]Department of Neurology, Fujian Medical University attached Union Hospital, Fuzhou, China. [5]West China Second University Hospital, Sichuan University, No.20,Third Section, Renmin Nan Lu, Chengdu, Sichuan 610041, People's Republic of China. [6]Chengdu City, China.

References
1. Depression. NIMH. May 2016.
2. Berto P, D'Ilario D, Ruffo P, Di Virgilio R, Rizzo F. Depression: cost-of-illness studies in the international literature, a review. J Ment Health Policy Econ. 2000;3(1):3–10.
3. Kessler RC, Aguilar-Gaxiola S, Alonso J, Chatterji S, Lee S, Ormel J, et al. The global burden of mental disorders: an update from the WHO world mental health (WMH) surveys. Epidemiol Psychiatr Soc. 2009;18(1):23–33.
4. World Health Organization. Depression fact sheet. Genewa: WHO; 2014. retrieved from http://www.who.int/mediacentre/factsheets/fs369/en/ March2014
5. Gotlib IH, Hammen CL. Psychological aspects of depression: toward a cognitiveinterpersonal integration. Clinl. Psychol Rev. 1994;14(1):90.
6. Collins PY, Patel V, Joestl SS, March D, Insel TR, Daar AS, et al. Grand challenges in global mental health. Nature. 2011;475(475):27–30.
7. Kendler KS, Thornton LM, Gardner CO. Stressful life events and previous episodes in the etiology of major depression in women: an evaluation of the "kindling" hypothesis. Am J Psychiatry. 2000;157(8):1243–51.
8. Belsher G, Costello CG. Relapse after recovery from unipolar depression: a critical review. Psychol Bull. 1988;104(1):84–96.
9. Kessing LV, Hansen MG, Andersen PK, Angst J. The predictive effect of episodes on the risk of recurrence in depressive and bipolar disorders – a life-long perspective. Acta Psychiatr Scand. 2004;109(109):339–44.
10. Katon W, Rutter C, Ludman EJ, Von Korff M, Lin E, Simon G, et al. A randomized trial of relapse prevention of depression in primary care. Arch of Gen Psychiatry. 2001;58(3):241–7.
11. Judd LL, Akiskal HS, Zeller PJ, Paulus M, Leon AC, Maser JD, et al. Psychosocial disability during the long-term course of unipolar major depressive disorder. Arch Gen Psychiatry. 2000;57(4):375–80.
12. Geddes JR, Carney SM, Davies C, Furukawa TA, Kupfer DJ, Frank E, et al. Relapse prevention with antidepressant drug treatment in depressive disorders: a systematic review. Lancet. 2003;361(9358):653–61.
13. Nieuwstraten C, Labiris NR, Holbrook A. Systematic overview of drug interactions with antidepressant medications. Can J Psychiatr. 2006;51(5):300–16.
14. Moret C, Isaac M, Briley M. Problems associated with long-term treatment with selective serotonin reuptake inhibitors. J Psychopharmacol. 2009;23(8):967–74.
15. Viguera AC, Baldessarini RJ, Friedberg J. Discontinuing antidepressant treatment in major depression. Harv Rev Psychiatry. 1998;5(6):293–306.
16. Anderson IM, Tomenson BM. Treatment discontinuation with selective serotonin reuptake inhibitors compared with tricyclic antidepressants: a meta analysis. BMJ. 1995;310(6992):1433–8.
17. Simon GE, Von Korff M, Rutter PLA, Peterson DA. Treatment process and outcomes for managed care patients receiving new antidepressant prescriptions from psychiatrists and primary care physicians. Arch Gen Psychiatry. 2001;58(4):395–401.
18. Ten Doesschate MC, Bockting CL, Schene AH. Adherence to continuation and maintenance antidepressant use in recurrent depression. J Affect Disorder. 2009;115(1–2):167–70.
19. Raue PJ, Schulberg HC, Heo M, Klimstra S, Bruce ML. Patients' depression treatment preferences and initiation, adherence, and outcome: a randomized primary care study. Psychiatr Serv. 2009;60(3):337–43.
20. Kocsis JH, Leon AC, Markowitz JC, Manber R, Arnow B, Klein DN, et al. Patient preference as a moderator of outcome for chronic forms of major depressive disorder treated with nefazodone, cognitive behavioral analysis system of psychotherapy, or their combination. J Clin Psychiatry. 2009;70(3):354–61.
21. Mergl R, Henkel V, Allgaier AK, Kramer D, Hautzinger M, Kohnen R, et al. Are treatment preferences relevant in response to serotonergic antidepressants and cognitive behavioral therapy in depressed primary patients? Results from a randomized controlled trial including a patients' choice arm. Psychother Psychosom. 2011;80(1):39–47.
22. Gortner ET, Gollan JK, Dobson KS, Jacobson NS. Cognitive-behavioral treatment for depression: relapse prevention. J Consult Clin Psychol. 1998;66(2):377–84.
23. Hollon SD, Stewart MO, Strunk D. Enduring effects for cognitive behavior therapy in the treatment of depression and anxiety. Annu Rev of Psychol. 2006;57(1):285–315.
24. Beck JS. Cognitive behavior therapy: basics and beyond (2nd ed.). J Autism Dev Disord. 2011;17(1):81–93.
25. Benjamin CL, Puleo PLA, Settipani CA, Brodman DM, Edmunds JM, Cummings PLA, et al. History of cognitive-behavioral therapy in youth. Child Adolesc Psychiatr Clin N Am. 2011;20(2):179–89.
26. Bockting CL, Schene AH, Spinhoven P, Koeter MW, Wouters LF, Huyser J, et al. Preventing relapse/recurrence in recurrent depression with cognitive therapy: a randomized controlled trial. J Consult Clin Psychol. 2005;73(4): 647–57.
27. Kuyken W, Hayes R, Barrett B, Byng R, Dalgleish T, Kessler D, et al. The effectiveness and cost-effectiveness of mindfulness-based cognitive therapy compared with maintenance antidepressant treatment in the prevention of depressive relapse/recurrence: results of a randomised controlled trial (the PREVENT study). Health Technol Assess. 2015;19(73):1–124.
28. Teasdale JD, Segal ZV, Williams JM, Ridgeway VA, Soulsby JM, Lau MA. Prevention of relapse/recurrence in major depression by mindfulness-based cognitive therapy. J Consult Clin Psychol. 2000;68(4):615–23.
29. Williams JM, Kuyken W. Mindfulness-based cognitive therapy: a promising new approach to preventing depressive relapse. Br J Psychiatry. 2012;200(5):359–60.
30. Nolen-Hoeksema S. Responses to depression and their effects on the duration of depressive episodes. J Abnorm Psychol. 1991;100(4):569–82.
31. Segal ZV, Williams JMG, Teasdale JD. Mindfulness-based cognitive therapy for depression (2nd ed.). J Can Acad Child Adolesc Psychiatry. 2013;22(4):328–9.
32. Ma SH, Teasdale JD. Mindfulness-based cognitive therapy for depression: replication and exploration of differential relapse prevention effects. J Consult Clin Psychol. 2004;72(1):31–40.
33. Post RM. Transduction of psychosocial stress into the neurobiology of recurrent affective disorder. Am J Psychiatry. 1992;149(8):999–1010.
34. Segal ZV, Williams JMG, Teasdale JD. Mindfulness-based cognitive therapy for depression: a new approach to preventing relapse. New York: Guilford Press; 2002.
35. Piet J, Hougaard E. The effect of mindfulness-based cognitive therapy for prevention of relapse in recurrent major depressive disorder: a systematic review and meta-analysis. Clin Psychol Rev. 2011;31(6):1032–40.
36. Clarke K, Mayowilson E, Kenny J, Pilling S. Can non-pharmacological interventions prevent relapse in adults who have recovered from depression? A systematic review and meta-analysis of randomised controlled trials. Clin Psychol Rev. 2015;39:58–70.
37. van der Velden AM, Kuyken W, Wattar U, Crane C, Pallesen KJ, Dahlgaard J, et al. A systematic review of mechanisms of change in mindfulness-based cognitive therapy in the treatment of recurrent major depressive disorder. Clin Psychol Rev. 2015;37:26–39.
38. Liberati A, Altman DG, Tetzlaff J, Mulrow C, Gotzsche PC, Ioannidis JP, et al. The PRISMA statement for reporting systematic reviews and meta-analyses of studies that evaluate health care interventions: explanation and elaboration. BMJ. 2009;339:b2700.
39. Moher D, Liberati A, Tetzlaff J, Altman DG, PRISMA Group. Preferred reporting items for systematic reviews and meta-analyses: the PRISMA statement. PLoS Med. 2009;6(7):e1000097.
40. Zimmerman M, McGlinchey JB, Posternak MA, Friedman M, Attiullah N, Boerescu D. How should remission from depression be defined? The depressed patient's perspective. Am J Psychiatry. 2006;163(1):148–50.

41. Frank E, Prien RF, Jarrett RB, Keller MB, Kupfer DJ, Lavori PW, et al. Conceptualization and rationale for consensus definitions of terms in major depressive disorder. Arch Gen Psychiatry. 1991;48(9):851.
42. Higgins JPT, Green S, editors. Cochrane handbook for systematic reviews of interventions version 5.1.0 [updated march 2011]. The Cochrane collaboration, 2011. Available from www.cochrane-handbook.org.
43. Tierney JF, Stewart LA, Ghersi D, Burdett S, Sydes MR. Practical methods for incorporating summary time-to-event data into meta-analysis. Trials. 2007;8:16.
44. Bockting CL, Spinhoven P, Wouters LF, Koeter MW, Schene AH, DELTA Study Group. Long-term effects of preventive cognitive therapy in recurrent depression: a 5.5-year follow-up study. J Clin Psychiatry. 2009; 70(12):1621–8.
45. Bondolfi G, Jermann F, der Linden MV, Gexfabry M, Bizzini L, Rouget BW, et al. Depression relapse prophylaxis with mindfulness-based cognitive therapy: replication and extension in the swiss health care system. J Affect Disord. 2010;122(3):224–31.
46. Fava GA, Grandi S, Zielezny M, Canestrari R, Morphy MA. Cognitive behavioral treatment of residual symptoms in primary major depressive disorder. Am J Psychiatry. 1994;151(9):1295–9.
47. Fava GA, Grandi S, Zielezny M, Rafanelli C, Canestrari R. Four-year outcome for cognitive behavioral treatment of residual symptoms in major depression. Am J Psychiatry. 1996;153(7):945–7.
48. Fava GA, Rafanelli C, Grandi SO, Canestrari R, Morphy MA. Six-year outcome for cognitive behavioral treatment of residual symptoms in major depression. Am J Psychiatry. 1998;155(10):1443–5.
49. Fava G, Rafanelli CS, Conti S, Belluardo P. Prevention of recurrent depression with cognitive behavioral therapy: preliminary findings. Arch Gen Psychiatry. 1998;55(9):816–20.
50. Fava GA, Ruini C, Rafanelli C, Finos L, Conti S, Grandi S. Six-year outcome of cognitive behavior therapy for prevention of recurrent depression. Am J Psychiatry. 2004;161(10):1872–6.
51. Godfrin KA, van Heeringen C. The effects of mindfulness-based cognitive therapy on recurrence of depressive episodes, mental health and quality of life: a randomized controlled study. Behav Res Ther. 2010;48(8):738–46.
52. Holländare F, Anthony SA, Randestad M, Tillfors M, Carlbring P, Andersson G, et al. Two-year outcome of internet-based relapse prevention for partially remitted depression. Behav Res Ther. 2013;51(11):719–22.
53. Kuyken W, Byford S, Taylor RS, Watkins E, Holden E, White K, et al. Mindfulness-based cognitive therapy to prevent relapse in recurrent depression. J Consult Clin Psychol. 2008;76(6):966–78.
54. Paykel ES, Scott J, Teasdale JD, Johnson AL, Garland A, Moore R, et al. Prevention of relapse in residual depression by cognitive therapy: a controlled trial. Arch Gen Psychiatry. 1999;56(9):829–35.
55. Segal ZV, Bieling P, Young T, Macqueen G, Cooke R, Martin L, et al. Antidepressant Monotherapy versus sequential pharmacotherapy and mindfulness-based cognitive therapy, or placebo, for relapse prophylaxis in recurrent depression. Arch Gen Psychiatry. 2010;67(12):1256–64.
56. Stangier U, Hilling C, Heidenreich T, Risch AK, Barocka A, Schlösser R, et al. Maintenance cognitive-behavioral therapy and manualized psychoeducation in the treatment of recurrent depression: a multicenter prospective randomized controlled trial. Am J Psychiatry. 2013;170(6):624–32.
57. Teismann T, von Brachel R, Hanning S, Grillenberger M, Hebermehl L, Hornstein I, et al. A randomized controlled trial on the effectiveness of a rumination-focused group treatment for residual depression. Psychother Res. 2014;24(1):80–90.
58. Wilkinson P, Alder N, Juszczak E, Matthews H, Merritt C, Montgomery H, et al. A pilot randomised controlled trial of a brief cognitive behavioural group intervention to reduce recurrence rates in late life depression. Int J Geriatr Psychiatry. 2009;24(1):68–75.
59. Williams JM, Crane C, Barnhofer T, Brennan K, Duggan DS, Fennell MJ, et al. Mindfulness-based cognitive therapy for preventing relapse in recurrent depression: a randomized dismantling trial. J Consult Clin Psychol. 2014; 82(2):275–86.
60. Beck AT, Rush AJ, Shaw BF, Emery G. Cognitive therapy of depression. New York: Guilford Press; 1979.
61. Beshai S, Dobson KS, Bockting CL, Quigley L. Relapse and recurrence prevention in depression: current research and future prospects. Clin Psychol Rev. 2011;31(8):1349–60.
62. Bockting CL, Hollon SD, Jarrett RB, Kuyken W, Dobson K. A lifetime approach to major depressive disorder: the contributions of psychological interventions in preventing relapse and recurrence. Clin Psychol Rev. 2015;41:16–26.
63. Spruance SL, Reid JE, Grace M, Samore M. Hazard ratio in clinical trials. Antimicrob Agents Chemother. 2004;48(8):2787–92.
64. Gelenberg AJ, Freeman MP, Markowitz JC, Rosenbaum JF, Thase ME, Trivediet MH, et al. Practice guideline for the treatment of patients with major depressive disorder (3rd ed): American Psychiatric Association.

A pilot feasibility randomised controlled trial of an adjunct brief social network intervention in opiate substitution treatment services

Ed Day[1,2*], Alex Copello[1,3], Jennifer L. Seddon[1,3], Marilyn Christie[4], Deborah Bamber[4], Charlotte Powell[4], Carmel Bennett[1], Shabana Akhtar[1], Sanju George[1], Andrew Ball[4], Emma Frew[5], Ilias Goranitis[5] and Nick Freemantle[6]

Abstract

Background: Approximately 3% of people receiving opioid substitution therapy (OST) in the UK manage to achieve abstinence from prescribed and illicit drugs within three years of commencing treatment. Involvement of families and wider social networks in supporting psychological treatment may be an effective strategy in facilitating recovery, and this pilot study aimed to evaluate the impact of a social network-focused intervention for patients receiving OST.

Methods: A two-site, open feasibility trial randomised patients receiving OST for at least 12 months but still reporting illicit opiate use in the past 28 days to one of three treatments: 1) treatment as usual (TAU), 2) Brief Social Behaviour and Network Therapy (B-SBNT) + TAU, or 3) Personal Goal Setting (PGS) + TAU. The two active interventions consisted of 4 sessions. There were 3 aims: 1) test the feasibility of recruiting OST patients to a trial of B-SBNT, and following them up over 12 months; 2) test the feasibility of training clinicians to deliver B-SBNT; 3) test whether B-SBNT reduces heroin use 3 and 12 months after treatment, and to explore potential mediating factors. The primary outcome for aim 3 was number of days of heroin use in the past month, and a range of secondary outcome measures were specified in advance (level of drug dependence, mental health, social satisfaction, therapist rapport, treatment satisfaction, social network size and support).

Results: A total of 83 participants were randomised, and 70 (84%) were followed-up at 12 months. Fidelity analysis of showed that B-SBNT sessions were clearly distinguishable from PGS and TAU sessions, suggesting it was possible to train clinical staff to an adequate level of competence.
No significant differences were found between the 3 intervention arms in the primary or secondary outcome measures. Attendance at psychosocial treatment intervention sessions was low across all three arms (44% overall).

Conclusions: Patients receiving OST can be recruited into a trial of a social network-based intervention, but poor attendance at treatment sessions makes it uncertain whether an adequate dose of treatment was delivered. In order to achieve the benefits of psychosocial interventions, further work is needed to overcome poor engagement.
(Continued on next page)

* Correspondence: Edward.Day@kcl.ac.uk
[1]Birmingham and Solihull Mental Health NHS Foundation Trust, c/o Dept of Psychiatry, The Barberry 25 Vincent Drive, Edgbaston, Birmingham B152FG, UK
[2]Addictions Department, Institute of Psychiatry, Psychology & Neuroscience, King's College London, London, UK
Full list of author information is available at the end of the article

(Continued from previous page)

Keywords: Randomised controlled trial, Social networks, Social behaviour and network therapy (SBNT), Heroin use, Opioid substitution therapy

Background

The first decade of the twenty-first century saw a step change in the size and scope of treatment services for illicit drug users in England, with increased financial investment leading to a doubling of the number of people in treatment in the period 2000–2005 alone [1]. The political drive behind this change was a desire to reduce criminal activity, but with a newly-elected UK Government in 2010 came a change in direction. Since then there has been more focus on 'recovery', with a national strategy requiring treatment agencies to focus on increasing the number of patients leaving their service abstinent from all illicit and prescribed drugs, in good mental and physical health, and with improved quality of life [2]. Supporters of this approach noted that this goal was rarely achieved, with only 3% of people reporting abstinence within three years of starting opiate substitution treatment (OST) in one study in Scotland [3]. Treatment services often focused on medication to the exclusion of effective psychosocial interventions for the opiate dependent population [4], and one large-scale attempt to evaluate Cognitive Behavioural Therapy in OST clinics identified major training and organisational barriers [5].

The social environment can directly support and reinforce drug use, particularly if a majority of an individual's social network is made up of other drug users [6–9]. One potential strategy to support abstinence from illicit drugs is to encourage patients of OST services to end all contact with drug-using peers. However, this is unlikely to happen if no alternative social contact or support is available, and so psychosocial treatment approaches have begun to focus on building links to individuals and groups who provide competitive reinforcement for abstinence. When this is done successfully, the development of new positive social supports is associated with a reduced risk of relapse to heroin and other drug use and better overall outcomes [10–14].

The important role of families and communities in recovery from drug use has been emphasised in recent treatment policy in England [15, 16], with the National Treatment Agency for Substance Misuse (NTA) signalling its enthusiasm for involving families and other social network members in the treatment process (pp. 15) [17]. However, despite support for change from both researchers and policy makers, drug treatment agencies tend to focus on the individual rather than the family or wider community. Further work is needed to develop and evaluate treatment interventions that aim to build social support for change in substance use and other behaviours, but also to understand the barriers to implementing such an approach. In an increasingly pressured financial environment, psychosocial interventions must be feasible in routine clinical practice and acceptable to both service users and clinicians. They must also move beyond merely targeting changes in drug use, but focus on the pursuit of the wider goal of recovery, including mental and physical health, employment and quality of life [18]).

We report the findings of a pilot trial with the aim of implementing, observing and assessing the efficacy of a social-network intervention (Brief-Social Behaviour and Network Therapy – B-SBNT) for both opiate substitution treatment patients and their social network members. This paper reports on three of the trial's main objectives:

1. To test the feasibility of recruiting patients engaged in drug treatment services for at least a year but still reporting heroin use to a trial of B-SBNT, and following them up over 12 months.
2. To test the feasibility of training NHS clinicians with no previous experience of working with social network members to deliver a brief social network-driven intervention (B-SBNT).
3. To test whether B-SBNT reduces heroin use 3 and 12 months after treatment, and to explore potential mediating factors.

The full study evaluation also included a comprehensive economic evaluation which has been published elsewhere [19, 20].

Method

Design

This early phase open pilot study had a pragmatic, multicentre, randomised parallel group design, comparing a 4-session social network intervention (B-SBNT) with an individually-based personal goal setting intervention of equivalent intensity (PGS), and with treatment as usual (TAU). It targeted patients receiving OST for more than 12 months but still reporting opiate use in the preceding 28 days, and was conducted within three National

Health Service (NHS) community drug treatment teams in two UK regions; the West Midlands (Solihull and Birmingham) and the East Midlands (Leicester).

Intervention

Participants allocated to either of the active treatment groups received an intervention as an adjunct to usual care, delivered by a different therapist to the participant's usual drug worker.

1. Treatment as usual (TAU):

In the control arm participants received usual care with no additional therapy sessions. The treatment services allowed the clinicians to utilise a therapeutic style of their choice for working with patients, and TAU sessions did not follow a treatment manual. Some drug workers had been exposed to goal setting and SBNT techniques as part of their previous training and development. However, previous evaluation in these services had shown that TAU sessions occurred between weekly and fortnightly, lasted an average of 45 min, and focussed on case management, signposting of other services, and other activities such as medication issues [21]. Therefore TAU would consist of interventions that were both less structured and less frequent than the two active treatments.

2. Brief Social Behaviour and Network Therapy (B-SBNT) ± TAU:

Social Behaviour and Network Therapy (SBNT) is built on the idea that social support for change is central to resolving substance dependence and seeks to involve close friends and family as part of the treatment process [22]. The approach was shown to be effective and cost--effective in the large UK Alcohol Treatment Trial (UKATT) [23, 24]. Subsequently, therapists from community drug services in Birmingham were trained to deliver the intervention at a two-day training workshop and then guided by a written manual and supervision using video-recordings of sessions. An evaluation concluded that it was feasible to train 12 therapists to deliver SBNT, with the participating patients reporting a reduction in drug use and improved family and social relationships at the 3-month follow-up point [25].

Originally SBNT was developed as an 8-session intervention, although in reality 64% of the UKATT sample ($n = 320$) received no more than 4 sessions [26]. Some of the most important components occur during the early part of the treatment e.g. drawing a social network diagram; contacting and inviting people; reviewing communication and interactions with significant network members. The original intervention manual [25] was therefore adapted for the current study using a four session format, and is hereafter referred to as Brief Social Behaviour and Network Therapy (B-SBNT). The most effective components of the SBNT intervention [26] were combined with elements of node-link mapping [27] to facilitate the training and delivery of the intervention. The therapist worked with the patient to draw a 'social network diagram' during the first session in order to identify potential social support for change that could be drawn upon in later sessions [28]. Network members identified by the participant were then approached and invited to take part in treatment sessions, and the therapist used elements of communication skill development, coping behaviours and the development of joint activities to support the development of a network-supported relapse management plan. B-SBNT was delivered by a trained clinician that wasn't the patient's usual key worker. Participants were invited to attend four 50-min B-SBNT sessions over a period of 6 weeks, in addition to TAU sessions with their usual keyworker. They were asked to nominate at least one 'network' member who would then be actively encouraged to participate in subsequent sessions.

3. Personal Goal Setting (PGS) ± TAU:

PGS involved an additional active component to usual care through a structured process of setting personal goals and monitoring their attainment. This arm was included to control for the intensity of treatment in the B-SBNT arm and the process of receiving the intervention from a different therapist. PGS consisted of four 50-min sessions over a period of 6 weeks delivered according to a purpose designed manual [29] by a trained clinician. It was based on the principles of node-link mapping [27] and included a review of the participant's current situation and future aspirations, the development of SMART (Specific, Measurable, Agreed-upon, Realistic, Time-limited) goals, and monitoring and feedback on progress in achieving these goals.

Treatment monitoring and fidelity

To ensure that B-SBNT and PGS were delivered with sufficient fidelity, all trial therapists were required to participate in monthly supervision meetings with research clinicians. Each therapeutic session with the therapist was audio recorded, with a proportion randomly selected for fidelity assessment using the UKATT Process Rating Scale [30].

Staff recruitment & training

As the aim of the study was to test the feasibility of training staff to deliver a social network intervention, no attempt was made to randomly select therapists and clinicians volunteered to participate. They were trained using the process adopted in previous SBNT pilot work [25], with an initial one-day training session to introduce the key concepts and procedures involved in each treatment intervention. All staff delivering B-SBNT were then required to pilot the methods with one clinical case prior to the commencement of the trial. Monthly 90-min group supervision sessions were provided for both active treatment conditions, and clinicians brought node-link maps developed in the session to guide discussion.

Participant recruitment & randomisation

Inclusion and exclusion criteria

Each potential participant had to (1) be 18 years or older; (2) have been prescribed OST (methadone or buprenorphine) continuously for the past 12 months; (3) report use of heroin on one or more days in the previous 28 days; (4) give informed consent to participation. The only reason for exclusion was a severe co-morbid mental or physical health issue that prevented an individual from participating in treatment sessions. Any such cases were discussed with clinicians at the time of screening.

The Treatment Outcome Profile (TOP) assessment is completed every 3–6 months for all patients receiving specialist substance misuse treatment in England [31], and includes questions about use of illicit opiates. These data are stored as part of the patient's electronic record unless the patient has refused consent to share this information, and so the research team were able to identify individuals that met the study inclusion criteria by reviewing the case record every 6 weeks. A list of potential participants was given to clinical staff in each participating team, and the patient was given an initial overview and written information about the study at their next routine appointment with their usual clinician. If the patient expressed an interest they were contacted by a researcher who provided further information and invited them to sign a consent form. Patients were randomised and allocated to treatment intervention following completion of the baseline interview. A dynamic randomisation algorithm was used, minimizing differences in the numbers allocated to each experimental group [32]. As this was an open trial, randomisation was not stratified by investigational site as this would not be properly concealed, and was done using a secure, remote randomisation service independent of the research team.

Assessments

Assessment was conducted before treatment randomisation (baseline), and at 3 and 12 months post-baseline. Sociodemographic data was only collected at baseline, and included age, sex, ethnicity, employment status, and living situation. Ten other instruments were administered at all three time points, and further details are given in the study protocol [33].

(i) Illicit drug use: section B of the Maudsley Addiction Profile (MAP) [34] was used to quantify the number of days on which heroin, cocaine, benzodiazepine or alcohol was used in the previous 28 days, and the average amount of use of each drug on each using day. A urine sample was taken to test for heroin, methadone, buprenorphine, cocaine and benzodiazepines.

(ii) Health risk behaviour: section C of the MAP [34] to quantify the number of days on which drugs were injected in the previous 28 days.

(iii) Drug-related problems: section E of the MAP [34] was used to quantify the number of days of work and acquisitive crime in the previous 28 days.

(iv) Severity of drug dependence: the Leeds Dependence Questionnaire (LDQ) [35] is validated in drug users and is composed of 10 questions that are summed to give a maximum score of 30. A higher score indicates greater dependence.

(v) Psychological functioning: measured using three domains of the Clinical Outcome in Routine Evaluation (CORE-OM) scale [36] (a) well-being (4 items); (b) symptoms (12 items: 4 depression, 4 anxiety, 2 trauma, 2 physical); (c) functioning (12 items – 4 general functioning, 4 functioning in social relationships, 4 functioning in close relationships). Each item is scored between 0 and 4, and a mean score is reported for each domains.

(vi) Social functioning: the Social Satisfaction Questionnaire (SSQ) [37] is an 8-item self-complete questionnaire that measures perceived social problems. The maximum score is 24, and higher scores represent greater satisfaction with housing, finances or relationships.

(vii) Motivation to change behaviour: the Readiness to Change Questionnaire–Treatment Version (RTCQ-TV) [38] is a 15-item questionnaire that allows the assignment of substance users to one of the stages described in Prochaska and DiClemente's model of change (i.e. Precontemplation, Contemplation or Action) [39].

(viii) Social network structure and function: the Important People Drug & Alcohol Interview (IPDA) [14] is a researcher-administered instrument that requires respondents to provide the first name and relationship of up to 10 members of their social network who have been important to them in the previous three months. For each network member identified the respondent then rates their frequency of contact, importance, general support, frequency of use of drugs or alcohol, and their reaction to the participant's substance use and treatment.

(ix) General social support: the Interpersonal Support Evaluation List (ISEL) [40] is a self-completion instrument that requires the participant to rate 40 statements about the availability of possible social resources. Four 10-item subscales are then generated, measuring 'Tangible' support, 'Appraisal' support, 'Self-esteem' support, and 'Belonging' support. Each subscale is scored between 0 and 30, where a higher score indicates a greater perception of support.

(x) Therapeutic engagement: the 36 items that make up the Engagement section of the Client Evaluation of Self and Treatment (CEST) [41] were completed by the participant, with each item scored between 1 and 5. This generated 4 sub-scale scores representing 'Treatment Participation', 'Treatment Satisfaction', 'Counselling Rapport', and 'Peer Support'.

Sample size

As this was a pilot feasibility study, a formal sample size calculation was not appropriate. However, by using a recruitment goal of 120 participants (i.e. 40 in each treatment arm), we calculated that if the proportion of patients that stopped taking heroin in the B-SBNT group was 0.3 (e.g. 30%), this would produce an approximate 95% confidence interval of 0.18–0.44 (e.g. 18% to 44%) for this estimate. Alternatively, if the proportion was found to be 0.1 (e.g. 10%), an approximate 95% confidence interval would be 0.01–0.19 (e.g. 1% to 19%).

Data analysis

Trial outcome analysis

Data was analysed according to the intention-to-treat principle; all randomised participants were included in the analysis irrespective of whether they stayed in the trial or not, with missing data treated as failing to achieve the outcome. The major analyses were pre-specified in a statistical analysis plan completed prior to database lock. Analyses were conducted in SAS 9.2 or above (www.sas.com/software/sas9). The primary outcome measure was the number of days that the participant had used heroin in the previous 28 days. The primary analyses compared B-SBNT with the other two arms (PGS and TAU), and subjects were analysed using a generalised mixed model with Gaussian mixed error structures, including experimental group as an explanatory classification variable. The therapists were included as random effects [42]. Analysis of continuous secondary outcomes was conducted using analogous statistical models, including changes in level of injecting drug use, criminal activity, psychological symptoms, severity of drug dependence, motivation for drug abstinence, social satisfaction, therapeutic engagement, social network structure and function, and general social support.

Session rating

Each audio-recorded treatment session was rated by the two independent raters (CB and SA) using a standardised measure of fidelity for SBNT developed for the UK Alcohol Treatment Trial (UKATT) [30]. Inter-rater reliability was assessed using a two-way mixed, consistency, average-measures Intra Class Correlations (ICC) [43] to assess the degree that coders provided consistency in their ratings of the frequency and quality items across sessions.

Results

Sample

The study began in NHS services in the metropolitan areas of Solihull and Leicester. However, the service in Leicester underwent a re-commissioning process early in the trial period which led to a large reorganisation that drew resources away from the study. Staff were uncertain of their jobs throughout the trial period, and the disruption to clinical services hampered screening and recruitment. As a result, the Leicester site managed only 32% of its target of 60 participants, whereas Solihull recruited 90%. A further site (Birmingham) was added to compensate for this shortfall, but the overall recruitment level fell short of the target level at a total of 83 opiate dependent patients. Figure 1 shows a flow diagram for the trial, consistent with the Consolidated Standards of Reporting Trials (CONSORT) 2010 statement [44].

Participants were randomly allocated to SBNT+TAU ($n = 26$), PGS + TAU ($n = 27$) or TAU only ($n = 30$). The primary outcome was illicit opiate use, measured by urine screen and participant self-report. In addition, participants completed secondary outcome measures at baseline ($n = 83$), 3-months ($n = 74$) and 12-months ($n = 70$) post-treatment.

Study aims

1. To test the feasibility of recruiting patients engaged in drug treatment services for at least a year but still reporting heroin use to a trial of B-SBNT, and follow them up over 12 months.

The mean age of the sample was 37 years (range 25–61), and 72 (87%) participants were male. The participants were predominantly white British ($n = 69$, 83%), unmarried ($n = 75$, 90%), and unemployed ($n = 63$, 76%). Seventeen (21%) had been receiving OST for between 12 and 24 months, 40 (48%) between 25 and 60 months, and 25 (30%) for over 5 years. Most ($n = 51$, 61%)

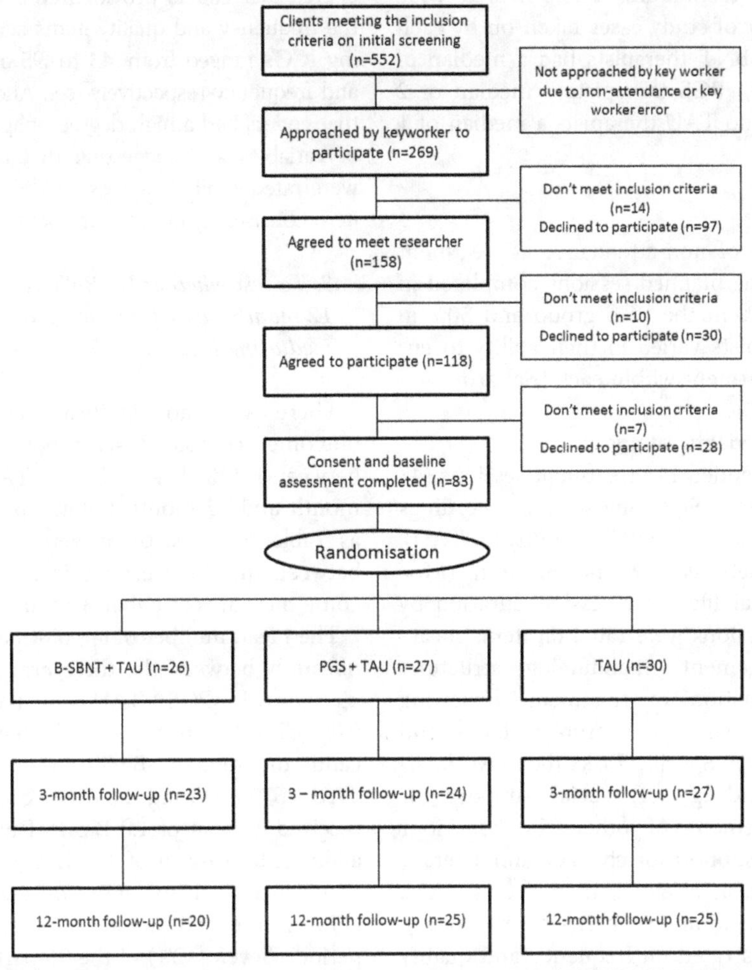

Fig. 1 Flow diagram for the trial, consistent with the Consolidated Standards of Reporting Trials (CONSORT) 2010 statement

expressed a goal of being abstinent from all opiates (prescribed and illicit) within 12 months. Seventy six of the participants (82%) were prescribed methadone solution and 7 (18%) buprenorphine sublingual tablets. The median dose of methadone was 60 mg/day (range 14 to 106), and the median dose of buprenorphine was 8 mg (range 6 to 16 mg).

Trial engagement & participation

A total of 1524 patients were treated in the 3 services during the period of study, and just over a third (552, 36%) were prescribed OST and reported opiate use in the past month according to the latest TOP. The protocol required the patient's regular key worker to approach patients meeting the inclusion criteria to enquire about their interest in participating in the study. Just under half (269, 49%) were approached, of which 118 (21%) were willing/able to discuss entering the trial, and 83 (15%) consented to participate. Reasons for refusal included not wishing to participate in research, not wanting extra treatment sessions, or having other commitments such as work or family that prevented regular attendance.

Research follow-up

Once recruited to the study, the retention rate was good (84% at 12-months), and the system of tracing participants by accessing their patient records, contacting their GP or pharmacist, or liaising with their drug worker was effective.

2. To test the feasibility of training NHS clinicians with no previous experience of working with social network members to deliver a brief social network-driven intervention (B-SBNT).

Training

Clinicians were asked to volunteer to be trial therapists, and 16 were trained in the 2 intervention arms (7 B-SBNT, 9 PGS). The attendance rate at the monthly group supervision sessions was 66%, and clinicians presented cases using node-link maps generated in sessions and discussed specific techniques. There was a wide variation in the number of study cases taken on by each trained therapist, but SBNT therapists had a median of 2 cases (range 1 to 12), PGS therapists a median of 2 cases (range 1 to 10), and TAU therapists a median of 1 case (range 1 to 4).

Participant engagement

There was a high level of non-attendance at treatment sessions, with 49% of the planned sessions completed in the B-SBNT group, 27% in the PGS group and 50% in the TAU group. Therapists varied in their ability to engage participants in treatment within each trial arm.

Session recordings and fidelity ratings

Overall, participants attended 115 treatment sessions (47 BSBNT, 29 PGS, 39 TAU). Sixty one session recordings were available for analysis (26 BSBNT, 20 PGS, 4 TAU). The sessions lasted between 19 and 67 min (M = 34.4 min; see Additional file 1 for session duration by study arm). Therapy sessions were rated on items measuring Session Management (maintaining structure, agenda setting, explanation of treatment, reviewing inter-session change, consistency of problem focus, and end of sessions summary), Specific Tasks (homework, alternatives to drinking/drug use, social support for change-general, involvement of others in behaviour change and identifying support for change), and Therapist Style (therapist as task oriented, therapist as active agent for change, collaboration, interpersonal focus). Each of these items was rated on frequency and quality on Likert scales ranging from 0 to 4. Additionally, raters recorded the type of treatment maps that were completed during sessions. Additional file 2 shows the average ratings for item frequency, quality and number of maps used per session by study arm. Both raters gave higher frequency and quality ratings for B-SBNT session than for PGS or TAU sessions. A greater number of maps were completed in PGS sessions than in B-SBNT sessions, while a greater number of maps was completed in both active study arms compared to TAU.

Each session was rated by the two independent raters. Inter-rater reliability was assessed using a two-way mixed, consistency, average-measures Intra Class Correlations (ICC; McGraw & Wong, 1996) to assess the degree that coders provided consistency in their ratings of the frequency and quality items across sessions. The resulting ICC's ranged from .43 to .95 and .41 to .93 for quality and frequency respectively (see Additional file 3), indicating that coders had a high degree of agreement for the majority of variables and suggesting that the majority of variables were rated similarly across coders (poor consistency for the item consistency of problem focus only).

3. To test whether B-SBNT reduces heroin use 3 and 12 months after treatment, and to explore potential mediating factors.

There were no significant changes in the primary outcome (combined self-report + objective drug use) between B-SBNT +TAU, GS + TAU, and TAU only at 3-month and 12-month follow-up (see Table 1). Likewise, as Table 2 shows, there were no significant differences between the three groups in any of the secondary outcome measures at either 3-months or 12-months.

The mean number of appointments offered differed significantly between the three arms of the study (B-SBNT +TAU = 6.2, PGS + TAU = 4, TAU = 2, F = 30.11, $p <$ 0.001), but the mean rates of attendance were not significantly different (B-SBNT+TAU = 54%, PGS + TAU = 49%, TAU = 63%). During the 6-week study period participants received a mean of 1.8 B-SBNT and 1.1 PGS sessions, in addition to a mean of 1.3 TAU sessions, representing an attendance rate of 44% overall. Sixteen participants (19.2%) attended no sessions at all during the study period. Eleven (42%) of the 26 participants randomised to B-SBNT brought a network member to a session (7 for 1 session, 1 for 2 sessions and 3 for 3 sessions), compared with none in the PGS and one in the TAU groups.

As the focus of the intervention was on changing social support for recovery from opiate dependence, the IPDA data are explored in more detail. For the whole sample, the median number of people considered important with whom they had contact in the preceding 90 days was 5 (range 2–10). Family members were the most frequently named group (median = 3.2, range 0–10), followed by friends (1.4, 0–6), members of the recovery community (0.5, 0–4), and co-workers (0.2, 0–4). Nearly 80% (66/83) could name 4 'very important people', and none of this sub-group accepted or

Table 1 Differences in the primary outcome measure between the three trial arms

	Median days abstinent from heroin				
	Baseline	3 months	12 months	Relative risk (95% CI) vs TAU 3 months	Relative risk (95% CI) vs TAU 12 months
B-SBNT	15	18	17	0.96 (0.79–1.17)	0.96 (0.78–1.17)
PGS	18	18	18	0.93 (0.77–1.13)	1.00 (0.83–1.20)
TAU	20	23	25		

Table 2 Differences in the secondary outcome measure between the three trial arms

Item	SBNT ($n = 26$)			PGS ($n = 27$)			TAU ($n = 30$)		
	Baseline	3 months	12 months	Baseline	3 months	12 months	Baseline	3 months	12 months
Days abstinent from heroin, median (IQR)	15 (8,24)	18 (2,22)	17 (11,23)	18 (8,24)	18 (8,20)	18 (8,27)	20 (12,26)	23 (14,26)	25 (14,27)
LDQ total, median (IQR)	14 (8,17)	9 (5,16)	10 (6.6,16)	11 (5,15)	6 (5,12)	7 (4,10)	7 (2,13)	6 (3,12)	5 (2,13)
CORE									
Wellbeing, median (IQR)	2 (2,3)	2 (0.8,2.5)	2 (1.3,2.9)	2 (1,2)	1.6 (0.8,2.1)	1.5 (0.8,2)	2 (1,2)	1.3 (0.8,2)	1.5 (0.8,2.3)
Symptoms, median (IQR)	2 (2,3)	2.1 (0.9,2.9)	2.4 (1.1,2.6)	2 (1,2)	1.3 (1,2.3)	1.5 (0.8,2)	2 (1,3)	1.3 (1,2.3)	1.6 (0.8,2.3)
Functioning, median (IQR)	2 (2,3)	1.8 (1.2,2.6)	2.2 (1,2.7)	2 (1,2)	1.5 (1.1,2)	1.6 (0.8,2)	2 (1,2)	1.5 (1.1,2.1)	1.2 (0.8,1.9)
SSQ total, median (IQR)	23 (19,26)	24 (22,28)	24 (19.5,27)	22 (18,25)	23 (19,24)	22 (20,26)	23 (20,27)	24 (20,28)	24 (22,27)
CEST									
Counselling rapport, median (IQR)	40 (38,43)	41 (38,43)	39 (35,46)	39 (36,42)	39 (38,42)	40 (39,42)	40 (39,43)	40 (39,44)	41 (40,48)
Peer support, median (IQR)	32 (28,40)	30 (26,38)	30 (25,37)	30 (28,34)	30 (28,32)	30 (26,34)	32 (28,38)	32 (26,36)	36 (28,38)
Treatment participation, median (IQR)	38 (33,39)	38 (36,39)	38 (31,42)	37 (35,38)	37 (35,38)	38 (35,40)	38 (34,41)	39 (37,42)	41 (40,47)
Treatment satisfaction, median (IQR)	39 (35,41)	40 (36,43)	40 (35,40)	39 (37,41)	39 (37,41)	40 (36,42)	40 (39,43)	40 (39,44)	41 (40,47)
ISEL									
Appraisal, median (IQR)	16 (15,19)	17 (15,18)	18 (14,21)	16 (14,18)	18 (16,20)	18 (16,20)	16 (15,18)	18 (17,20)	18 (16,20)
Belonging, median (IQR)	17 (14,19)	16 (14,18)	17 (14,19.5)	15 (13,17)	17 (15,19.5)	16 (14.5,19.5)	17 (15,18)	17 (16,20)	18 (15,21.5)
Self-esteem, median (IQR)	14 (12,17)	14 (13,15)	13.5 (12,16.5)	14 (12,16)	15 (14,17)	15 (14,18)	16 (13,18)	15 (14,18)	15 (14,20)
Tangible, median (IQR)	17 (13,19)	16 (14,19)	16 (14,19.5)	15 (14,19)	16 (15,19)	18 (14.5,19.5)	16 (14,18)	16 (14,17)	17.5 (15.5,21)
IPDA									
Index 1-network size (IQR)	−0.42 (−0.66,0.24)	0.07 (−0.83,0.83)	−0.29 (−0.74,1.01)	− 0.18 (− 0.66,0.64)	−0.14 (− 0.83,0.65)	0.12 (− 0.74,0.49)	0.24 (− 0.18,1.0)	0.07 (− 0.83,1.18)	0.12 (− 0.29,0.84)
Index 2–daily network size (IQR)	− 0.50 (−1.06,0.06)	− 0.10 (− 0.58,0.37)	−0.49 (− 0.76,0.06)	−0.06 (− 0.50,1.18)	−0.10 (− 0.58,0.37)	−0.49 (− 0.49,0.61)	−0.22 (− 0.50,0.06)	−0.50 (− 0.50,0.62)	0.06 (− 0.49,0.61)
Index 3-importance (IQR)	−0.14 (− 0.65,0.62)	0.17 (− 0.33,0.75)	−0.12 (− 0.58,0.67)	−0.02 (− 1.08,1.25)	−0.01 (− 0.89,0.94)	−0.12 (− 0.62,0.38)	−0.02 (− 0.86,1.25)	−0.01 (− 0.43,0.75)	0.38 (− 0.12,1.14)
Component 1: substance involvement (IQR)	−0.40 (− 0.93,0.05)	−0.35 (− 0.83,0.62)	−0.28 (− 0.79,1.14)	−0.06 (− 0.44,0.67)	−0.24 (− 0.51,0.34)	−0.37 (− 0.84,0.16)	−0.24 (− 0.75,0.85)	−0.49 (− 0.66,0.47)	−0.07 (− 0.58,0.57)
Component 2: general/ treatment support (IQR)	0.14 (− 0.56,0.66)	−0.04 (− 0.48,0.57)	0.24 (− 0.58,0.66)	−0.49 (− 1.03, 0.30)	−0.10 (− 0.50,0.74)	−0.14 (− 0.83,0.43)	0.48 (− 0.35,1.02)	0.09 (− 0.17,0.77)	0.34 (− 0.30,0.82)
Component 3-support for substance use (IQR)	0.16 (− 0.86,0.89)	0.25 (− 0.75,0.82)	0.48 (− 0.72,1.37)	0.34 (− 0.86,0.89)	0.08 (−0.75,0.68)	− 0.51 (− 0.94,0.90)	0.02 (− 0.86,0.72)	0.07 (− 1.02,0.57)	−0.51 (− 0.94,0.68)
RCQ-TV, median (IQR)	4.5 (4,7)	5 (4,6)	4 (4,7)	4 (3,5)	4 (3,5)	4 (4,6)	4.5 (4,6)	4 (4,6)	5 (4,7)

encouraged drug use. A clear majority of the reported network (84%) supported the participant attending drug treatment services. Heavy drug users made up just 7% of the reported network, and a median of 4 out of 5 network members named were totally abstinent from illicit drugs.

Discussion

The National Institute for Health and Care Excellence (NICE) has highlighted the limits of the evidence base for psychosocial treatments for heroin dependence, but also noted the promise of family and social network interventions [45]. Here an attempt was made to specifically adapt the SBNT intervention to make it more suitable for use within drug treatment services by using the elements found to be most important in the process of change [26]. Although it was possible to train clinical staff to an adequate level of competence (fidelity analysis of the audiotapes showed that B-SBNT sessions were clearly distinguishable from the PGS and TAU sessions), and to follow-up a high proportion (84%) of study participants for 12 months, the study highlights two major challenges to implementation of this feasibility study in UK treatment services.

The first relates to organisational barriers to conducting research with this population in OST services in England. The current national policy of re-tendering the contract to provide treatment services [46, 47] means that the service provider may change every three years. Not only is this disruptive to patients and staff, but it also presents a significant impediment to conducting clinical research. One site in this trial was unaffected by re-commissioning during the trial period and recruited 90% of its target in the available time; the other underwent a re-commissioning process three months after the study started and recruited a third of its target. The need to compete to win a new contract possibly drew vital resources away from the clinical 'front line' and distracted otherwise motivated clinicians from their research role. As substance use disorders have come to be understood as chronic illnesses that require a chronic disease management model, so continuity of treatment provision becomes more important [48]. In a review of the evidence base for Recovery Oriented Systems of Care, White highlights stability in terms of funding, organizational ownership and workforce is a key measure of quality [49].

The second challenge concerns the potential participants' reluctance to engage in psychosocial therapy. The population under study was the most intractable group in treatment i.e. opiate dependent individuals who had received OST at flexible dosing levels for at least one year but had not stopped using heroin. Many had been receiving OST at a therapeutic dose for at least 5 years and were still reporting heroin use on more than half of the preceding 28 days, in addition to regular use of crack cocaine. Across the three sites 552 patients met the eligibility criteria, but only 83 (15%) started the study. Overall 155 (28%) patients refused the offer of participating when they were initially assessed or failed to attend the assessment appointment. This reflects the difficulty of making contact with patients of UK OST services, but also their reluctance to receive interventions in addition to an OST prescription. Less than two-thirds of the sample (51/83) saw their goal of treatment to be abstinent from both illicit (i.e. heroin) and prescribed (i.e. OST) opiates in the next year, with the rest either unsure of their goal ($n = 9$) or aiming for abstinence from illicit opiates only ($n = 23$). Nearly 20% of the participants did not attend any treatment sessions during the study period, although there was some evidence once engaged the social network intervention was more likely to be completed (8 (30.7%) B-SBNT cases completed the full 4-session program compared to 2 (7.4%) PGS participants).

The benefits of OST in this population are well documented [50], but the effect of additional psychosocial treatment is not clear [4]. There is a body of evidence that shows that adding more service produces better outcomes [51–53], but when specific psychosocial interventions are added the evidence base is not as strong [54]. This study found no difference in any measure between the three treatment arms. This mirrors recent findings in prescription opioid dependence where the addition of counselling to OST made no difference to drug related outcomes [55], and in treatment-refractory opioid dependent individuals where there was no evidence for the superiority of a cognitive behavioural intervention over an active comparison condition [56]. Another study cited loss of hope as a reason for non-attendance at counselling sessions [57]. This was a feasibility study of a promising intervention, and the next planned step was to move to a larger, adequately powered trial. However, for this study to lead to a definitive trial it would have needed to provide an indication of positive change in the main outcome measure for the social network intervention. Incomplete recruitment meant a lack of power to determine potentially small effects, and it is also likely that the 'dose' of social network treatment administered was inadequate to change behaviour in a group with such complex and enduring needs. During the 6-week study period participants attended less than 50% of the treatment sessions offered to them (active intervention or routine appointments), and less than half of the B-SBNT cases involved a social network member in a treatment session.

Orford has called for a shift in the way addiction research is conducted, with less emphasis on studying named interventions and more focus on studying change processes within the broader, longer-acting systems of which treatment is part [58]. Previous research has shown that some patients benefit from OST without the need for additional non-medical treatment, whereas others only benefit when an adequate dose of psychosocial intervention is added [53, 59]. Rates of abstinence-based recovery are low in this population, and McKay has argued that treatments need to link patients to reinforcers that will make continued abstinence more appealing [60]. Interventions that extend beyond the individual to the family and wider social network are a good way of doing this. However, in order to increase the amount of exposure to therapeutic components it may be necessary to incorporate 'evidence based practices' (EBPs) into routine care [61], rather than trying to deliver a whole new additional intervention package. A greater emphasis on finding suitable reinforcers for participation may be needed, and contingency management strategies have shown promise in this population [62, 63]. The variability in therapist involvement in this trial also reminds us that there should also be a greater focus on studying therapist factors in existing treatment staff, and future attempts might start by integrating social network-orientated thinking into a whole team approach.

Conclusions

This study has shown that promising interventions to harness social network support for change are feasible in the OST population, and staff can be trained to deliver them. However, further work is required to tailor the intervention to this population, possibly through the addition of more potent reinforcers to attend therapy sessions. It has also highlighted the need for a stable workforce and organizational structure within which to deliver elements of a chronic care model.

Additional files

Additional file 1: Minimum, maximum, and mean session duration in minutes by trial arm. A comparison of the treatment session lengths between the three trial arms.

Additional file 2: Mean ratings for item frequency, quality and number of maps used per session by study arm. Each audio-recorded treatment session was rated by two independent raters using a standardised measure of fidelity for SBNT. This file presents data from this measure, as well as information about the number of node-link maps produced in each session.

Additional file 3: Inter-rater reliability for frequency and quality ratings. Each session was rated by the two independent raters, and inter-rater reliability was assessed using Intra Class Correlations to assess the degree that coders provided consistency in their ratings of the frequency and quality items across sessions.

Abbreviations

B-SBNT: Brief Social Behaviour and Network Therapy; CEST: Client Evaluation of Self and Treatment; CONSORT: Consolidated standards of reporting trials; CORE-OM: Clinical outcome in routine evaluation – outcome measure; EBP: Evidence-based practice; ICC: Intra class correlation; IPDA: Important people drugs and alcohol; IQR: Inter-quartile range; ISEL: Interpersonal support evaluation list; LDQ: Leeds dependence questionnaire; MAP: Maudsley addiction profile; NHS: National Health Service; NICE: National Institute for Health and Care Excellence; NTA: National treatment agency; OST: Opioid substitution therapy; PGS: Personal goal setting; RTCQ-TV: Readiness to change questionnaire – treatment version; SBNT: Social behaviour and network therapy; SMART: Specific, measurable, agreed-upon, realistic, time-limited; SSQ: Social satisfaction questionnaire; TAU: Treatment as usual; TOP: Treatment outcome profile; UKATT: UK alcohol treatment trial

Acknowledgements

The authors are grateful to Rob Herson and Jason Turner for acting as service user advisors on the trial management group from both the family member (RH) and the patient (JT) perspective.

Funding

This paper presents independent research funded by the National Institute for Health Research (NIHR) under its Research for Patient Benefit (RfPB) Programme (Grant Reference Number PB-PG-0610-22392). The views expressed are those of the author(s) and not necessarily those of the NHS, the NIHR or the Department of Health. The funding body had no role in the design of the study beyond organising peer review as part of the process of obtaining funding. The funding body had no role in the collection, analysis, and interpretation of data or in writing the manuscript.

Authors' contributions

ED is the chief investigator for the project. ED, AC and JS drafted the manuscript. ED, AC, MC, SG, AB, EF and NF contributed to the design of the study. JS coordinated the implementation of the project. JS, DB, CP, CB, SA & IG were involved in the collection and analysis of the data. NF was the trial statistician. All authors read and approved the final manuscript.

Consent for publication

Not applicable.

Competing interests

The authors declare that they have no competing interests.

Author details

[1]Birmingham and Solihull Mental Health NHS Foundation Trust, c/o Dept of Psychiatry, The Barberry 25 Vincent Drive, Edgbaston, Birmingham B152FG, UK. [2]Addictions Department, Institute of Psychiatry, Psychology & Neuroscience, King's College London, London, UK. [3]School of Psychology, The University of Birmingham, Birmingham, UK. [4]Leicester City Drug and Alcohol Service, Leicester, UK. [5]Health Economics Unit, College of Medical and Dental Sciences, University of Birmingham, Birmingham, UK. [6]Institute of Clinical Trials and Methodology, University College London, London, UK.

References

1. Best D, George S, Day E. The development of the drug treatment system in England. In: Day E, editor. Clinical topics in addiction. London: RCPsych; 2007. p. 14–28.
2. HM Government. Drug strategy 2010. Reducing demand, restricting supply, building recovery: supporting people to live a drug free life. London: Home Office; 2010.

3. McKeganey N, Bloor M, Robertson M, Neale J, MacDougall J. Abstinence and drug abuse treatment: results from the drug outcome research in Scotland study. Drugs Educ Prev Policy. 2006;13(6):537–50.
4. Day E, Mitcheson L. Psychosocial interventions in OST services: does the evidence provide a case for optimism or nihilism? Addiction. 2017;113(8):1329–36.
5. Drummond DC, Kouimtsidis C, Reynolds M, Russell I, Godfrey C, McCusker M, Coulton S, Parrott S, Davis P, Tarrier N et al: The effectiveness and cost effectiveness of cognitive behaviour therapy for opiate misusers in methadone maintenance treatment: a multicentre randomised controlled trial (UKCBTMM). Final report to the Department of Health Research and Development Directorate. In. London: Department of Health; 2004.
6. Best D, Hernando R, Gossop M, Sidwell C, Strang J. Getting by with a little help from your friends, the impact of peer networks on criminality in a cohort of treatment-seeking drug users. Addict Behav. 2003;28:597–603.
7. Gogineni A, Stein M, Friedmann PD. Social relationships and intravenous drug use among methadone maintenance patients. Drug Alcohol Depend. 2001;64:47–53.
8. Latkin C, Mandell W, Oziemkowska M, Celentano D, Vlahov D, Ensminger M, Knowlton A. Using social network analysis to study patterns of drug use among urban drug users at high risk for HIV/AIDS. Drug Alcohol Depend. 1995;38(1):1–9.
9. Schroeder JR, Latkin CA, Hoover DR, Curry AD, Knowlton AR, Celentano DD. Illicit drug use in one's social network and in one's neighbourhood predicts individual heroin and cocaine use. Ann Epidemiol. 2001;11:389–94.
10. Cohen S, Lichtenstein E. Partner Behaviours that support quitting smoking. J Consult Clin Psychol. 1990;58(3):304–9.
11. Goehl L, Nunes E, Quitkin F, Hilton I. Social networks and methadone treatment outcome: the costs and benefits of social ties. Am J Drug Alcohol Abuse. 1993;19(3):251–62.
12. Havassy BE, Wasserman DA, Hall SM. Social relationships and abstinence from cocaine in an American treatment sample. Addiction. 1995;90:699–710.
13. Wasserman DA, Stewart AL, Delucchi KL. Social support and abstinence from opiates and cocaine during opioid maintenance treatment. Drug Alcohol Depend. 2001;65:65–75.
14. Zywiak WH, Neighbors CJ, Martin RA, Johnson JE, Eaton CA, Rohsenow DJ. The important people drug and alcohol interview: psychometric properties, predictive validity, and implications for treatment. J Subst Abus Treat. 2009;36:321–30.
15. Centre for Social Justice. Green paper on criminal justice and addiction. London: The Centre for Social Justice; 2010.
16. National Treatment Agency for Substance Misuse. NTA policy on involvement of users and family members. London: NTA; 2008.
17. National Treatment Agency for Substance Misuse. NTA business plan 2010–11. London: NTA; 2010.
18. The Betty Ford Institute Consensus Panel. What is recovery? A working definition from the Betty ford institute. J Subst Abus Treat. 2007;33:221–8.
19. Goranitis I, Coast J, Day E, Copello A, Freemantle N, Frew E. Maximizing health or sufficient capability in economic evaluation? A methodological experiment of treatment for drug addiction. Med Decis Mak. 2017;37(5):498–511.
20. Goranitis I, Coast J, Day E, Copello A, Freemantle N, Seddon J, Bennett C, Frew E. Measuring health and broader well-being benefits in the context of opiate dependence: the psychometric performance of the ICECAP-A and the EQ-5D-5L. Value Health. 2016;19:820–8.
21. Best D, Day E, Morgan B, Oza T, Copello A, Gossop M. What treatment means in practice: an analysis of the delivery of evidence-based structured interventions in criminal justice drug treatment services in Birmingham, England. Addict Res Theory. 2009;17(6):678–87.
22. Copello A, Orford J, Hodgson R, Tober G, Barrett C. Social behaviour and network therapy - basic principles and early experiences. Addict Behav. 2002;27(3):345–66.
23. UKATT Research Team. Effectiveness of treatment for alcohol problems: findings of the randomised UK alcohol treatment trial (UKATT). BMJ. 2005;331(7516):541–4.
24. UKATT Research Team. Cost effectiveness of treatment for alcohol problems: findings of the randomised UK alcohol treatment trial (UKATT). BMJ. 2005;331(7516):544–8.
25. Copello A, Williamson E, Orford J, Day E. Implementing and evaluating social behaviour and network therapy in drug treatment practice in the UK: a feasibility study. Addict Behav. 2006;31(5):802–10.
26. Dale V, Coulton S, Godfrey C, Copello A, Hodgson R, Heather N, Orford J, Raistrick D, Slegg G, Tober G, et al. Exploring treatment attendance and its relationship to outcome in a randomized controlled trial of treatment for alcohol problems: secondary analysis of the UK alcohol treatment trial (UKATT). Alcohol Alcohol. 2011;46(5):592–9.
27. Dansereau DF, Simpson DD. A picture is worth a thousand words: the case for graphic representations. Prof Psychol. 2009;40(1):104–10.
28. Day E. Building bridges to positive social identities: the social network diagram and opiate substitution treatment. In: Buckingham SA, Best D, editors. Addiction, Behavioural change and social identity. Abingdon: Routledge; 2017.
29. Day E, Best D, Bartholomew NG, Dansereau DF, Simpson DD. The BTEI care planning manual: mapping achievable goals. In: Routes to recovery. London: National Treatment Agency for Substance Misuse; 2008.
30. Tober G, Clyne W, Finnegan O, Farrin A, Russell I, UKATT Research Team. Validation of a scale for rating the delivery of psycho-social treatments for alcohol dependence and misuse: the UKATT process rating scale (PRS). Alcohol Alcohol. 2008;43(6):675–82.
31. Marsden J, Farrell M, Bradbury C, Dale-Perera A, Eastwood B, Roxborough M, Taylor S. Development of the treatment outcomes profile. Addiction. 2008; 103:1450–60.
32. Pocock SJ. Clinical trials: a practical approach. Chichester: John Wiley & Sons; 1983.
33. Day E, Copello A, Seddon J, Christie M, Bamber D, Powell C, George S, Ball A, Frew E, Freemantle N. Pilot study of a social network intervention for heroin users in opiate substitution treatment: study protocol for a randomized controlled trial. Trials. 2013;14(1):264.
34. Marsden J, Gossop M, Stewart D, Best D, Farrell M, Strang J. The Maudsley addiction profile: development and user manual. London: National Addiction Centre/Institute of Psychiatry; 1998.
35. Raistrick D, Bradshaw J, Tober G, Weiner J, Allison J, Healey C. Development of the Leeds dependence questionnaire (LDQ): a questionnaire to measure alcohol and opiate dependence in the context of a treatment evaluation package. Addiction. 1994;89:563–72.
36. Evans C, Connell J, Barkham M, Margison F, McGrath G, Mellor-Clark J, Audin K. Towards a standardized brief outcome measure: psychometric properties and utility of the CORE-OM. Br J Psychiatry. 2002;180:51–60.
37. Raistrick D, Tober G, Heather N, Clark JA. Validation of the social satisfaction questionnaire for outcome evaluation in substance use disorders. Psychiatr Bull. 2007;31:333–6.
38. Heather N, Luce A, Peck D, Dunbar B, James I. Development of a treatment version of the readiness to change questionnaire. Addict Res. 1999;7(1):63–83.
39. Prochaska JO, DiClemente CC. Transtheoretical therapy: toward a more integrative model of change. Psychother Theory Res Pract Train. 1982;19(3): 276–88.
40. Cohen S, Mermelstein R, Kamarck T, Hoberman HM. Measuring the functional components of social support. In: Sarason IG, Sarason BR, editors. Measuring the functional components of social support. London: Springer; 1985. p. 73–94.
41. Joe GW, Broome KM, Rowan-Szal GA, Simpson DD. Measuring patient attributes and engagement in treatment. J Subst Abus Treat. 2002;22:183–96.
42. SAS Institute Inc. Chapter 6: introduction to mixed Modelling procedures. In: SAS/STAT 92 User's guide (second edition). Cary: SAS Institute Inc.; 2009. p. 127–40.
43. KO MG, Wong SP. Forming inferences about some intraclass correlation coefficients. Psychol Methods. 1996;1(1):30–46.
44. Schulz KF, Altman DG, Moher D, Group ftC. CONSORT 2010 statement: updated guidelines for reporting parallel group randomised trials. BMJ. 2010;340:c332.
45. National Collaborating Centre for Mental Health. Drug misuse: psychosocial interventions. London: British Psychological Society & The Royal College of Psychiatrists; 2008.
46. Drummond C. Cuts to addiction services are a false economy. In: The bmj opinion, vol. 2017: BMJ; 2017.
47. Mohammadi D. Addiction Services in England: in need of an intervention. Lancet Psychiatry. 2014;1:421–2.
48. AT ML, Starrels JL, Tai B, Gordon AJ, Brown R, Ghitza U, Gourevitch M, Stein J, Oros M, Horton T, et al. Can substance use disorders be managed using the chronic care model? Review and recommendations from a NIDA consensus group. Public Health Rev. 2013;35(2):8.
49. White WL. Recovery management and recovery-oriented systems of care: scientific rationale and promising practices. Northeast Addiction Technology Transfer Center: Pittsburgh; 2008.

50. Connock M, Juarez-Garcia A, Jowett S, Frew E, Liu Z, Fry-Smith A, Day E, Linzeris N, Roberts T, Burls A, et al. Methadone and Buprenorphine for the Management of Opioid Dependence: a systematic review and economic evaluation. Health Technol Assess. 2006;11(9):1–171.
51. Ball JC, Ross A. The effectiveness of methadone maintenance treatment: patients, progress, services and outcomes. New York: Springer-Verlag; 1991.
52. Kraft MK, Rothbard AB, Hadley TR, AT ML, Asch DA. Are supplementary services provided during methadone maintenance really cost-effective? Am J Psychiatr. 1997;154(9):1214–9.
53. AT ML, Hagan TA, Levine M, Gould F, Meyers K, Bencivengo M, Durell J. Supplemental social services improve outcomes in public addiction treatment. Addiction. 1998;93(10):1489–99.
54. Amato L, Minozzi S, Davoli M, Vecchi S. Psychosocial combined with agonist maintenance treatments versus agonist maintenance treatments alone for treatment of opioid dependence. Coch Database Syst Rev. 2011;10: CD004147.
55. Weiss RD, Potter JS, Fiellin DA, Byrne M, Connery HS, Dickinson W, Gardin J, Griffin LM, Gourevitch MN, Haller DL, et al. Adjunctive counseling during brief and extended Buprenorphine-Naloxone treatment for prescription Opioid dependence: a 2-phase randomized controlled trial. Arch Gen Psychiatry. 2011;68(12):1238–46.
56. Otto MW, Hearon BA, RK MH, Calkins AW, Pratt E, Murray HW, Safren SA, Pollack MH. A randomized, controlled trial of the efficacy of an interoceptive exposure-based CBT for treatment-refractory outpatients with opioid dependence. J Psychoactive Drugs. 2014;46(5):402–11.
57. Darker C, Sweeney B, El Hassan H, Kelly A, O'Connor S, Smyth B, Barry J. Non-attendance at counselling therapy in cocaine-using methadone-maintained patients: lessons learnt from an abandoned randomised controlled trial. Ir J Med Sci. 2012;181(4):483–9.
58. Orford J. Asking the right questions in the right way: the need for a shift in research on psychological treatments for addiction. Addiction. 2008;103(6): 875–85.
59. Schwartz RP, Kelly SM, O'Grady KE, Gandhi D, Jaffe JH. Randomized trial of standard methadone treatment compared to initiating methadone without counseling: 12-month findings. Addiction. 2012;107:943–52.
60. McKay JR. Making the hard work of recovery more attractive for those with substance use disorders. Addiction. 2017;112(5):751–7.
61. Manuel JK, Hagedorn HJ, Finney JW. Implementing evidence-based psychosocial treatment in specialty substance use disorder care. Psychol Addict Behav. 2011;25(2):225–37.
62. Weaver T, Metrebian N, Hellier J, Pilling S, Charles V, Little N, Poovendran D, Mitcheson L, Ryan F, Bowden-Jones O, et al. Use of contingency management incentives to improve completion of hepatitis B vaccination in people undergoing treatment for heroin dependence: a cluster randomised trial. Lancet. 2015;384(9938):153-63.
63. Lussier JP, Heil SH, Mongeon JA, Badger GJ, Higgins ST. A meta-analysis of voucher-based reinforcement therapy for substance use disorders. Addiction. 2006;101(2):192–203.

Permissions

All chapters in this book were first published in PSYCHIATRY, by BioMed Central; hereby published with permission under the Creative Commons Attribution License or equivalent. Every chapter published in this book has been scrutinized by our experts. Their significance has been extensively debated. The topics covered herein carry significant findings which will fuel the growth of the discipline. They may even be implemented as practical applications or may be referred to as a beginning point for another development.

The contributors of this book come from diverse backgrounds, making this book a truly international effort. This book will bring forth new frontiers with its revolutionizing research information and detailed analysis of the nascent developments around the world.

We would like to thank all the contributing authors for lending their expertise to make the book truly unique. They have played a crucial role in the development of this book. Without their invaluable contributions this book wouldn't have been possible. They have made vital efforts to compile up to date information on the varied aspects of this subject to make this book a valuable addition to the collection of many professionals and students.

This book was conceptualized with the vision of imparting up-to-date information and advanced data in this field. To ensure the same, a matchless editorial board was set up. Every individual on the board went through rigorous rounds of assessment to prove their worth. After which they invested a large part of their time researching and compiling the most relevant data for our readers.

The editorial board has been involved in producing this book since its inception. They have spent rigorous hours researching and exploring the diverse topics which have resulted in the successful publishing of this book. They have passed on their knowledge of decades through this book. To expedite this challenging task, the publisher supported the team at every step. A small team of assistant editors was also appointed to further simplify the editing procedure and attain best results for the readers.

Apart from the editorial board, the designing team has also invested a significant amount of their time in understanding the subject and creating the most relevant covers. They scrutinized every image to scout for the most suitable representation of the subject and create an appropriate cover for the book.

The publishing team has been an ardent support to the editorial, designing and production team. Their endless efforts to recruit the best for this project, has resulted in the accomplishment of this book. They are a veteran in the field of academics and their pool of knowledge is as vast as their experience in printing. Their expertise and guidance has proved useful at every step. Their uncompromising quality standards have made this book an exceptional effort. Their encouragement from time to time has been an inspiration for everyone.

The publisher and the editorial board hope that this book will prove to be a valuable piece of knowledge for researchers, students, practitioners and scholars across the globe.

List of Contributors

Gabriella Gobbi, Eduard Dumitrescu, Maykel F. Ghabrash, John Tabaka and Nicolas A. Nuñez
Department of Psychiatry, Neurobiological Psychiatry Unit, McGill University Health Center (MUHC), McGill University, Room 220, 1033 Pine Avenue West,, Montreal, QC, Canada
Department of Psychiatry, Mood Disorder Clinic, McGill University Health Center, McGill University, Montreal, QC, Canada

Marilyn Christie, Deborah Bamber, Charlotte Powell and Andrew Ball
Leicester City Drug and Alcohol Service, Leicester, UK

Emma Frew and Ilias Goranitis
Health Economics Unit, College of Medical and Dental Sciences, University of Birmingham, Birmingham, UK

Nick Freemantle
Institute of Clinical Trials and Methodology, University College London, London, UK

Stefano Comai
Department of Psychiatry, Neurobiological Psychiatry Unit, McGill University Health Center (MUHC), McGill University, Room 220, 1033 Pine Avenue West, Montreal, QC, Canada
Division of Neuroscience, San Raffaele Scientific Institute and Vita-Salute University, Milan, Italy

Linda Booij
Department of Psychiatry, Neurobiological Psychiatry Unit, McGill University Health Center (MUHC), McGill University, Room 220, 1033 Pine Avenue West, Montreal, QC, Canada
Department of Psychology, Concordia University and Sainte-Justine Hospital Research Center, University of Montréal, Montréal, QC, Canada

Marie Saint-Laurent, Stephen Vida, Theodore Kolivakis, Allan Fielding, Nancy Low and Pablo Cervantes
Department of Psychiatry, Mood Disorder Clinic, McGill University Health Center, McGill University, Montreal, QC, Canada

Yuankai Zhu, Liqiang Zhou, Yunfeng Han, Tao Yin, Zhaoting Cheng, Guopeng Zhang, Yanxia Shen and Jing Chen
Department of Nuclear Medicine, Tongji Hospital, Tongji Medical College, Huazhong University of Science and Technology, Wuhan, Hubei Province 430030, China

Jinming Li
Department of Nuclear Medicine, Tongji Hospital, Tongji Medical College, Huazhong University of Science and Technology, Wuhan, Hubei Province 430030, China
Department of Nuclear Medicine, Renmin Hospital of Wuhan University, Wuhan, Hubei Province 430060, China

Yuan Yang
Department of Neurology, Tongji Hospital, Tongji Medical College, Huazhong University of Science and Technology, Wuhan, Hubei Province 430030, China

Santushi D. Amarasuriya
Department of Medical Humanities, Faculty of Medicine, University of Colombo, 25, Kynsey Road, Colombo 8, Sri Lanka
Centre for Mental Health, Melbourne School of Population and Global Health, University of Melbourne, 207 Bouverie Street, Parkville, VIC 3010, Australia

Anthony F. Jorm and Nicola J. Reavley
Centre for Mental Health, Melbourne School of Population and Global Health, University of Melbourne, 207 Bouverie Street, Parkville, VIC 3010, Australia

Zongchang Li
Department of Psychiatry, the Second Xiangya Hospital, Central South University, Changsha, Hunan, China
Laboratory of Medical Genetics, School of Life Sciences, Central South University, Changsha, Hunan, China

Dong Wang, Jun Zhou and Xiaoqian Ma
Department of Psychiatry, the Second Xiangya Hospital, Central South University, Changsha, Hunan, China
Mental Health Institute, the Second Xiangya Hospital, Central South University, Changsha, Hunan, China

Jinsong Tang and Xiaogang Chen
Department of Psychiatry, the Second Xiangya Hospital, Central South University, Changsha, Hunan, China
Mental Health Institute, the Second Xiangya Hospital, Central South University, Changsha, Hunan, China
National Clinical Research Center on Mental Disorders, Changsha, Hunan, China
National Technology Institute on Mental Disorders, Changsha, Hunan, China
Hunan Key Laboratory of Psychiatry and Mental Health, Changsha, Hunan, China

Sandipan Bhattacharjee and David Rhys Axon
Department of Pharmacy Practice and Science, College of Pharmacy, The University of Arizona, 1295 North Martin Avenue, Tucson, AZ 85721, USA

Majed Al Yami and Sawsan Kurdi
Health Outcomes & PharmacoEconomic Research (HOPE) Center, College of Pharmacy, The University of Arizona, Tucson, AZ, USA

Saima Awan
Addictions Division, Centre for Addiction and Mental Health (CAMH), 33 Russell Street, Office T519, Toronto, ON M5S 2S1, Canada

Peter Voore
Addictions Division, Centre for Addiction and Mental Health (CAMH), 33 Russell Street, Office T519, Toronto, ON M5S 2S1, Canada
Division of Brain and Therapeutics, Department of Psychiatry, University of Toronto, Toronto, ON, Canada

Tony P. George
Addictions Division, Centre for Addiction and Mental Health (CAMH), 33 Russell Street, Office T519, Toronto, ON M5S 2S1, Canada
Institute for Medical Science, University of Toronto, Toronto, ON, Canada
Division of Brain and Therapeutics, Department of Psychiatry, University of Toronto, Toronto, ON, Canada

Andriy V. Samokhvalov
Addictions Division, Centre for Addiction and Mental Health (CAMH), 33 Russell Street, Office T519, Toronto, ON M5S 2S1, Canada
Institute for Medical Science, University of Toronto, Toronto, ON, Canada
Institute for Mental Health Policy Research, CAMH, Toronto, ON, Canada
Division of Brain and Therapeutics, Department of Psychiatry, University of Toronto, Toronto, ON, Canada

Bernard Le Foll
Addictions Division, Centre for Addiction and Mental Health (CAMH), 33 Russell Street, Office T519, Toronto, ON M5S 2S1, Canada
Institute for Medical Science, University of Toronto, Toronto, ON, Canada
Institute for Mental Health Policy Research, CAMH, Toronto, ON, Canada
Division of Brain and Therapeutics, Department of Psychiatry, University of Toronto, Toronto, ON, Canada
Campbell Family Mental Health Research Institute, Toronto, ON, Canada

Jürgen Rehm
Addictions Division, Centre for Addiction and Mental Health (CAMH), 33 Russell Street, Office T519, Toronto, ON M5S 2S1, Canada
Institute for Medical Science, University of Toronto, Toronto, ON, Canada
Institute for Mental Health Policy Research, CAMH, Toronto, ON, Canada
Division of Brain and Therapeutics, Department of Psychiatry, University of Toronto, Toronto, ON, Canada
Campbell Family Mental Health Research Institute, Toronto, ON, Canada
Division of Adult Psychiatry and Health Systems, Department of Psychiatry, University of Toronto, Toronto, ON, Canada
Dalla Lana School of Public Health, University of Toronto, Toronto, ON, Canada
Institute for Clinical Psychology and Psychotherapy, Technische Universität Dresden, Dresden, Sachsen, Germany
WHO Collaborating Centre on Mental Health and Addiction, Toronto, ON, Canada

Charlotte Probst
Institute for Mental Health Policy Research, CAMH, Toronto, ON, Canada
Institute for Clinical Psychology and Psychotherapy, Technische Universität Dresden, Dresden, Sachsen, Germany
WHO Collaborating Centre on Mental Health and Addiction, Toronto, ON, Canada

B. Olivan-Blázquez and Y. López-del-Hoyo
Department of Psychology and Sociology, University of Zaragoza, Violante de Hungria 23, 50009 Zaragoza, Spain
Research Network on Preventive Activities and Health Promotion (Red de Investigación en Actividades Preventivas y Promoción de la Salud - RedIAPP), Barcelona, Spain
Promosam Network, Red de Excelencia PSI2014-56303-REDT PROMOSAM: (Investigación en procesos, mecanismos y tratamientos psicológicos para la promoción de la salud mental), Economy and Competitiveness Ministry, Madrid, Spain

J. Montero-Marin
Research Network on Preventive Activities and Health Promotion (Red de Investigación en Actividades Preventivas y Promoción de la Salud - RedIAPP), Barcelona, Spain
Promosam Network, Red de Excelencia PSI2014-56303-REDT PROMOSAM: (Investigación en procesos, mecanismos y tratamientos psicológicos para la promoción de la salud mental), Economy and Competitiveness Ministry, Madrid, Spain

Weiqing Liu
Department of Psychiatry, First Affiliated Hospital of Kunming Medical University, Kunming, Yunnan, China

Therese Wirback, Jette Möller and Karin Engström
Department of Public Health Sciences, Karolinska Institutet, Solnavägen 1E, 113 65 Stockholm, Sweden

Jan-Olov Larsson
Department of Women's and Children's Health, Karolinska Institutet, Tomtebodavägen 18A, 171 77 Stockholm, Sweden

J. Garcia-Campayo
Research Network on Preventive Activities and Health Promotion (Red de Investigación en Actividades Preventivas y Promoción de la Salud - RedIAPP), Barcelona, Spain
Promosam Network, Red de Excelencia PSI2014-56303-REDT PROMOSAM: (Investigación en procesos, mecanismos y tratamientos psicológicos para la promoción de la salud mental), Economy and Competitiveness Ministry, Madrid, Spain
Aragones Health Service, Zaragoza, Spain
Department of Medicine and Psychiatry, University of Zaragoza, Zaragoza, Spain

M. García-Toro
Research Network on Preventive Activities and Health Promotion (Red de Investigación en Actividades Preventivas y Promoción de la Salud - RedIAPP), Barcelona, Spain
Institut Universitari d'Investigació en Ciències de la Salut (IUNICS), Universitat de les Illes Balears (UIB), Palma de Mallorca, Spain

E. Vicens-Pons
Research Network on Preventive Activities and Health Promotion (Red de Investigación en Actividades Preventivas y Promoción de la Salud - RedIAPP), Barcelona, Spain
Departamento de Psiquiatría, Parc Sanitari San Joan de Déu, Sant Boi de Llobregat, Spain

M. J. Serrano-Ripoll and A. Castro-Gracia
Institut Universitari d'Investigació en Ciències de la Salut (IUNICS), Universitat de les Illes Balears (UIB), Palma de Mallorca, Spain

M. C. Sarasa-Bosque
Aragones Health Service, Zaragoza, Spain

J. M. Mendive-Arbeloa
Institut Català de la Salut, Barcelona, Spain

Julie Calonge
Université de Toulouse III, F-31000 Toulouse, France

Emmanuelle Bougon and Laurent Schmitt
Université de Toulouse III, F-31000 Toulouse, France
CHU Toulouse, Service de Psychiatrie eSt Psychologie, Psychiatrie, F-31000 Toulouse, France

Juliette Salles
Université de Toulouse III, F-31000 Toulouse, France
CHU Toulouse, Service de Psychiatrie eSt Psychologie, Psychiatrie, F-31000 Toulouse, France
CHU Toulouse, Service d'addictologie clinique, urgences réanimation médecine, F-31000 Toulouse, France

Nicolas Franchitto
Université de Toulouse III, F-31000 Toulouse, France
CHU Toulouse, Service d'addictologie clinique, urgences réanimation médecine, F-31000 Toulouse, France

Ti Lu and Cheng-Ho Chang
Department of Psychiatry, Kaohsiung Veterans General Hospital, No.386, Dajhong 1st Rd., Zuoying Dist., Kaohsiung City 813, Taiwan

Li-Yu Hu
Department of Psychiatry, Taipei Veterans General Hospital, Taipei, Taiwan
Center for Geriatrics and Gerontology, Kaohsiung Veterans General Hospital, Kaohsiung, Taiwan
School of Medicine, National Yang-Ming University, Taipei, Taiwan

Chia-Jen Liu
School of Medicine, National Yang-Ming University, Taipei, Taiwan
Division of Hematology and Oncology, Department of Medicine Taipei Veterans General Hospital, Taipei, Taiwan

Tzeng-Ji Chen
School of Medicine, National Yang-Ming University, Taipei, Taiwan
Department of Family Medicine, Taipei Veterans General Hospital, Taipei, Taiwan

Yu-Wen Hu
School of Medicine, National Yang-Ming University, Taipei, Taiwan
Cancer Center, Taipei Veterans General Hospital, Taipei, Taiwan

Chiu-Mei Yeh
Department of Family Medicine, Taipei Veterans General Hospital, Taipei, Taiwan

Pan-Ming Chen
Department of Psychiatry, Yuanshan & Su-ao Branch, Taipei Veterans General Hospital, Yilan, Taiwan

Shyh-Chyang Lee
Department of Information Management, Chia Nan University of Pharmacy & Science, Tainan, Taiwan
Department of Orthopedics, Chiayi Branch, Taichung Veterans General Hospital, Chiayi, Taiwan

Aixia Zhang, Ning Sun, Chunxia Yang, Gaizhi Li, Zhifen Liu, Yanfang Wang and Kerang Zhang
Department of Psychiatry, First Hospital of Shanxi Medical University, Taiyuan 030001, People's Republic of China

Lijun Kang
Department of Psychiatry, First Hospital of Shanxi Medical University, Taiyuan 030001, People's Republic of China
Shanxi Medical University, Taiyuan 030001, People's Republic of China

Penghong Liu
Shanxi Medical University, Taiyuan 030001, People's Republic of China

Jingxu Chen, Hongmei Chen, Ligang Zhang, Juyan Li, Ran Li, Shaoli Wang, Yunlong Tan and Fude Yang
Beijing Hui-Long-Guan Hospital, Peking University, Beijing 100096, China

Junhui Feng
Jining Psychiatric Hospital, Jining 272051, China

Ian Wilson, Alison Jones and Xu-Feng Huang
Illawarra Health and Medical Research Institute and School of Medicine, University of Wollongong, Wollongong, NSW 2522, Australia

Changjun Teng, Hui Ma, Yarong Tan, Xin Wu, Chengbin Guan, Huifen Qiao, Jijun Li, Chun Wang and Ning Zhang
Nanjing Brain Hospital Affiliated to Nanjing Medical University, Nanjing 210029, People's Republic of China

Jing Zhou
Nanjing PuKou Central Hospital, Nanjing 211800, People's Republic of China

Yuan Zhong
School of Psychology, Nanjing Normal University, Nanjing 210024, People's Republic of China

Rita A. Maroun and Lisa A. Thackeray
Faculty of Brain and Language Sciences, University College London, London, UK
Anna Freud National Centre for Children and Families (AFNCCF), London, UK

Nick Midgley
The Child Attachment and Psychological Therapies Research Unit (ChAPTRe), University College London and Anna Freud National Centre for Children and Families, London, UK

Qing Zhang and Huitzong Tsai
Department of Psychiatry, Second Affiliated Hospital, Zhejiang University College of Medicine, Hangzhou, China

Bing Pan
Department of Psychiatry, Second Affiliated Hospital, Zhejiang University College of Medicine, Hangzhou, China
Department of Clinical Psychology and Psychiatry/ School of Public Health, Zhejiang University College of Medicine, Zhejiang 310058, Hangzhou, China

Bingren Zhang and Wei Wang
Department of Clinical Psychology and Psychiatry/ School of Public Health, Zhejiang University College of Medicine, Zhejiang 310058, Hangzhou, China

Robert Lundqvist
Research and Innovation Unit, Luleå, Norrbotten Region, Sweden

Yingjun Xi, Xue Wang, Yaqiong Li, Yuyang He and Jiong Luo
The National Clinical Research Center for Mental Disorders & Beijing key Laboratory of Mental Disorders, Beijing Anding Hospital, Capital Medical University, No. 5 Ankang Lane, Dewai Avenue, Xicheng District, Beijing 100088, China

Runsen Chen
The National Clinical Research Center for Mental Disorders & Beijing key Laboratory of Mental Disorders, Beijing Anding Hospital, Capital Medical University, No. 5 Ankang Lane, Dewai Avenue, Xicheng District, Beijing 100088, China
Department of Psychiatry, University of Oxford, Oxford, UK

Louise Öhlund
Sunderby Research Unit, Department of Clinical Sciences, Division of Psychiatry, Umeå University, Umeå, Sweden

Ursula Werneke
Sunderby Research Unit, Department of Clinical Sciences, Division of Psychiatry, Umeå University, Umeå, Sweden
Sunderby Hospital - Psychiatry, 97180 Luleå, Sweden

Michael Ott
Department of Public Health and Clinical Medicine, Division of Medicine, Umeå University, Umeå, Sweden

Sofia Oja
Department of Psychiatry, Sunderby Hospital, Luleå, Sweden

Malin Bergqvist
Department of Psychiatry, Piteå Älvdals Hospital, Piteå, Sweden

Mikael Sandlund and Ellinor Salander Renberg
Department of Clinical Science, Division of Psychiatry, Umeå University, Umeå, Sweden

Rajnish Mago
Simple and Practical Mental Health, Philadelphia, PA, USA

Andrea Fagiolini
University of Siena Medical Center, Siena, Italy

Emmanuelle Weiller
H. Lundbeck A/S, Valby, Denmark

Catherine Weiss
Otsuka Pharmaceutical Development & Commercialization, Inc., Princeton, NJ, USA

Zuojie Zhang
Department of Pharmacy, Evidence-based Pharmacy Center, West China second hospital, Sichuan University, Chengdu, China
Key Laboratory of Birth Defects and Related Diseases of Women and Children (Sichuan University), Ministry of Education, Chengdu, China
West China School of Pharmacy, Sichuan University, Chengdu, China

Lingli Zhang
Department of Pharmacy, Evidence-based Pharmacy Center, West China second hospital, Sichuan University, Chengdu, China
Key Laboratory of Birth Defects and Related Diseases of Women and Children (Sichuan University), Ministry of Education, Chengdu, China
West China Second University Hospital, Sichuan University, No.20,Third Section, Renmin Nan Lu, Chengdu, Sichuan 610041, People's Republic of China Chengdu City, China

Guorong Zhang and Jianing Jin
West China School of Pharmacy, Sichuan University, Chengdu, China

Zhenyang Zheng
Department of Neurology, Fujian Medical University attached Union Hospital, Fuzhou, China

Carmel Bennett, Shabana Akhtar and Sanju George
Birmingham and Solihull Mental Health NHS Foundation Trust, c/o Dept of Psychiatry, The Barberry 25 Vincent Drive, Edgbaston, Birmingham B152FG, UK

Ed Day
Birmingham and Solihull Mental Health NHS Foundation Trust, c/o Dept of Psychiatry, The Barberry 25 Vincent Drive, Edgbaston, Birmingham B152FG, UK
Addictions Department, Institute of Psychiatry, Psychology & Neuroscience, King's College London, London, UK

Alex Copello and Jennifer L. Seddon
Birmingham and Solihull Mental Health NHS Foundation Trust, c/o Dept of Psychiatry, The Barberry 25 Vincent Drive, Edgbaston, Birmingham B152FG, UK
School of Psychology, The University of Birmingham, Birmingham, UK

Index

www.ingramcontent.com/pod-product-compliance
Lightning Source LLC
LaVergne TN
LVHW080650210926
848485LV00003B/355